Critical Role of PET in Assessing Age Related Disorders

Editors

ABASS ALAVI
BABAK SABOURY
ALI GHOLAMREZANEZHAD

PET CLINICS

www.pet.theclinics.com

Consulting Editor
ABASS ALAVI

January 2023 • Volume 18 • Number 1

ELSEVIER

1600 John F. Kennedy Boulevard • Suite 1800 • Philadelphia, Pennsylvania, 19103-2899

http://www.pet.theclinics.com

PET CLINICS Volume 18, Number 1
January 2023 ISSN 1556-8598, ISBN-13: 978-0-323-96054-0

Editor: John Vassallo (j.vassallo@elsevier.com)
Developmental Editor: Karen Solomon

PET Clinics (ISSN 1556-8598) is published quarterly by Elsevier Inc., 360 Park Avenue South, New York, NY 10010-1710. Months of issue are January, April, July, and October. Periodicals postage paid at New York, NY, and additional mailing offices. Subscription prices per year are $275.00 (US individuals), $500.00 (US institutions), $100.00 (US students), $304.00 (Canadian individuals), $563.00 (Canadian institutions), $100.00 (Canadian students), $297.00 (foreign individuals), $563.00 (foreign institutions), and $140.00 (foreign students). To receive student and resident rate, orders must be accompanied by name of affiliated institution, date of term, and the signature of program/residency coordinator on institution letterhead. Orders will be billed at individual rate until proof of status is received. Foreign air speed delivery is included in all Clinics subscription prices. All prices are subject to change without notice. POSTMASTER: Send address changes to PET Clinics, Elsevier Health Sciences Division, Subscription Customer Service, 3251 Riverport Lane, Maryland Heights, MO 63043. **Customer Service: 1-800-654-2452 (U.S. and Canada); 314-447-8871 (outside U.S. and Canada). Fax: 314-447-8029. E-mail: journalscustomerservice-usa@elsevier.com (for print support); journalsonlinesupport-usa@elsevier.com (for online support).**

Reprints. For copies of 100 or more of articles in this publication, please contact the Commercial Reprints Department, Elsevier Inc., 360 Park Avenue South, New York, NY 10010-1710. Tel.: 212-633-3874; Fax: 212-633-3820; E-mail: reprints@elsevier.com.

PET Clinics is covered in MEDLINE/PubMed (Index Medicus).

Contributors

CONSULTING EDITOR

ABASS ALAVI, MD, MD (Hon), PhD (Hon), DSc (Hon)
Professor of Radiology and Neurology, Director of Research Education, Division of Nuclear Medicine, Department of Radiology, Hospital of the University of Pennsylvania, Perelman School of Medicine, University of Pennsylvania, Philadelphia, Pennsylvania, USA

EDITORS

ABASS ALAVI, MD, MD (Hon), PhD (Hon), DSc (Hon)
Professor of Radiology and Neurology, Director of Research Education, Division of Nuclear Medicine, Department of Radiology, Hospital of the University of Pennsylvania, Perelman School of Medicine, University of Pennsylvania, Philadelphia, Pennsylvania, USA

BABAK SABOURY, MD MPH
Department of Radiology and Imaging Sciences, Clinical Center, National Institutes of Health, Bethesda, Maryland, USA

ALI GHOLAMREZANEZHAD, MD
Department of Diagnostic Radiology, Keck School of Medicine of USC, University of Southern California, Los Angeles, California, USA

AUTHORS

HAMID ABDOLLAHI, PhD
Department of Integrative Oncology, BC Cancer Research Institute, Vancouver, Canada

MARIAM ABOIAN, MD, PhD
Assistant Professor, Department of Radiology, Yale School of Medicine, New Haven, Connecticut, USA

ABASS ALAVI, MD, MD (Hon), PhD (Hon), DSc (Hon)
Professor of Radiology and Neurology, Director of Research Education, Division of Nuclear Medicine, Department of Radiology, Hospital of the University of Pennsylvania, Perelman School of Medicine, University of Pennsylvania, Philadelphia, Pennsylvania, USA

ABDULLAH AL-ZAGHAL, MD
The Russell H. Morgan Department of Radiology, Johns Hopkins School of Medicine, Baltimore, Maryland, USA

SANDIP BASU, MBBS, DRM, DNB, MNAMS
Radiation Medicine Centre, Bhabha Atomic Research Centre, Tata Memorial Hospital Annexe, Homi Bhabha National Institute, Mumbai, India

TOBIAS BÄUERLE, MD
Department of Radiology, Friedrich-Alexander University Erlangen-Nürnberg (FAU) and University Hospital Erlangen, Erlangen, Germany

SANDRA E. BLACK, MD
Departments of Neurology and Medicine, Sunnybrook Health Sciences Centre, University of Toronto, Toronto, Ontario, Canada

KATARINA CHIAM
Division of Engineering Science, University of Toronto, Toronto, Ontario, Canada

GLORIA C. CHIANG, MD
Associate Professor, Department of Radiology, Weill Cornell Medicine, NewYork-Presbyterian Hospital, New York, New York, USA

THOMAS G. CLIFFORD, MD
Keck School of Medicine of USC, University of Southern California, Los Angeles, California, USA

MICHAEL T. COLLINS, MD
National Institute of Dental and Craniofacial Research, National Institutes of Health, Bethesda, Maryland, USA

PATRICK DEBS, MD
The Russell H. Morgan Department of Radiology, Johns Hopkins School of Medicine, Baltimore, Maryland, USA

LIESL EIBSCHUTZ, MS
Keck School of Medicine of USC, University of Southern California, Los Angeles, California, USA

FARAZ FARHADI, BS
Radiology and Imaging Sciences, Clinical Center, National Institutes of Health, Bethesda, Maryland, USA; Geisel School of Medicine at Dartmouth, Hanover, New Hampshire, USA

ANA M. FRANCESCHI, MD PhD
Associate Professor, Department of Radiology, Northwell Health/Donald and Barbara Zucker School of Medicine at Hofstra/Northwell, Lenox Hill Hospital, New York, New York, USA

VINCENT C. GAUDET, PhD
Department of Electrical and Computer Engineering, University of Waterloo, Waterloo, Ontario, Canada

ALI GHOLAMREZANEZHAD, MD
Department of Diagnostic Radiology, Keck School of Medicine of USC, University of Southern California, Los Angeles, California, USA

ALI GUERMAZI, MD, PHD
Department of Radiology, VA Boston Healthcare System, West Roxbury, Massachusetts, USA

JESS HAN
Keck School of Medicine of USC, University of Southern California, Los Angeles, California, USA

MOHAMED JARRAYA, MD
Department of Radiology, Massachusetts General Hospital, Harvard Medical School, Boston, Massachusetts, USA

SANAZ KATAL, MD, MPH
Independent Researcher, St Vincent's Hospital Medical Imaging Department, Melbourne, Victoria, Australia

FELIKS KOGAN, PhD
Department of Radiology, Stanford University, Stanford, California, USA

PHILLIP H. KUO, MD, PhD
Professor, Departments of Medical Imaging, Medicine, Biomedical Engineering, University of Arizona, Tucson, Arizona, USA

HUI CHONG LAU, MD
Department of Medicine, Crozer-Chester Medical Center, Upland, Pennsylvania, USA

LOUIS LEE, MASc
Department of Electrical and Computer Engineering, University of Waterloo, Waterloo, Ontario, Canada

SARVESH LOHARKAR, MBBS, MD
Radiation Medicine Centre, Bhabha Atomic Research Centre, Tata Memorial Hospital Annexe, Homi Bhabha National Institute, Mumbai, India

MARIA LY, MD, PhD
Division of Neuroradiology, Mallinckrodt Institute of Radiology, Washington University in St. Louis, St Louis, Missouri, USA

GEORGE MATCUK, MD
Cedars-Sinai Medical Center, Los Angeles, California, USA

MICHAEL A. MORRIS, MD
Radiology and Imaging Sciences, Clinical Center, National Institutes of Health, Bethesda, Maryland, USA

RIZWAN NASEER, MD
Department of Medicine, Crozer-Chester Medical Center, Upland, Pennsylvania, USA

SZE JIA NG, MD
Department of Medicine, Crozer-Chester Medical Center, Upland, Pennsylvania, USA

MOOZHAN NIKPANAH, MD
Radiology and Imaging Sciences, Clinical Center, National Institutes of Health, Bethesda, Maryland, Department of Radiology, University of Alabama, Birmingham, Alabama, USA

CHARLES C. OSAMOR III, BSA
National Institute of Dental and Craniofacial Research, National Institutes of Health, Bethesda, Maryland, USA

SRIRAM S. PARAVASTU, BS
National Institute of Dental and Craniofacial Research, National Institutes of Health, Bethesda, Maryland, USA

ARMAN RAHMIM, PhD
Department of Integrative Oncology, BC Cancer Research Institute, Vancouver, Canada; Department of Radiology, University of British Columbia, Vancouver, Canada

JAYASAI R. RAJAGOPAL, BA
Radiology and Imaging Sciences, Clinical Center, National Institutes of Health, Bethesda, Maryland, USA

CYRUS A. RAJI, MD, PhD
Division of Neuroradiology, Mallinckrodt Institute of Radiology, Department of Neurology, Washington University in St. Louis, St. Louis, Missouri, USA

WILLIAM Y. RAYNOR, MD
Department of Radiology, Hospital of the University of Pennsylvania, Philadelphia, Pennsylvania, USA; Department of Radiology, Rutgers Robert Wood Johnson Medical School, New Brunswick, New Jersey, USA

FRANK W. ROEMER, MD
Department of Radiology, Boston University School of Medicine, Boston, Massachusetts, USA; Department of Radiology, Friedrich-Alexander University Erlangen-Nürnberg (FAU) and University Hospital Erlangen, Erlangen, Germany

MICHELLE ROYTMAN, MD
Assistant Professor, Department of Radiology, Weill Cornell Medicine, NewYork-Presbyterian Hospital, New York, New York, USA

BABAK SABOURY, MD, MPH
Radiology and Imaging Sciences, Clinical Center, National Institutes of Health, Bethesda, Maryland, USA

SIMRAN SANDHU
College of Health and Human Development, Pennsylvania State University, University Park, Pennsylvania, USA

AARON J. SHEPPARD, BS
National Institute of Dental and Craniofacial Research, National Institutes of Health, Bethesda, Maryland, USA

ISAAC SHIRI, PhD
Division of Nuclear Medicine and Molecular Imaging, Geneva University Hospital, Geneva, Switzerland

LILJA B. SOLNES, MD, MBA
The Russell H. Morgan Department of Radiology, Johns Hopkins School of Medicine, Baltimore, Maryland, USA

SUNITA NITIN SONAVANE, MBBS, DRM, DNB, MNAMS
Radiation Medicine Centre, Bhabha Atomic Research Centre, Tata Memorial Hospital Annexe, Homi Bhabha National Institute, Mumbai, India

MATTHEW SPANO, MD
Department of Radiology, Weill Cornell Medicine, NewYork-Presbyterian Hospital, New York, New York, USA

KIM TAUBMAN, MD
St Vincent's Hospital Medical Imaging Department, Melbourne, Victoria, Australia

EREN M. VEZIROGLU, MS
Geisel School of Medicine at Dartmouth, Hanover, New Hampshire, USA

JOSHUA WARD, BS
Division of Neuroradiology, Mallinckrodt Institute of Radiology, Washington University in St. Louis, St Louis, Missouri, USA

THOMAS J. WERNER, MS
Department of Radiology, Hospital of the University of Pennsylvania, Philadelphia, Pennsylvania, USA

NATALIA M. WOJNOWSKI, BS
National Institute of Dental and Craniofacial Research, National Institutes of Health,

Bethesda, Maryland, USA; Northwestern
University Feinberg School of Medicine,
Chicogo, Illinois, USA

HABIB ZAIDI, PhD
Division of Nuclear Medicine and Molecular
Imaging, Geneva University Hospital, Geneva,
Switzerland; Department of Nuclear Medicine
and Molecular Imaging, University of
Groningen, University Medical Center

Groningen, Groningen, Netherlands;
Department of Nuclear Medicine, University of
Southern Denmark, Odense, Denmark;
Geneva University Neurocenter, Geneva
University, Geneva, Switzerland

KATHERINE A. ZUKOTYNSKI, MD, PhD
Departments of Medicine and Radiology,
McMaster University, Hamilton, Ontario,
Canada

Contents

Osteoporosis is a metabolic bone disorder that leads to a decline in bone microarchitecture, predisposing individuals to catastrophic fractures. The current standard of care relies on detecting bone structural change; however, these methods largely miss the complex biologic forces that drive these structural changes and response to treatment. This review introduces sodium fluoride (18F-NaF) positron emission tomography/computed tomography (PET/CT) as a powerful tool to quantify bone metabolism. Here, we discuss the methods of 18F-NaF PET/CT, with a special focus on dynamic scans to quantify parameters relevant to bone health, and how these markers are relevant to osteoporosis.

Osteoarthritis is a common cause of pain and morbidity resulting in heavy economic burden and large societal costs. Although cross-sectional imaging and in particular MR imaging have largely contributed to a better understanding of the complexity of this complex disease, especially in large joints such as the hip and knee joints, metabolic information of the subchondral bone and periarticular synovial environment has been consistently suggested to provide valuable supplemental information to morphologic and compositional MR imaging. The aim of this narrative review is to provide an overview of the role of the hybrid PET imaging in osteoarthritis with particular focus on PET/MR imaging.

Fluorodeoxyglucose (FDG) PET/computed tomography (CT) is a valuable diagnostic modality in the work-up of patients with suspected inflammatory myopathy. Sarcopenia and metabolic muscle activity on staging FDG PET/CT has been shown to correlate with overall survival in certain oncologic settings. Knowledge of the physiologic FDG uptake in skeletal muscles and optimization of imaging protocols are key for proper image analysis.

Back pain is a common health complaint that contributes globally to medical burden and costs, particularly in elderly populations. Nuclear medicine techniques using PET tracers offer diagnostic information about various spine disorders, including malignant, degenerative, inflammatory, and infectious diseases. Herein, the authors briefly review applications of PET in the evaluation of spine disorders in elderly patients.

This communication gives a short review of clinical utilities of PET/computed-tomography (CT) imaging in bone and joint infections. PET/CT imaging provides additional information over conventional modalities by providing information regarding disease extent in the bone as well as whole body, giving an idea of active pathology at the molecular level, and response evaluation. The roles of fluorodeoxyglucose have been examined in multiple indications, particularly in osteomyelitis, prosthetic joint infections, diabetic foot, and systemic diseases with skeletal involvement. The role of PET/CT imaging using other tracers like 18F-sodium fluoride, gallium-68 citrate, 18F-fluorodeoxyglucose-labeled WBCs, and futuristic PET/MR have been also discussed shortly.

Assessment of molecular changes by PET has introduced a new paradigm in atherosclerosis imaging, which has traditionally relied on anatomic changes visualized by conventional angiography or computed tomography. The use of 18F-fluorodeoxyglucose (FDG) to identify atherosclerotic changes in the vessel wall was first described more than 2 decades ago. Since then, PET tracers targeting macrophage activity, neoangiogenesis, smooth muscle activity, and other aspects of atherogenic changes have been proposed. The evolving roles of PET tracers including frontrunners FDG and 18F-sodium fluoride, which show arterial wall inflammation and microcalcification, respectively, are discussed

PET/computed tomography (CT) studies can be potentially useful in elderly thyroid carcinoma patients for exploring the disease biology, especially in metastatic setting and thereby directing appropriate therapeutic management on case-to-case basis, adopting nuclear theranostics, and disease prognostication. With the availability of multiple PET radiopharmaceuticals, it would be worthwhile to evolve and optimally use FDG and the other non-fluorodeoxyglucose and investigational PET/CT tracers as per the clinical situation and need and thereby define their utilities in a given case scenario. In this regard, (I) differentiated thyroid carcinoma (DTC) including radioiodine refractory disease, poorly differentiated thyroid cancer (PDTC) and TENIS, (II) medullary thyroid carcinoma (MTC), (III) anaplastic carcinoma and (IV) Primary thyroid lymphoma (PTL) should be viewed and dealt separately.

more quantitative assessments of disease. We then identify some major challenges associated with longitudinal studies including the need for improved data collection and increased data sharing, limitations of current algorithms for studying longitudinal data, a need for the development of performance metrics that include a macro-scalar component, and ethical considerations for patient based studies. Finally, we offer some observations and recommendations for advancing medical imaging practice and research while integrating macro-scale considerations.

Advancing age significantly affects the structural and functional characteristics of organs and tissues, including the peripheral nervous system (PNS) and musculoskeletal system. PET molecular imaging systems offer the ability to assess the metabolic and quantitative effects due to nerve and muscle injuries, which has the potential to impact clinical management of aged subjects. Here, we aim to describe some features of molecular imaging PET systems using different tracers and methods of imaging in musculoskeletal disorders and peripheral neuropathies commonly seen in elderly patients.

PET CLINICS

SERIES OF RELATED INTEREST

Advances in Clinical Radiology
Available at: Advancesinclinicalradiology.com
MRI Clinics of North America
Available at: MRI.theclinics.com
Neuroimaging Clinics of North America
Available at: Neuroimaging.theclinics.com
Radiologic Clinics of North America
Available at: Radiologic.theclinics.com

THE CLINICS ARE AVAILABLE ONLINE!
Access your subscription at:
www.theclinics.com

PROGRAM OBJECTIVE
The goal of the *PET Clinics* is to keep practicing radiologists and radiology residents up to date with current clinical practice in positron emission tomography by providing timely articles reviewing the state of the art in patient care.

TARGET AUDIENCE
Practicing radiologists, radiology residents, and other health care professionals who provide patient care utilizing radiologic findings.

LEARNING OBJECTIVES
Upon completion of this activity, participants will be able to:
1. Review the effects of PET imaging on disorders associated with aging.
2. Discuss the need for additional research into the use of PET imaging in the evaluation, diagnosis, and management of age-related disorders.
3. Recognize PET imaging as a useful tool for detecting, diagnosing, prognosis, decision-making, and managing age-related disorders.

ACCREDITATION
The Elsevier Office of Continuing Medical Education (EOCME) is accredited by the Accreditation Council for Continuing Medical Education (ACCME) to provide continuing medical education for physicians.

The EOCME designates this journal-based CME activity for a maximum of 12 *AMA PRA Category 1 Credit*(s)™. Physicians should claim only the credit commensurate with the extent of their participation in the activity.

All other health care professionals requesting continuing education credit for this enduring material will be issued a certificate of participation.

DISCLOSURE OF CONFLICTS OF INTEREST
The EOCME assesses conflict of interest with its instructors, faculty, planners, and other individuals who are in a position to control the content of CME activities. All relevant conflicts of interest that are identified are thoroughly vetted by EOCME for fair balance, scientific objectivity, and patient care recommendations. EOCME is committed to providing its learners with CME activities that promote improvements or quality in healthcare and not a specific proprietary business or a commercial interest.

The planning committee, staff, authors, and editors listed below have identified no financial relationships or relationships to products or devices they or their spouse/life partner have with commercial interest related to the content of this CME activity:
Hamid Abdollahi, PhD; Mariam Aboian, MD, PhD; Abass Alavi, MD, MD (Hon), PhD (Hon), DSc (Hon); Abdullah Al-Zaghal, MD; Sandip Basu, MD; Tobias Bäuerle, MD; Sandra E. Black, MD; Katarina Chiam; Gloria C. Chiang, MD; Thomas G. Clifford, MD; Michael T. Collins, MD; Patrick Debs, MD; Liesl Eibschutz; Faraz Farhadi; Ana M. Franceschi, MD, PhD; Vincent C. Gaudet, PhD; Ali Gholamrezanezhad, MD; Ali Guermazi, MD, PhD; Jess Han; Mohamed Jarraya, MD; Sanaz Katal, MD, MPH; Feliks Kogan, PhD; Mohana Manoj Krishnamoorthy; Phillip H. Kuo, MD, PhD; Hui Chong Lau, MD; Louis Lee; Sarvesh Loharkar, MD; Maria Ly, MD, PhD; George R. Matcuk, MD; Rizwan Naseer, MD; Sze Jia Ng, MD; Moozhan Nikpanah, MD; Charles C. Osamor III; Sriram S. Paravastu; Arman Rahmim, PhD; Jayasai R. Rajagopal; Cyrus A. Raji, MD, PhD; William Y. Raynor, MD; Frank W. Roemer, MD; Michelle Roytman, MD; Babak Saboury, MD, MPH; Simran Sandhu; Aaron J. Sheppard; Isaac Shiri; Lilja B. Solnes, MD, MBA; Sunita Nitin Sonavane, MBBS; Matthew Spano, MD; Kim Taubman, MBBS; Doreen Thomas-Payne, MSN, BSN, RN, PMHNP-BC; Eren M. Veziroglu, MS; Joshua Ward; Thomas J. Werner, MS; Natalia M. Wojnowski; Habib Zaidi, PhD; Katherine A. Zukotynski, MD, PhD

UNAPPROVED/OFF-LABEL USE DISCLOSURE
The EOCME requires CME faculty to disclose to the participants:
1. When products or procedures being discussed are off-label, unlabelled, experimental, and/or investigational (not US Food and Drug Administration [FDA] approved); and
2. Any limitations on the information presented, such as data that are preliminary or that represent ongoing research, interim analyses, and/or unsupported opinions. Faculty may discuss information about pharmaceutical agents that is outside of FDA-approved labelling. This information is intended solely for CME and is not intended to promote off-label use of these medications. If you have any questions, contact the medical affairs department of the manufacturer for the most recent prescribing information.

TO ENROLL
To enroll in the *PET Clinics* Continuing Medical Education program, call customer service at 1-800-654-2452 or sign up online at http://www.theclinics.com/home/cme. The CME program is available to subscribers for an additional annual fee of USD 254.00

METHOD OF PARTICIPATION
In order to claim credit, participants must complete the following:
1. Complete enrolment as indicated above.

2. Read the activity.
3. Complete the CME Test and Evaluation. Participants must achieve a score of 70% on the test. All CME Tests and Evaluations must be completed online.

CME INQUIRIES/SPECIAL NEEDS

For all CME inquiries or special needs, please contact elsevierCME@elsevier.com.

Preface
Graying Population: Role of PET in Age-Related Disorders

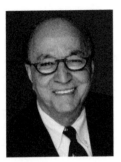
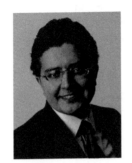
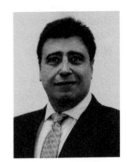

Abass Alavi, MD, PhD (Hon), DSc (Hon)   Babak Saboury, MD, MPH   Ali Gholamrezanezhad, MD

Editors

The rapidly increasing, aging population is one of the major challenges of the health care systems across the globe. According to the World Health Organization, the proportion of the world's population over 60 years will nearly double from 12% in 2015 to 22% in 2050. Also, aging is considered one of the main risk factors for different human diseases and disorders. The health world is facing serious challenges in responding to age-related human ailments. Health expenditures substantially grow past age 50. Other than its financial burden, cooccurrence of several chronic health-related conditions (multimorbidity) in the elderly makes their management more challenging. Furthermore, development of subclinical pathologic conditions in various body organs of the elderly population, even in the absence of clinically detectable disease, leads to substantial health-related disabilities in the long run.

Clinical imaging is an integral component of management of various diseases and disorders in elderly subjects. Among all imaging modalities, PET/computed tomography (CT) plays a paramount role among various diagnostic modalities in this population for several reasons: (1) PET/CT provides advantages of combining molecular data with those of structural alterations in many settings; (2) PET is more sensitive than CT and MR imaging in detecting early disease; and (3) PET provides accurate quantitative results and therefore allows assessment of disease activity following various interventions.

Based on the global experience gained during the past two decades, applications of PET/CT in the elderly population have exponentially risen worldwide. This substantial rise has occurred despite some difficulties that were encountered in imaging elderly patients due to their frailty and ability to cooperate during image acquisition. The introduction of simultaneous total body PET imaging will allow overcoming this shortcoming in the future.

The fact that during the last two decades, the number of published research studies about the rapidly evolving role of PET/CT and PET/MR imaging in the senior population has increased steadily, motivated us to assemble this special issue of *PET*

PET Clin 18 (2023) xv–xvi
https://doi.org/10.1016/j.cpet.2022.10.003
1556-8598/23/© 2022 Published by Elsevier Inc.

Clinics on this topic. In this issue, we provide comprehensive scientific communications about age-related disorders, such as osteoporosis, osteoarthritis, spine disorders, infections and age-related inflammation, atherosclerosis, cognitive impairment and dementia, and cerebrovascular disease. We believe that applications of PET in the elderly will expand substantially in the future due to the advent of novel radiotracers and advanced imaging modalities.

Abass Alavi, MD, PhD (Hon), DSc (Hon)
Division of Nuclear Medicine
Department of Diagnostic Radiology
University of Pennsylvania School of Medicine
Hospital of the University of Pennsylvania
3400 Spruce Street
Philadelphia, PA 19104, USA

Babak Saboury, MD, MPH
Radiology and Imaging Sciences
Clinical Center
National Institutes of Health
10 Center Drive
Bethesda, MD 20892, USA

Ali Gholamrezanezhad, MD
Department of Radiology
Keck School of Medicine
University of Southern California
1520 San Pablo Street
Los Angeles, CA 90333, USA

E-mail addresses:
Abass.Alavi@pennmedicine.upenn.edu (A. Alavi)
Babak.Saboury@nih.gov (B. Saboury)
ali.gholamrezanezhad@med.usc.edu
(A. Gholamrezanezhad)

Emerging Role of ¹⁸F-NaF PET/Computed Tomographic Imaging in Osteoporosis
A Potential Upgrade to the Osteoporosis Toolbox

Aaron J. Sheppard, BSª, Sriram S. Paravastu, BSª,
Natalia M. Wojnowski, BSª,ᶜ, Charles C. Osamor III, BSAª,
Faraz Farhadi, BSᵇ,ᵈ, Michael T. Collins, MDª, Babak Saboury, MD, MPHᵇ,*

KEYWORDS

- Osteoporosis • Sodium fluoride (¹⁸F-NaF) PET/CT • Bone mineral density • Bone Turnover
- Bone Metabolism

KEY POINTS

- While measuring bone mineral content via dual-energy x-ray absorptiometry (DXA) and other modalities has proven useful in clinical management of osteoporosis, these modalities largely miss the complex biology that describe the pathophysiology of osteoporosis.
- The fluoride ion of ¹⁸F-NaF exchanges for a hydroxyl group of hydroxyapatite, making ¹⁸F-NaF PET/computed tomography (CT) a useful tool to measure newly synthesized bone mineral and offers a 3D view of bone metabolism.
- Several methods exist for utilizing ¹⁸F-NaF PET/CT scans, with each their own advantages, limitations, and challenges.
- Dynamic scans and kinetic modeling offer a more robust measurement of bone metabolism and provide estimates of bone perfusion and bone extracellular volume that can help characterize bone health.
- Despite current challenges, ¹⁸F-NaF PET/CT has already demonstrated to be a sensitive readout for response to osteoporosis treatment, as well as significantly correlated with more invasive measures of bone turnover.

INTRODUCTION

Osteoporosis is the most common metabolic bone disorder, with an estimated prevalence of 13.1% to 27.1% of women and 3.3% to 5.7% of men over the age of 50 affected.[1,2] As a systemic skeletal disease, osteoporosis results in bone fragility with increased risk for fracture, primarily due to disintegration of the bone microarchitecture leading to a decrease in bone mineral density (BMD) and a loss of trabecular connectivity.[3–5] This deterioration of bone structure is the result of an aberrant bone remodeling process.

ª National Institute of Dental and Craniofacial Research, National Institutes of Health, 30 Convent Drive, Building 30, Room 228, Bethesda, MD 20892-4320, USA; ᵇ Radiology and Imaging Sciences, Clinical Center, National Institutes of Health, 10 Center Drive, Bethesda, MD 20892-4320, USA; ᶜ Northwestern University Feinberg School of Medicine, 420 East Superior Street, Chicago, IL 60611, USA; ᵈ Geisel School of Medicine at Dartmouth, 1 Rope Ferry Road, Hanover, NH 03755, USA
* Corresponding author. 10 Center Drive, Bethesda, MD 20892.
E-mail address: babak.saboury@nih.gov

PET Clin 18 (2023) 1–20
https://doi.org/10.1016/j.cpet.2022.09.001
1556-8598/23/© 2022 Elsevier Inc. All rights reserved.

Normal bone remodeling consists of the replacement of old bone with new bone through the process of bone resorption and bone formation (by osteoclasts and osteoblasts, respectively). In a healthy adult, the amount of bone resorbed and formed is tightly regulated. From childhood to early adulthood, the rate of bone formation exceeds resorption with BMD peaking in the third decade of life.[2,4,6] After this point, the balance shifts to favor bone resorption, and BMD slowly declines throughout the lifespan of a normal adult, with a period of accelerated bone loss around the time of menopause in women.[6,7] In patients with osteoporosis, the degree of bone resorption is even greater than the degree of formation that takes place during normal aging. Osteoporosis is defined by BMD that is ≤ 2.5 standard deviations below peak bone mass for an age- and sex-matched control group.[5,8]

Biological Players in Osteoporosis

Bone mass is the net sum of bone formation and bone resorption. Both arms of the process have been targeted in osteoporosis treatment. Drugs that promote formation (eg, parathyroid hormone analogues) are known as anabolic agents, and those that inhibit resorption are known as antiresorptive agents (eg, denosumab and bisphosphonates).[4,9] Although the cause of osteoporosis can be simply understood by an imbalance between the relative rates of bone formation and resorption, the molecular biology involved is complex. The molecular interactions between osteoprotegerin (OPG), receptor activator of nuclear factor kappa-B ligand (RANKL), and the receptor activator of nuclear factor kappa-B (RANK) are a well-studied aspect of bone remodeling (shown by the bolded arrows in **Fig. 1**).[5,10,11] RANKL on the surface of osteoprogenitors/osteoblasts binds and activates the osteoclast RANK receptor, which subsequently upregulates nuclear factor kappa-B to kick-start osteoclast differentiation. Osteoblasts also secrete OPG, which acts as a decoy receptor for RANKL and leads to decreased RANKL/RANK interactions.[5] Therefore, the relative levels of OPG and RANKL production contribute to more bone formation or resorption, respectively. Given this relationship, co-opting the interaction between RANKL and RANK (on the osteoclast cell surface) with the drug denosumab, a monoclonal antibody against RANKL that blocks RANKL–RANK interaction, is one of the main weapons in osteoporosis therapy armamentarium.[11,12]

There are many other factors regulating bone formation and remodeling, as summarized in **Fig. 1**. Briefly, it is recognized that osteocytes also play a key role in regulating bone remodeling and response to mechanical loading. In addition, the osteocyte is increasingly recognized as playing roles in osteoblast and osteoclast function as well as mineral homeostasis, responding to and secreting several factors such as RANKL and FGF23, as shown in **Fig. 1**.[13,14,16] A major contributor to osteoporosis is the decrease in estrogen seen in postmenopausal women.[17,18] Estrogen has numerous effects on bone remodeling through interactions with the estrogen receptors (ERs). The decline of estrogen has been shown to increase osteoblast apoptosis, increase pro-resorptive cytokines such as interleukin-6 (IL-6), interleukin-1 (IL-1), tumor necrosis factor-α (TNF-α), monocyte colony-stimulating factor, and prostaglandin E2, which act to create an inflammatory environment and increased osteoclastic activity[19] (**Fig. 1**). Much like the RANKL/RANK interaction, the ERs have been targets for osteoporosis therapy, either through estrogen or estrogen-like molecules including selective ER modifiers that have various actions depending on their activity at certain ER subtypes.[20,21] Several other targets are emerging as potential causes and treatments of osteoporosis, including micro ribonucleic acids (miRNAs), long noncoding RNAs (lncRNA), circular RNAs (cirRNA), reactive oxygen species (ROS), and small molecular inhibitors.[19,22]

As previously mentioned, the normal skeleton peaks in BMD around the third decade and then gradually declines until the end of life.[2,23] This decrease in the bone formation/resorption ratio leads to the gradual decrease in BMD, bone strength, and an increase in fractures. It is also clear that an individual's genetic background plays a major role in both bone mass and bone strength, accounting for up to 50% of the determination of fracture risk[5,24–27] (**Fig 2**).

Additive to an individual's underlying genetic risk for osteoporosis, are numerous environmental factors including lactose allergies (poor calcium intake), underlying medical conditions predisposing to vitamin D deficiency (gastrointestinal disorders), corticosteroid treatment, chronic inflammation, and nutrient deficiencies have all been shown to affect the biological interactions illustrated by **Fig. 1** and linked to osteoporosis.[5,18] The current guidelines to screen women over 65 and men over 70 is merely sufficient to detect an already deteriorated skeleton, and largely misses the biological complexities that come before it.[2,17] Although the current guidelines and tools are largely cost-effective and aid in stratifying patients based on fracture risk, they miss the complex metabolic interactions that may augment the ability to characterize bone health and better manage osteoporosis.[2]

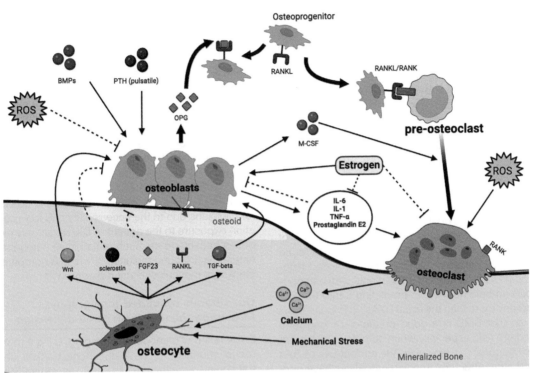

Fig. 1. Bone modeling and remodeling are tightly regulated processes, involving the interactions between osteoblast, osteoclasts, and osteocytes. The molecular interactions illustrated here provide a brief overview of known regulating factors of bone metabolism. For simplicity, osteoblasts can increase osteoclast activity by producing receptor activator of nuclear factor kappa-B ligand (RANKL) and monocyte colony-stimulating factor (M-CSF). Other factors that increase osteoclast resorption include interleukin-1 (IL-1), interleukin-6 (IL-6), tumor necrosis factor-α (TNFα), prostaglandin E2, and reactive oxygen species (ROS). Estrogen leads to a suppression of these inflammatory cytokines and ROS while also directly stimulating osteoblasts and inhibiting osteoclasts. Further, osteoblasts can decrease osteoclast activity by secreting osteoprotegerin (OPG). Factors that increase osteoblast activity include bone morphogenic proteins (BMPs), parathyroid hormone (PTH, pulsatile secretion), transforming growth factor-β (TGF-β), and wingless-related integration site (Wnt) proteins. Osteocytes also receive signals from the environment, mechanical stress, and local calcium to regulate osteoblast and osteoclast function via previously mentioned factors.[5,12–15] FGF23, Fibroblast Growth Factor-23. (Image created with BioRender.com)

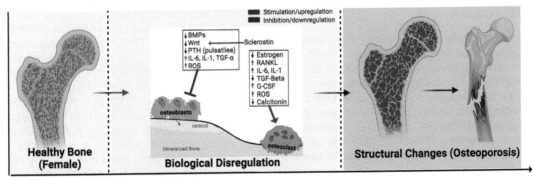

Fig. 2. Early in life, the rate of bone formation exceeds the rate of bone resorption, allowing BMD to peak in the third decade of life (green panel). After this peak, BMD slowly declines with age. In osteoporosis, the decline in BMD is much more pronounced and is preceded by complex biological dysregulation (yellow panel). Many factors have been linked to an increase in osteoclast and decrease in osteoblast activity (green *arrows* signify stimulation or upregulation, and red *arrows* signify inhibition or downregulation, which kick-starts a subsequent decline in bone architecture red panel). (Image created with BioRender.com)

Impact of Osteoporosis and Current Management

It was estimated that around 12.3 million people in the United States over the age of 50 have osteoporosis, and nearly 30% of individuals who suffer a hip fracture die within 1 year.[28] There is a potential therapeutic window of opportunity to take steps to prevent morbidity from osteoporotic fractures by detecting early changes in bone metabolism. Given the significant degree of morbidity and mortality associated with osteoporotic hip fractures, it is clear that there is a great need for a better predictor for these catastrophic fractures.[29,30] Many clinical groups are recognizing the lack of clinical usefulness in repeated dual-energy X-ray absorptiometry (DXA) scans for the monitoring and prediction of fractures[31–33] In fact, Hillier and colleagues found that 8 years of follow-up DXA scans provided insignificant value to the care of patients with osteoporosis and did not help in predicting future fracture risk any more than the *initial* DXA.[32] It is clear, however, that BMD is a good predictor of long-term fracture risk, especially when combined with other risk factors.[2,9,34] However, the current use of DXA and other structural imaging modalities have poor temporal resolution (predict fracture within a 10 year period), do not allow us to catch bone deterioration early, and miss a lot of heterogeneity that could help to more accurately predict fractures.

As an adjunct to the standard, newer imaging techniques and using radiopharmaceuticals such as ^{18}F-sodium fluoride (^{18}F-NaF) PET/computed tomography (CT) may provide an additional layer of information that could not only aid in detecting changes in bone metabolism and remodeling but also better understand microarchitectural changes in bone.

CURRENT IMAGING MODALITIES IN OSTEOPOROSIS

This review briefly discusses the current imaging modalities available for screening, diagnosing, and managing osteoporosis. First, we will discuss DXA and newer modalities that assess bone structure. Finally, the authors discuss nuclear medicine technology that allows us to incorporate bone metabolic information with bone architecture. Most importantly, ^{18}F-NaF PET/CT will be discussed as a powerful tool for assessing skeletal metabolism and health.[35]

Dual-energy X-ray absorptiometry: Current screening method

Osteoporosis is most commonly evaluated by calculating a patient's BMD using DXA (**Fig 3**) to find the bone mineral content for a region of interest (ROI).[3] Two different X-ray beams, one low-photon and one high-photon energy, are passed through a ROI (commonly the hip and lumbar spine) to create a pixel-by-pixel map of BMD.[36] The United States Preventive Services Task Force currently recommends all women over the age of 65 years, and men over 70, to be screened for osteoporosis with bone measurement testing via DXA.[37] The diagnosis of osteoporosis is given when a patient's BMD falls into a T-score of −2.5 or lower. Osteopenia, the precursor to osteoporosis, is characterized by a T-score between −1.0 and −2.5. DXA remains a popular modality for clinicians due to the accessibility and low radiation exposure to the patient. A DXA scan only exposes patients to as much radiation as 3 hours of natural background radiation,[38] which is comparable with a musculoskeletal radiograph.[39]

Quantitative computed tomography: Measuring the density in three-dimension

In the realm of osteoporosis imaging, CT is a more robust modality for analyzing bone cortical and trabecular architecture as well as quantifying BMD. CT can provide information on the three-dimensional (3D) structure of bone, allowing assessment of site-specific differences in structure that may better predict fracture risk.[41] Low-dose scan quantitative CT (qCT) is an imaging modality that relies on standard CT imaging and a phantom representing varying bone mineral concentrations as a standard. As the various mineral content of the phantom is known, the Hounsfield unit (HU) can be calibrated to reflect BMD, providing more accurate measures of BMD compared with using native HUs.[42] There has also been extensive research to develop "phantomless" methods of determining BMD.[43] Although BMD measurements obtained from using phantoms or internal calibration techniques have been shown to have variations from DXA-measured BMD, several groups have shown its effectiveness. A case–control study found that combining phantomless qCT BMD with finite element analysis could predict fractures with an area under the curve (AUC) of 0.692.[44] Another group found that qCT combined with FEA was just as effective as DXA in identifying patients at high risk for fracture.[43,45] Although it is possible to approximate BMD using these methods, it is difficult to precisely measure the BMD (**Fig. 4**).

Dual-energy computed tomography: Bone mineral density beyond the basics

Dual-energy CT (DECT) is an X-ray-based technology, similar to DXA, which collects two images at

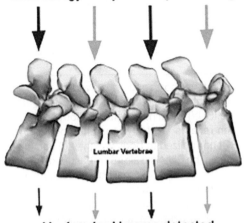

Dual energy X-ray beams pass through

Lumbar Vertebrae

Unabsorbed beams detected

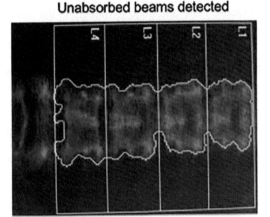

Fig. 3. Diagram of the function of a DXA scan and BMD calculation. Two different X-ray beams, one low-photon and one high-photon energy, are passed through a region of interest (commonly the lumbar spine) to create a pixel-by-pixel map of BMD. The cumulative BMD is then multiplied by the area for that region to get the Bone Mineral Content (BMC).[36] (*Adapted from* Berger A. Bone mineral density scans40. BMJ. 2002 Aug 31;325(7362):484.)

two different X-ray energies and measures tissue-specific attenuation along an X-ray spectrum.[43] The main advantage of the DECT-based BMD measurement is that there is no need for a phantom measurement, or internal calibrations, in order to measure BMD. Similarly to DXA, due to the dual spectrum of radiation emitted by the DECT machine, attenuation constants for both of the CT energies can be used to directly calculate the amount of calcium present in bone. Koch and colleagues recently found that DECT-derived BMD values were significantly different from qCT-based measurements and were repeatedly closer to the actual values of hydroxyapatite (HA).[46] Another advantage of DECT over DXA is the ability to see bones in 3D resolution, providing for improved assessment of the bone

architecture. There is a continual advancement of scanners and software packages that can allow a 3D view of BMD. Compared with qCT, DECT shows promise in the diagnosis and management of bone architecture, as well as density disorders without the use of phantoms for BMD approximation. DECT-derived BMD measurements have been recently shown to strongly predict 2-year fracture risk in patients with osteoporosis.[47,48] However, as with all X-ray-based modalities, the information gained from DECT is purely structural and does not convey physiologic information which is crucial to tracking bone disorders over time.

Metabolic Imaging with ¹⁸F-NaF PET/CT and ⁹⁹ᵐT-MDP SPECT/CT

The aforementioned imaging techniques work well for quantifying bone architecture, but as previously mentioned, there is a need for modalities that give insight to bone metabolic activity.

¹⁸F-NaF is a radiotracer that reflects skeletal metabolism and calcification.[49] It was introduced in 1962 for detection of osteogenic activity,[50] but it was not until the 1990s that NaF regained interest for bone scanning with the global increase in PET and PET/CT.[51] With a half-life of 110 minutes, ¹⁸F-NaF can be injected into the vein and visualized by PET/CT. ¹⁸F-NaF is able to diffuse across membranes and ¹⁸F incorporates into HA (representing bone remodeling) and is rapidly renally cleared.[49] For those reasons, along with the fact that PET scanners have superior resolution to single photon emission computed tomography (SPECT), ¹⁸F-NaF is the preferred radiotracer for bone metabolic activity over the older technetium 99m-methyl diphosphonate (⁹⁹ᵐT-MDP) SPECT/CT.[51-55] ¹⁸F-NaF PET has traditionally been used to detect metastatic bone disease, such as bone metastases from prostate cancer.[56,57] Given its ability to evaluate bone turnover at the molecular level, ¹⁸F-NaF-PET/CT has the potential to provide an alternative superior modality to imaging of metabolic bone disorders to track changes with higher sensitivity.[53]

Furthermore, there are several characteristics of ⁹⁹ᵐT-MDP which make it a poor radiotracer for osteoporosis. First, given it is a bisphosphonate, ⁹⁹ᵐT-MDP is not rapidly metabolized *in vivo* and relies heavily on renal clearance. This is an issue given renal function steadily declines with age, allowing more of the radiopharmaceutical to enter the bone compartment, thus overestimating osteoblastic activity.[58,59] In addition, ⁹⁹ᵐTcMDP binds to plasma proteins, which alters measurements, unlike with ¹⁸F-NaF PET imaging.[51] In addition, the half-life of ⁹⁹T-MDP is long compared with ¹⁸F-NaF, at around 6 hours. Thus, the radioactive

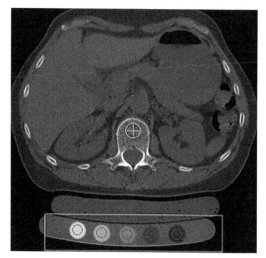

Fig. 4. Cross-section of human subject undergoing qCT of a lumbar vertebrae with a phantom (outlined by green rectangle) for calibration of Hounsfield units (HU) to bone mineral. Illustrated here with permission from Brett and colleagues[42] is a Cann–Genant phantom, which consists of five various concentrations of potassium phosphate-equivalent phases. Once calibrated to the phantom, the HU measurements can be used to estimate bone mineral content within a region of interest (lumbar spine here). From Brett AD, Brown JK. Quantitative computed tomography and opportunistic bone density screening by dual use of computed tomography scans. J Orthop Translat. 2015 Sep 15;3(4):178-184.

agent is in the body for longer periods of time and potentially subjecting the subject to greater amounts of radiation.[60]

The remainder of this review expounds on the methodology of ^{18}F-NaF PET/CT, as well as its ability to give metabolic insight as well as morphologic characteristics, which may aid in screening and managing osteoporosis.

[18]F-NaF PET/COMPUTED TOMOGRAPHY FOR BONE METABOLIC IMAGING

As alluded to, ^{18}F-NaF is a reliable measure for assessing bone metabolism. After the sodium and radiolabeled fluoride ions dissociate *in vivo*, the fluoride ion incorporates into the HA chemical structure as shown by Equation 1.[53] As fluoride can only be incorporated into sites of exposed, newly formed bone mineral, it is a direct measure of osteoblastic activity. However, as osteoblast activity is tightly coupled to osteoclast activity, the amount of ^{18}F-NaF incorporated into bone mineral is also a strong reflection of osteoclast activity and bone turnover.[51,53]

$$Ca_{10}(PO_4)_6(OH)_2 + 2F^- \rightarrow Ca_{10}(PO_4)_6F_2 + 2OH^-$$

(1)

There are two methods for quantifying ^{18}F-NaF uptake and bone turnover, with each having their own pros, cons, and clinical utility.

Clinical ^{18}F-NaF PET and Standardized Uptake Value

The first method, and most widely used in the clinic, entails calculating standardized uptake value (SUV) 60 minutes after radiotracer injection, which reflects ^{18}F-NaF concentration (kBq/mL) in a ROI normalized to body weight (kg) and injection activity. The SUV is a simple measure of bone turnover, where the SUV can be used as a relative measure of how much newly formed HA is available for the reaction expressed as Equation 1. This can provide useful information about bone metabolic state and bone formation. In the clinic, SUV measurements are routinely used to monitor or detect metastatic bone disease (ie, prostate cancer) and metabolic bone disease.[53,61] Static SUV measurements are advantageous as they allow for shorter scan times, making it more comfortable for the patient and less technically demanding on clinical staff.[61]

While very useful when studying or comparing longitudinal data from focal bone lesions, SUV measurements from ^{18}F-NaF PET is not the best measure when comparing a population with a systemic bone disorder (ie, osteoporosis and Paget's disease) to a healthy population, as SUV depends on plasma concentration (a point discussed later).[62,63] To get around this dependence on plasma concentrations, more robust, kinetic methods have been developed to better reflect bone metabolism and provide insights into morphologic characteristics **Fig. 5**.

Dynamic ^{18}F-NaF PET and Kinetic Modeling Parameters

By thinking of physiologic and biological systems from the viewpoint of kinetic modeling, there is an opportunity to translate PET images into meaningful physiologic parameters.[49,64,65] The foundation for kinetic modeling, as it relates to bone, comes from thinking about where the ^{18}F-NaF radiotracer is present from a microanatomical standpoint. Given that NaF freely diffuses across cell membranes and has high tissue extraction (low plasma protein binding), the flow of ^{18}F-NaF can be modeled by the transfer of radiotracer from the plasma into the bone environment, where there is then exchange between the bone extracellular fluid (ECF) and between the ECF and newly mineralized bone.[35,61] Further, the exchange between the unbound pool of ^{18}F-NaF and the newly mineralized bone depends on the tightly coupled interactions

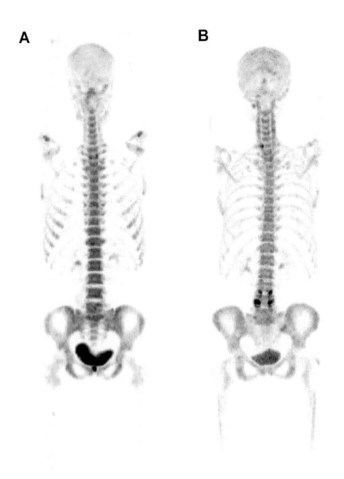

A

B

Fig. 5. (*A*) Is a maximum intensity projection (MIP) of a ^{18}F-NaF scan taken of a healthy 26-year-old woman with normal distribution of radiotracer throughout the skeleton. Although (*B*) is a scan of a 62-year-old woman, showing visible less ^{18}F-NaF incorporation at the lumbar spine and total hip, indicating the potential of ^{18}F-NaF PET to detect low levels of bone mineralization. (*From* Park PSU, Raynor WY, Sun Y, Werner TJ, Rajapakse CS, Alavi A. 18F-Sodium Fluoride PET as a Diagnostic Modality for Metabolic, Autoimmune, and Osteogenic Bone Disorders: Cellular Mechanisms and Clinical Applications. Int J Mol Sci. 2021;22(12).)[53]

of osteoblasts, osteoclasts, and osteocytes (see **Fig. 1**). This exchange of ^{18}F-NaF within the bone is illustrated in **Fig. 6**, where the plasma, ECF, and newly mineralized bone compartments are denoted by C_a, C1, and C2, respectively.

In the compartment model, the rate of transfer of ^{18}F-NaF from the arterial compartment to the ECF ($C_a \rightarrow$ C1) is denoted by K_1, also referred to as the plasma clearance of ^{18}F-NaF to the ECF, and has units of mL min^{-1} cm^{-3} (*meaning of these parameters discussed later*). The parameters k_2 and k_3 have units of min^{-1} and represent the rate of transfer from the ECF back to the plasma (C2 $\rightarrow$ C_a) and from the ECF to the newly mineralized bone (C1 $\rightarrow$ C2), respectively. Although the physiologic meaning of k_2 is not immediately clear (discussed later), k_3 is a valuable measure of the efficiency of ^{18}F-NaF uptake into the mineralized compartment. Further, k_4 also has units of min^{-1} and represents the backward rate of transfer of ^{18}F-NaF from the newly mineralized bone compartment to the ECF (C2 $\rightarrow$ C1).[66] Finally, it is important to not forget about total bone mineral, as the volume of newly mineralized bone depends on total bone that is

available to remodel. This entire model can be simplified into a two-compartment schematic (**Fig. 7**), commonly referred to as the Hawkins two-compartment bone model.[67]

Now with a working model for the transfer of ^{18}F-NaF throughout a bone ROI, the law of conservation of matter can be applied to each compartment to obtain the differential Equations 2 and 3.

$$\frac{dC_1}{dt} = K_1 C_a(t) - k_2 C_1(t) - k_3 C_1(t) + k_4 C_2(t) \tag{2}$$

$$\frac{dC_2}{dt} = k_3 C_1(t) - k_4 C_2(t) \tag{3}$$

Here, we have a solvable set of first-order differential equations. The solution to these equations (Equations 4 and 5) is two functions for the concentration of ^{18}F-NaF over time within the ECF and new bone mineral compartment [C_1(t) and C_2(t), respectively].

$$C_1(t) = C_a \left[A_{11} e^{-a_1(t)} + A_{12} e^{-a_2 t} \right] \tag{4}$$

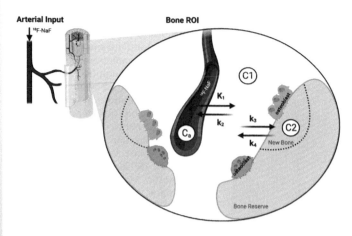

Fig. 6. ^{18}F-NaF is exchanged from the arterial compartment (labeled C_a) into an unbound extracellular compartment (ECF) (labeled C1). The ^{18}F-NaF within the unbound ECF is also exchanged between the newly mineralized bone compartment (labeled C2), which depends on the amount of new bone mineral available for incorporation of ^{18}F-NaF. K_1 describes the rate of transfer of radiotracer from arterial compartment to the ECF, with units of mL min^{-1}·cm^{-3}. k_2, k_3, and k_4 are the rate of transfer of radiotracer from ECF to the arterial compartment, from the ECF to the new bone mineral, and from the bone mineral back into the ECF space, respectively. (Image created with BioRender.com). Park, P.S.U.; Raynor, W.Y.; Sun, Y.; Werner, T.J.; Rajapakse, C.S.; Alavi, A. 18F-Sodium Fluoride PET as a Diagnostic Modality for Metabolic, Autoimmune, and Osteogenic Bone Disorders: Cellular Mechanisms and Clinical Applications. Int. J. Mol. Sci. 2021, 22, 6504. https://doi.org/10.3390/ijms22126504

$$C_1(t) = C_a A_{22} \left[e^{-a_1(t)} + e^{-a_2 t} \right] \quad (5)$$

Here, C_α is the initial spike in plasma concentration at time zero. A_{11}, A_{12}, A_{22}, α_1, and α_2 are the algebraic functions of parameters K_1, k_2, k_3, and k_4[65].

In PET, we do not know the parameters (K_1, k_2, k_3, or k_4). After all, this is the information we are trying to gain from the kinetic model. By measuring the SUVs within a ROI of bone at various time points, we are effectively creating the plot of $C_1(t) + C_2(t)$, which is defined as the tissue activity curve (TAC). C_a can also be plotted by measuring the SUV within an arterial ROI (ideally the artery that supplies the bone ROI) over a period of time. This is defined as the arterial input function (AIF). With knowledge of our kinetic model, computational methods and regression algorithms can be applied to the TAC and AIF to estimate the parameter values that best fit the compartmental model. Hawkins and colleagues proposed a method to measure plasma clearance of ^{18}F-NaF using 60-min dynamic ^{18}F-NaF PET scans, which are performed by acquiring multiple scans with increasing time frames over the protocol duration.[67] This method uses a nonlinear regression using the two-compartment kinetic model (described up to

this point) to estimate the four rate constants to describe the movement of ^{18}F-NaF between the compartments. The kinetic parameters can provide insightful bone physiology measures (**Table 1**).

K_1

Since the extraction efficiency of ^{18}F-NaF into the bone compartment from the arterial compartment is nearly 100%, the value of K_1 is a good estimate of bone perfusion and has been shown to be in agreement with ^{15}O-H$_2$O studies (the gold standard for blood flow studies).[66,68]

This perfusion parameter may be very useful in terms of osteoporosis, as bone perfusion is crucial to maintaining skeletal health.[69,70,77] Going back to osteoblast and osteoclast coupling, it is reasonable to conclude that decreased blood supply, and subsequent increase in catabolic molecules that may contribute to the increase in osteoclast activity. This is supported by studies that find low bone perfusion is correlated with greater bone loss and increased fracture risk.[71,78] It is also important to consider the ROI with higher blood flow. When blood flow is high, there is insufficient time for the ^{18}F-NaF to equilibrate with the tissue, thus K_1 can underestimate true bone perfusion in this

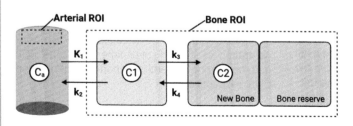

Fig. 7. The two-compartment model of bone (Hawkins model), a simplified schematic of **Fig. 7**. (Image created with BioRender.com)

Table 1
Kinetic parameters

Parameter	Units	Functional Definition	Biological Meaning
K_1	mL/min cm^3	Volume of ^{18}F-NaF cleared from plasma pool to ECF space per unit time per unit tissue volume [1]	Given extraction efficiency of ^{18}F-NaF is near 100% and is not bound to plasma proteins, K1 is closely related to bone blood flow (bone perfusion) [1,2] Clinical relevance/example: Low bone perfusion is significantly correlated with increased bone loss and increased fracture risk [3,4,5]
K_2	1/min	Rate of transfer of ^{18}F-NaF from the ECF space back to arterial compartment [1]	Measure of how efficiently ^{18}F-NaF moves back to the ECF space. Potentially reflects bone microarchitecture and capillary permeability Clinical relevance/example: Unclear. Some speculate that can give insight into bone morphology (more trabecular crowding in Paget's disease → more difficult for ^{18}F-NaF to exchange into arterial compartment) [6]. It may also correlate with capillary permeability [7]. A decrease in k_2 may also reflect ^{18}F-NaF trapped within cells of ECF space (F → HF → diffuse though cell membranes) [1,6]
K_3	1/min	Rate of transfer of ^{18}F-NaF from the ECF space to newly mineralized bone compartment.[1]	Direct reflection of mineralization rate and osteoblast activity, also is an indirect measure of osteoclast function, as both are intricately coupled. Clinical relevance/example: In study of teriparatide treatment, only k_3 showed significant ↑, suggesting it is a sensitive measure of expected increase in osteoblast activity [1,8].
K_4	1/min	Rate of transfer of ^{18}F-NaF form the newly mineralized none compartment back to the ECF space [1].	Represents a small fraction of ^{18}F-NaF that is weakly incorporated into exposed hydroxyapatite. Clinical relevance/example: Unclear. Near-zero value. Puri et al has shown that by neglecting its value, it underestimates ^{18}F-NaF clearance into none mineral (K_i).[1]

(continued on next page)

Parameter	Units	Functional Definition	Biological Meaning
Table 1 *(continued)*			
K_i	mL/min cm^3	Volume of ^{18}F-NaF cleared from plasma pool to newly mineralized bone per unit time per unit tissue volume, represented as none perfusion (K_1) multiplied by the fraction of ^{18}F-NaF that incorporates into bone mineral from ECF [1].	Most reported parameter. Referred to as bone metabolic flux and a measure of bone turnover. Directly related to bone perfusion (unlike k_3), as well as osteoblast activity. Clinical relevance/example: Significantly correlated with histomorphometry data for bone turnover, such as osteoblast per bone surface, osteoclast per bone surface, bone turnover rate, etc. [9]. Is significantly correlated with increased coupling of osteoblasts and osteoclasts [1].
K_1/k_2	mL/cm^3	Volume of distribution of ^{18}F-NaF within the ECF compartment per tissue volume [1].	For a skeletal region of interest, it describes the volume that is occupied by ECF space. As trabecular volume ↑'s, K/k_2 ↓'s [1]. Clinical relevance/example: Incorporates estimate of perfusion (K_1) and efficiency of ^{18}F-NaF to transfer back to arterial compartment (k_2) to give measure of how much tracer accumulates in ECF space. Gives insight into bone 3D structure. Bones with greater marrow space (vertebrae) have greater K_1/k_2 compared with bones with less marrow space (humerus) [7,10].

Data from [1],[66] [2],[68] [3],[69] [4],[70] [5],[71] [6],[72] [7],[73] [8],[49] [9],[74,75] [10].[76]

case. This is illustrated by the findings that K_1 is lower than expected in the lumbar spine, a tissue ROI that is highly metabolically active.[66,72] Therefore, K_1 can potentially give an extra layer of useful information about bone perfusion or a data point to better normalize other parameter measurements.

K_i

K_i is the most widely used and reported parameter and is calculated from Equation 6. Given the units of $k_3/(k_2+k_3)$ cancel, K_i has the same units as K_1 of mL min^{-1} mL^{-1}.

$$K_i = K_1\left(\frac{k_3}{k_2+k_3}\right) \qquad (6)$$

K_i is also referred to as the net plasma clearance of ^{18}F-NaF from the plasma to bone mineral.[66,79] Another way of thinking about K_i is that it is the volume of plasma cleared of ^{18}F-NaF per mL of bone per minute. This parameter is also widely referred to as a measure of bone turnover and bone metabolic flux.[79,80] Several groups have shown K_i

positively correlated with bone histomorphometric data of bone turnover, such as osteoblast per bone area, osteoclast per bone area, and bone formation rate (BFR), with r^2 values between +0.49 and +0.63.[74,75] Given that K_i is associated with both osteoblast and osteoclast activity, this parameter is best described as a measure of the coupling of bone remodeling processes and does not necessarily inform about the direction of bone formation, which depends on the relative rates of osteoblast and osteoclast activity. Therefore, calling K_i bone metabolic flux can be misleading since it does not tell you whether the mineral flux is positive or negative.

k_2, k_3, and k_4

In the two-compartment model, k_3 is the transfer of ^{18}F-NaF from the unbound ECF to the newly mineralized bone. k_3 may be the most direct measure of mineralization rate and osteoblast activity as it represents the transfer rate of tracer from the ECF to bone without the influence of other parameters. In a study of teriparatide treatment, only k_3 showed a significant increase, where no change was observed in K_1, k_2, and k_4, indicating k_3 was a sensitive measure of increased osteoblast function.[49] The true usefulness behind k_2 and k_4 is not fully understood. In Paget's disease, Cook and colleagues found that as k_3 increased, k_2 decreased, reflecting the increased bone turnover.[76] Also, it is thought k_2 may provide insight into bone morphology. For example, Paget's disease is accompanied by less marrow space (due to increased bone volume and crowding of trabecular space), and therefore the decrease in k_2 may be explained by the fact that it is more difficult for the tracer to return to the blood pool.[72,76] k_4 is the rate of ^{18}F-NaF flow from the new bone mineral to the ECF. Although many groups neglect this parameter due to its near zero value, others have shown that k_4 may provide important data when assessing overall kinetics.[81–83] The non-zero value for k_4 suggests that there is a small fraction of ^{18}F-NaF that is weakly bound to HA, and one study found that neglecting this value results in underestimation of K_i.[66]

K_1/k_2 as a measure of extracellular fluid volume

The ratio of K_1/k_2 has been proposed as a measure of the volume of distribution of ^{18}F-NaF within the ECF compartment. Assuming passive diffusion of fluoride between plasma and ECF, K_1/k_2 would represent the volume of total bone ROI occupied by ECF. However, this is not a great assumption, as fluoride is a small negatively charged molecule and is known to bind hydrogen to create HF, which can cross cell membranes.[66] Several groups have shown that K_1/k_2 is positively correlated with the amount of marrow space (ie, lumbar vertebrae trabecula displays higher relative K_1/k_2 than humoral bone).[72,84] In one study, Puri and colleagues argues that the reason K_i values at the hip were three-fold lower compared with the lumbar spine is due to the increase in K_1/k_2 seen at the spine. They found that there were significantly greater K_1/k_2 ratios at the lumbar vertebrae, suggesting more functioning red marrow and relatively greater levels of ^{18}F-NaF within the ECF.[83]

Interestingly, K_1/k_2 may also give some insight into the composition of the bone marrow.[66,69] For example, higher levels of marrow fat is negatively correlated with bone perfusion, as fat replaces healthy red marrow and decreases the effective trabecular ECF space. Thus, higher amounts of marrow fat would result in lower K_1/k_2 ratios. Given bone marrow fat is correlated with age and osteoporosis, this could be yet another important parameter, or means for making

sense of other measures such as K_i or SUVs of osteoporosis patients.[85]

A Simpler Method: Patlak Plot

One of the drawbacks of the Hawkins method is it requires complex computational methods. However, by assuming k_4 is negligible, and ^{18}F-NaF is irreversibly bound to the mineral compartment, the model can be simplified.[86,87] The mathematics simplify, allowing the clearance of ^{18}F-NaF to the bone mineral compartment (K_i) to be determined by a graphical approach. To do this, the measured positron emission tomography (PET) activity within the tissue ROI is divided by the plasma activity and plotted as a function of normalized time, which is the integral of the input curve from initial time of injection divided by the instantaneous plasma concentration.[65,81] The slope of this plot is equal to K_i **(Fig. 8)**.

This simplified approach is widely used as a measure of K_i, and several groups have shown that K_i from the Patlak method is highly correlated with K_i obtained with the Hawkins method.[86–91]

Making Sense of the Methods

It is important to call attention to the differences between the values obtained from SUVs, Patlak K_i, and Hawkins K_i.

Several groups have found that there is no obvious correlation between SUV measurements and age.[92,93] In fact, Kurata and colleagues found that the SUVmax in the humeral shaft was positively correlated with advanced age, but the SUVmax in the lumbar spine was negatively correlated with age.[92] It is likely that these differences are due to several factors, such as differences in regional blood flow and bone microarchitecture, in which case kinetic data could provide the most insight.[83,94] In addition, Blake and colleagues point out a potential limitation of SUV measurement being the fact that a finite amount of radiotracer must be distributed to bone throughout the body.[49] So, in systemic metabolic diseases such as Paget's disease and osteoporosis, there are multiple sites throughout the skeleton that are competing for ^{18}F-NaF, which competes for radiotracer.[49,95] Therefore, the SUV measurement may be underestimated at other sites throughout the skeleton.[49,62] To illustrate this point, a study of osteoporotic patients treated with teriparatide for 6 months found that the total plasma concentration of ^{18}F-NaF decreased by 21%, resulting in minimal change in SUV (3%). However, the K_i obtained from the dynamic scan saw a significant 24% increase.[62] Therefore, the kinetic analysis, if done meticulously, can remove the confounding

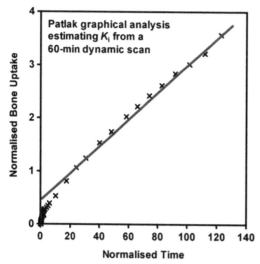

Fig. 8. The Patlak plot (used with permission from Blake and colleagues[88]) represents a graphical approach to solving for K_i, which is estimated by plotting the tissue concentration normalized to arterial concentration as a function of normalized time. Normalized time is the integral of the arterial input curve divided by the instantaneous plasma concentration.[81] (*From* Blake GM, Siddique M, Frost ML, Moore AE, Fogelman I. Quantitative PET Imaging Using (18)F Sodium Fluoride in the Assessment of Metabolic Bone Diseases and the Monitoring of Their Response to Therapy. PET Clin. 2012 Jul;7(3):275-91.)

influence of plasma concentration and provide perfusion status that can improve the conclusions made on analysis of ^{18}F-NaF PET data.

In a recent meta-analysis by Assiri and colleagues, it was found that the Patlak method had the lowest precision error and allowed for fewer study participants to show a significant treatment response.[87] K_i determined from the Hawkins method showed the highest precision error, which is explained by the high precision errors of each individual parameter (around 30% or greater each).[66] It can be reasoned that the Patlak method has the best sensitivity for clinical practice and research, but it can be argued that the variability of the other parameters (K_1, k_2, k_3, k_4, and so forth) can explain intersubject differences in bone characteristics that may be useful in predicting, or characterizing, bone health. Even with the Hawkins method, K_i has the least precision error of the parameters and is the most widely reported parameter to describe bone metabolism.[35]

^{18}F-NaF PET/COMPUTED TOMOGRAPHY AS AN ADJUNCT FOR SCREENING AND MONITORING OSTEOPOROSIS

To this point, we have reviewed the established methods of measuring bone turnover using ^{18}F-

NaF PET/CT. The aim being to deliver an overall understanding of how each method works, the insight that may come from the parameters as it relates to bone health, and the important considerations and nuances. This section presents the current evidence for why ^{18}F-NaF PET/CT may serve as a valuable upgrade to the available tools for managing osteoporosis.

A retrospective study of 139 patients (from CAMONA cohort) calculated a bone metabolism score (BMS) using ^{18}F-NaF-PET/CT. To do this, the authors segmented the entire femoral neck, and then created a subsegment only capturing the cortical and trabecular bone. The SUV within the segmented bone region was normalized by dividing it by the SUV of the entire femoral neck to create the BMS. They found that women over the age of 50 had a significantly lower BMS. Further, they noticed that patients who were classified as osteopenic ($-1 < T < -2.5$) had a wide spread of BMS, suggesting ^{18}F-NaF-PET/CT may be a valuable adjunct to DXA to provide insight into bone metabolism in the femoral neck and be useful for assessing fracture risk in patients where bone mineral density (BMD) provides inconclusive risk determination.[96] These findings echo other studies showing decreased SUV and K_i in osteoporosis patients[35] (**Fig. 9**).

However, should there be a decrease in ^{18}NaF PET signal in osteoporosis? After menopause, biological bone turnover markers (osteoclast markers) are *increased* by 90%, whereas bone formation markers are only *increased* by 45%.[5,97] As there is increased overall bone turnover and bone formation (just resorption outruns formation), one would expect an increased ^{18}F-NaF PET signal. However, the opposite is generally seen. To understand this, one must consider the resolution of PET/CT imaging. For standard CT scans done in clinical practice, the voxel size is around 2 mm^3, where the average trabecular thickness is 50 to 400 μm.[98] Thus, the signal detected by PET is the summation of bone turnover occurring within many bone remodeling units throughout the trabeculae. If the number of trabeculae decreased significantly and the metabolic activity did not change (amount of osteoclast–osteoblast activity per remodeling unit), then the signal would be decreased as there are less remodeling units per voxel. In another example more similar to osteoporosis (**Fig. 10**), there can be greater bone turnover per remodeling unit, but because there are less trabecular (less bone surface area for bone remodeling units), the signal on ^{18}F-NaF PET can be less per voxel.

Given that ^{18}F-NaF PET data are affected by bone microarchitecture, it is difficult to compare

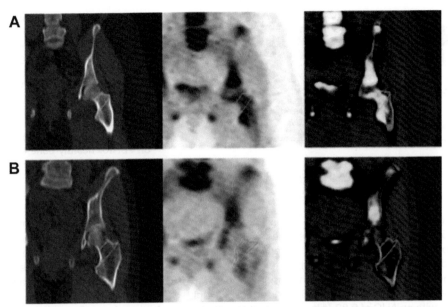

Fig. 9. (*A*) The coronal section of a CT scan (left), static 18F-NaF PET scan (middle), and a fusion of the two (right) at the left hip of a healthy, 25-year-old woman. (*B*) The same image sequence for a 62-year-old woman. Using the CT image to precisely segment the region of the femoral neck, the amount of radiotracer uptake within that commonly fractured region is easily quantified and can be used to track therapeutic response. (*From* Reilly CC, Raynor WY, Hong AL, et al. Diagnosis and Monitoring of Osteoporosis With 18F-Sodium Fluoride PET: An Unavoidable Path for the Foreseeable Future. *Semin Nucl Med.* 2018;48(6):535-540.)

the bone turnover data across populations with different bone morphology. There is a great need for further research to better understand how bone morphology affects 18F-NaF PET/CT data, so that it can be compared with healthy individuals. As mentioned, menopause is a major factor for developing osteoporosis. With the average age of menopause occurring at age 51 and the recommended screening age being 65, there is a potential 14-year window of metabolic change that is largely unmonitored leading up to the development of osteoporosis. Presumably, if an individual is in the early stages of osteoporosis (when bone microstructure is still normal relative to age-matched controls), 18F-NaF PET would show an increase in signal reflecting the increase in bone turnover (SUV and K_i). However, once microstructure declines, the 18F-NaF PET signal also declines, even though it is possible that there is an increase in bone turnover. If 18F-NaF PET data can be adjusted by bone architecture in the future, then it is possible that we will be capable of accurately monitoring relative bone turnover, which will improve monitoring disease progression and fracture risk prediction.[1,23,99]

The major outcome that clinicians aim to prevent in a patient with osteoporosis is bone fracture; however, many patients who sustain fractures do not meet the BMD T-score criteria for osteoporosis.[100–104] As previously alluded to,

repeat DXA scans provide little to no added benefit when assessing future fracture risk in patients with osteoporosis.[32] It is increasingly recognized that bone turnover markers, such as alkaline phosphatase (ALP), osteocalcin (OC), and carboxy terminal cross-linked telopeptide of type I collagen (CTX), are increased in people with high fracture risk.[105–109] In a prospective cohort of 435 women, subjects who had ALP and CTX levels in the highest quartile had a 2-fold increase in fractures, with relative risks of 2.4 and 2.3, respectively. Interestingly, Messa and colleagues has shown that the K_i from dynamic 18F-NaF PET is significantly correlated with global bone turnover markers ALP and parathyroid hormone (PTH) of patients with renal osteodystrophy ($r^2 = 0.81$ and $r^2 = 0.93$, respectively).[110] These markers only give a measure of global bone turnover, where 18F-NaF PET/CT adds the ability to measure bone turnover at site-specific locations with higher sensitivity which correlates with histomorphometric data.[52,74,110] In their study of 26 patients with end-stage renal disease and suspected renal osteodystrophy, Aaltonen and colleagues showed that K_i was significantly correlated with histomorphometric measures such as osteoblast per bone surface (OB/BS) ($r^2 = 0.49$), osteoclasts per bone surface (OC/BS) ($r^2 = 0.62$), BFR ($r^2 = 0.63$), and erosion surface per bone surface (ES/BS) ($r^2 = 0.57$).[74] Additional studies report an even higher

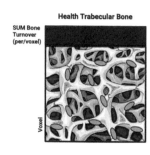
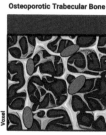

Health Trabecular Bone   **Osteoporotic Trabecular Bone**

SUM Bone Turnover (per/voxel)

No turnover — High turnover

Fig. 10. Red ovals represent bone remodeling units. The greater the intensity of red is, the higher the amount of bone turnover. When capturing ^{18}F-NaF PET data per voxel, the output SUV is equal to the sum of many bone remodeling units. For osteoporotic bone, with increased bone turnover (per bone remodeling unit), the sum of activity on PET can be less than the sum of activity on PET for healthy bone due to healthy bone having more bone surface area

per voxel. (Image created with BioRender.com)

correlation between K_i and BFR ($r^2 = 0.71$ and $r^2 = 0.65$).[110,111] Aaltonen and colleagues went on to show that K_i from ^{18}F-NaF PET alone was able to differentiate patients with low turnover versus non-low turnover (defined by histomorphometric analysis) with a sensitivity of 76% and specificity 78% with an AUC of 0.82.[74] It is important to note, these experiments were carried out on bone from the same disease state and likely similar microstructure. Thus, if ^{18}F-NaF PET data can be adjusted by bone microarchitecture, then it has the potential to be a powerful tool to noninvasively assess bone metabolism and potentially catch abnormal bone metabolism before it leads to structural change.

Further, there is a great need for future studies to investigate the added value of dynamic ^{18}F-NaF-PET/CT and kinetic parameters in fracture risk prediction. It is likely that the kinetic parameters (K_1, k_2, k_3, k_4, K_i, and K_1/k_2) may provide added information that can more reliably and accurately characterize bone status and fracture risk. From our literature review, there are no studies that integrate these parameters as a tool for characterizing bone in a way to predict bone fractures or predict structural change.

Monitoring Response to Treatment

One of the most promising applications for ^{18}F-NaF PET is monitoring response to therapy for osteoporotic patients. As structural changes of bone can take years to improve or decline with treatment, there is a need for an imaging technique with better sensitivity and temporal resolution to monitor response to treatment[112,113]

First-line treatment for osteoporosis is antiresorptive therapy with bisphosphonates that bind to HA binding sites on bone, stimulating apoptosis of osteoclasts and thereby inhibiting bone resorption. A study of 24 postmenopausal women with glucocorticoid-induced osteoporosis examined the effect of treatment with alendronate, a

bisphosphonate, on bone metabolism via ^{18}F-fluoride, demonstrated significant decreases in bone metabolism and turnover in the lumbar spine.[114] These metabolic changes are observed in ^{18}F-NaF PET before changes in ALP and BMD. In fact, SUV at the lumbar spine significantly decreased as early as 3 months, whereas ALP did not significantly change until 6 months, and BMD did not increase until 12 months.[114] Further, a study of 18 women with T-scores less than −2 treated with risedronate found similar findings to the prior study with K_i, net plasma clearance to bone mineral displaying a significant decrease as soon as 6 months of treatment on ^{18}F-fluoride PET.[94] To further illustrate the added sensitivity of dynamic ^{18}F-NaF PET/CT, this group also found that K_1 was not significantly affected by risedronate, whereas k_3/k_2+k_3 decreased by 18%.[115] This finding suggests the major effect of treatment was on the available sites for radiotracer disposition, clearly showing a decrease in osteoblast activity. It is clear that dynamic ^{18}F-NaF PET parameters can provide valuable measures to more accurately assess the desired treatment response of a therapeutic.

Studies have also been done to monitor response to treatment with teriparatide, a synthetic PTH analog that works by activating both osteoblasts and osteoclasts, with preferential activation of osteoblasts. Frost and colleagues randomized 27 osteopenic females ($−1 < T < −2.5$) into two groups, where one received calcium and vitamin D and the other received teriparatide along with calcium and vitamin D. They then performed 60-min dynamic ^{18}F-NaF PET scans at baseline and 12 months after treatment. They found that the teriparatide group had a significant increase in K_i at all ROIs analyzed, including the hip, lumbar spine, femoral shaft, and femoral shaft trabecular.[63] Interestingly, this same study performed DXA scans on the patients and found that BMD significantly increased at the lumbar spine, but only modestly increased at the hip and did not increase at the femoral neck ROI. This finding parallels the findings from clinical trials where teriparatide was shown to have the greatest increase in BMD at the lumbar spine and not significantly affect BMD at the hip.[116–118] By investigating further, other groups found that teriparatide actually decreased cortical density by increasing turnover within the cortical region of the femoral neck while at the same time increasing trabecular volume. Thus, DXA was unable to measure a difference in BMD due to these opposing effects, despite great overall bone anabolic activity.[116] On mechanical testing, the mechanical strength of the femoral neck ROI increased; however, this increase in biomechanical strength was only observed at either 18 or 24 months.[116,117] Therefore, these findings suggest that teriparatide effect on bone structure can take up to 2 years, where the study by Frost and colleagues was able to report a significant increase in bone anabolic activity as early as 12 months. This further supports the ability of ^{18}F-NaF PET to predict future bone structure and architecture, suggesting it is the optimal biomarker for observing treatment response to teriparatide.

SUMMARY

Osteoporosis is a metabolic bone disorder characterized by a dysregulation of osteoblast, osteoclasts, and osteocytes that leads to a fragile skeleton. The current standard of characterizing osteoporosis by bone density and structural architecture at particular ROIs is incapable of capturing this complex bone biology. These structural approaches (namely DXA) have their pitfalls in reliably predicting fractures. Patients with the same T-score have different rates of fracture, and fractures in non-hip and non-vertebral bones are collectively more common in osteoporotic patients.[119] This is concerning and highlights the need for a more sensitive imaging modality to better assess and categorize patients for fracture risk. ^{18}F-NaF-PET is a promising imaging modality for early detection and monitoring of metabolic bone disorders that alter bone biology. ^{18}F-NaF-PET can be used as a tool to assess bone turnover and aid in characterizing bone morphology, as well as a tool to monitor response to treatment. Here, we have laid out the various methods of ^{18}F-NaF PET/CT for assessing bone turnover. Although they each have their limitations, SUV measurements from a static ^{18}F-NaF PET/CT scan is likely the easiest and most clinically applicable method to capture bone turnover throughout the skeleton. These static scans can sensitively assess longitudinal

progression of bone metabolism and treatment response. Dynamic ^{18}F-NaF PET/CT and kinetic parameter estimation is a more technically challenging technique but may provide more useful research data, including estimates of bone perfusion, insights into ECF space volume, and osteoblast activity. Even more powerful is the fact that all kinetic parameters can be measured voxel-by-voxel within a larger ROI such as the femoral neck. This high-resolution mapping of bone turnover has great potential by not only the ability to reconstruct a 3D view of bone turnover but also assess treatment response, which may have spatial heterogeneity. Further research must continue to explore ways to refine kinetic ^{18}F-NaF PET/CT data in a way that is clinically useful and comparable across heterogeneous populations. Nevertheless, ^{18}F-NaF PET/CT may prove to be a much needed upgrade to the osteoporosis toolbox in the near future.

CLINICS CARE POINTS

- Osteoporosis is the most common metabolic bone disorder that is characterized by a disintegration of bone microarchitecture, predisposing individuals to devastating fractures followed by severe loss of quality of life.

- While a diagnosis of osteoporosis can be made by a bone mineral density reading, the underlying cause of this structural change is extremely complex and diverse, consisting of a myriad of biological factors that tip the scale of bone metabolism to favor resorption.

- Here, we introduce [18]NaF PET/computed tomography as an emerging tool that adds the ability to measure bone metabolism, which has already been shown to monitor response to osteoporosis treatment more sensitively compared to DEXA and other structural modalities.

- With the continual advancement of PET technologies and the application of kinetic modeling in the research setting, 18NaF PET/computed tomography has the potential to provide an in vivo assay for bone turnover and other useful parameters related to osteoporosis pathophysiology, including bone perfusion and extracellular fluid volume

- Taken together, [18]NaF PET/computed tomography may emerge as an invaluable clinical readout for characterizing bone health and allow for more sensitive monitoring and screening for osteoporosis.

DISCLOSURE

This research was supported by the Intramural Research Program of the NIH Clinical Center and National Institute of Dental and Craniofacial Research. The opinions expressed in this publication are the author's own and do not reflect the view of the National Institutes of Health, the Department of Health and Human Services, or the United States government. This work was also made possible by the NIH Medical Research Scholars Program, which is a public-private partnership supported jointly by the NIH and generous contributions to the Foundation for the NIH from the Doris Duke Charitable Foundation, the American Association for Dental Research, the Colgate-Palmolive Company, alumni of student research programs, and other individual supporters via contributions to the Foundation for the National Institutes of Health.

REFERENCES

1. Sarafrazi N. Osteoporosis or low bone mass in older adults: United States, 2017-2018. Centers Dis Control Prev 2021. https://doi.org/10.15620/cdc:103477.
2. Viswanathan M, Reddy S, Berkman N, et al. Screening to prevent osteoporotic fractures: Updated evidence report and Systematic review for the US preventive Services Task Force. JAMA 2018;319(24):2532–51.
3. Compston JE, McClung MR, Leslie WD. Osteoporos Lancet 2019;393(10169):364–76.
4. Barnsley J, Buckland G, Chan PE, et al. Pathophysiology and treatment of osteoporosis: challenges for clinical practice in older people. Aging Clin Exp Res 2021;33(4):759–73.
5. Eastell R, O'Neill TW, Hofbauer LC, et al. Postmenopausal osteoporosis. Nat Rev Dis Primers 2016;2:16069.
6. Berger C, Langsetmo L, Joseph L, et al. Change in bone mineral density as a function of age in women and men and association with the use of antiresorptive agents. CMAJ 2008;178(13):1660–8.
7. Lindgren E, Karlsson MK, Lorentzon M, et al. Bone traits Seem to develop also during the third decade in life-normative cross-Sectional data on 1083 men aged 18-28 years. J Clin Densitom 2017;20(1):32–43.
8. World Health Organization. Assessment of fracture risk and its application to screening for postmenopausal osteoporosis : report of a WHO study group [meeting held in rome from 22 to 25 june 1992]. World Health Organization; 1994. Available at: https://apps.who.int/iris/handle/10665/39142. Accessed August 19, 2022.
9. Kanis JA, Cooper C, Rizzoli R, et al. Scientific advisory board of the European Society for clinical and economic aspects of osteoporosis (ESCEO) and the committees of Scientific advisors and national Societies of the international osteoporosis foundation (IOF). European guidance for the diagnosis and management of osteoporosis in postmenopausal women. Osteoporos Int 2019;30(1):3–44.
10. Eriksen EF. Cellular mechanisms of bone remodeling. Rev Endocr Metab Disord 2010;11(4):219–27.
11. Kong YY, Yoshida H, Sarosi I, et al. OPGL is a key regulator of osteoclastogenesis, lymphocyte development and lymph-node organogenesis. Nature 1999;397(6717):315–23.
12. Matsumoto T, Endo I. RANKL as a target for the treatment of osteoporosis. J Bone Miner Metab 2021;39(1):91–105.
13. Han Y, You X, Xing W, et al. Paracrine and endocrine actions of bone-the functions of secretory proteins from osteoblasts, osteocytes, and osteoclasts. Bone Res 2018;6:16.
14. Guo YC, Yuan Q. Fibroblast growth factor 23 and bone mineralisation. Int J Oral Sci 2015;7(1):8–13.
15. Eastell R, Szulc P. Use of bone turnover markers in postmenopausal osteoporosis. Lancet Diabetes Endocrinol 2017;5(11):908–23.
16. Bolamperti S, Villa I, Rubinacci A. Bone remodeling: an operational process ensuring survival and bone mechanical competence. Bone Res 2022;10(1):48.
17. Arceo-Mendoza RM, Camacho PM. Postmenopausal osteoporosis: latest guidelines. Endocrinol Metab Clin North Am 2021;50(2):167–78.
18. Armas LAG, Recker RR. Pathophysiology of osteoporosis: new mechanistic insights. Endocrinol Metab Clin North Am 2012;41(3):475–86.
19. Gao Y, Patil S, Jia J. The development of molecular biology of osteoporosis. Int J Mol Sci 2021;22(15). https://doi.org/10.3390/ijms22158182.
20. Ettinger B, Black DM, Mitlak BH, et al. Reduction of vertebral fracture risk in postmenopausal women with osteoporosis treated with raloxifene: results from a 3-year randomized clinical trial. Multiple Outcomes of Raloxifene Evaluation (MORE) Investigators. JAMA 1999;282(7):637–45.
21. Noh JY, Yang Y, Jung H. Molecular mechanisms and emerging therapeutics for osteoporosis. Int J Mol Sci 2020;21(20). https://doi.org/10.3390/ijms21207623.
22. Yang Y, Yujiao W, Fang W, et al. The roles of miRNA, lncRNA and circRNA in the development of osteoporosis. Biol Res 2020;53(1):40.
23. Demontiero O, Vidal C, Duque G. Aging and bone loss: new insights for the clinician. Ther Adv Musculoskelet Dis 2012;4(2):61–76.

24. Xu Y, Ma J, Xu G, et al. Recent advances in the epigenetics of bone metabolism. J Bone Miner Metab 2021;39(6):914–24.

25. Ralston SH, Uitterlinden AG. Genetics of osteoporosis. Endocr Rev 2010;31(5):629–62.

26. Zhu X, Bai W, Zheng H. Twelve years of GWAS discoveries for osteoporosis and related traits: advances, challenges and applications. Bone Res 2021;9(1):23.

27. Rozenberg S, Bruyère O, Bergmann P, et al. How to manage osteoporosis before the age of 50. Maturitas 2020;138:14–25.

28. Curry SJ, Krist AH, Owens DK, et al, US Preventive Services Task Force. Screening for osteoporosis to prevent fractures: US preventive Services Task Force recommendation Statement. JAMA 2018; 319(24):2521–31.

29. Guzon-Illescas O, Perez Fernandez E, Crespí Villarias N, et al. Mortality after osteoporotic hip fracture: incidence, trends, and associated factors. J Orthop Surg Res 2019;14(1):203.

30. Menéndez-Colino R, Alarcon T, Gotor P, et al. Baseline and pre-operative 1-year mortality risk factors in a cohort of 509 hip fracture patients consecutively admitted to a co-managed orthogeriatric unit (FONDA Cohort). Injury 2018;49(3):656–61.

31. Ebeling PR, Nguyen HH, Aleksova J, et al. Secondary osteoporosis. Endocr Rev 2022;43(2):240–313.

32. Hillier TA, Stone KL, Bauer DC, et al. Evaluating the value of repeat bone mineral density measurement and prediction of fractures in older women: the study of osteoporotic fractures. Arch Intern Med 2007;167(2):155–60.

33. Sollmann N, Löffler MT, Kronthaler S, et al. MRI-based quantitative osteoporosis imaging at the spine and femur. J Magn Reson Imaging 2021; 54(1):12–35.

34. Black DM, Cauley JA, Wagman R, et al. The ability of a single BMD and fracture history assessment to predict fracture over 25 Years in postmenopausal women: the study of osteoporotic fractures. J Bone Miner Res 2018;33(3):389–95.

35. Reilly CC, Raynor WY, Hong AL, et al. Diagnosis and monitoring of osteoporosis with 18F-sodium fluoride PET: an Unavoidable Path for the foreseeable future. Semin Nucl Med 2018;48(6):535–40.

36. Blake GM, Fogelman I. Technical principles of dual energy x-ray absorptiometry. Semin Nucl Med 1997;27(3):210–28.

37. Osteoporosis to prevent fractures: screening. Available at: https://www.uspreventiveservicestaskforce.org/uspstf/recommendation/osteoporosis-screening. Accessed May 10, 2022.

38. Damilakis J, Adams JE, Guglielmi G, et al. Radiation exposure in X-ray-based imaging techniques used in osteoporosis. Eur Radiol 2010;20(11):2707–14.

39. Akram S, Chowdhury YS. Radiation exposure of medical imaging. In: StatPearls. StatPearls Publishing; 2021. https://www.ncbi.nlm.nih.gov/pubmed/33351446.

40. Berger A. Bone mineral density scans. BMJ 2002; 325(7362):484.

41. Oei L, Koromani F, Rivadeneira F, et al. Quantitative imaging methods in osteoporosis. Quant Imaging Med Surg 2016;6(6):680–98.

42. Brett AD, Brown JK. Quantitative computed tomography and opportunistic bone density screening by dual use of computed tomography scans. J Orthop Translat 2015;3(4):178–84.

43. Tse JJ, Smith ACJ, Kuczynski MT, et al. Advancements in osteoporosis imaging, screening, and study of disease etiology. Curr Osteoporos Rep 2021;19(5):532–41.

44. Michalski AS, Besler BA, Burt LA, et al. Opportunistic CT screening predicts individuals at risk of major osteoporotic fracture. Osteoporos Int 2021; 32(8):1639–49.

45. Adams AL, Fischer H, Kopperdahl DL, et al. Osteoporosis and hip fracture risk from routine computed tomography scans: the fracture, osteoporosis, and CT Utilization study (FOCUS). J Bone Miner Res 2018;33(7):1291–301.

46. Koch V, Hokamp NG, Albrecht MH, et al. Accuracy and precision of volumetric bone mineral density assessment using dual-source dual-energy versus quantitative CT: a phantom study. Eur Radiol Exp 2021;5(1):43.

47. Gruenewald LD, Koch V, Martin SS, et al. Diagnostic accuracy of quantitative dual-energy CT-based volumetric bone mineral density assessment for the prediction of osteoporosis-associated fractures. Eur Radiol 2022;32(5):3076–84.

48. Wichmann JL, Booz C, Wesarg S, et al. Dual-energy CT-based phantomless in vivo three-dimensional bone mineral density assessment of the lumbar spine. Radiology 2014;271(3):778–84.

49. Blake GM, Puri T, Siddique M, et al. Site specific measurements of bone formation using [18F] sodium fluoride PET/CT. Quant Imaging Med Surg 2018;8(1):47–59.

50. Blau M, Nagler W, Bender MA. Fluorine-18: a new isotope for bone scanning. J Nucl Med 1962;3:332–4. Available at: https://www.ncbi.nlm.nih.gov/pubmed/13869926.

51. Raynor W, Houshmand S, Gholami S, et al. Evolving role of molecular imaging with 18F-sodium fluoride PET as a biomarker for calcium metabolism. Curr Osteoporos Rep 2016;14(4):115–25.

52. Blake GM, Siddique M, Frost ML, et al. Imaging of site specific bone turnover in osteoporosis using

positron emission tomography. Curr Osteoporos Rep 2014;12(4):475–85.

53. Park PSU, Raynor WY, Sun Y, et al. 18F-Sodium fluoride PET as a diagnostic modality for metabolic, Autoimmune, and osteogenic bone disorders: cellular mechanisms and clinical applications. Int J Mol Sci 2021;22(12). https://doi.org/10.3390/ijms22126504.

54. Zhang V, Koa B, Borja AJ, et al. Diagnosis and monitoring of osteoporosis with total-body 18F-sodium fluoride-PET/CT. PET Clin 2020;15(4):487–96.

55. Haim S, Zakavi R, Imamovic L, et al. Predictive Value of 18F-NaF PET/CT in the Assessment of Osteoporosis: Comparison with Dual-Energy X-Ray Absorptiometry (DXA). European Journal of Nuclear Medicine and Molecular Imaging 2017;44:S857.

56. Dyrberg E, Larsen EL, Hendel HW, et al. Diagnostic bone imaging in patients with prostate cancer: patient experience and acceptance of NaF-PET/CT, choline-PET/CT, whole-body MRI, and bone SPECT/CT. Acta Radiol 2018;59(9):1119–25.

57. Velez EM, Desai B, Jadvar H. Treatment response assessment of skeletal metastases in prostate cancer with 18F-NaF PET/CT. Nucl Med Mol Imaging 2019;53(4):247–52.

58. Moore AEB, Blake GM, Fogelman I. Quantitative measurements of bone remodeling using 99mTc-methylene diphosphonate bone scans and blood sampling. J Nucl Med 2008;49(3):375–82.

59. Wale DJ, Wong KK, Savas H, et al. Extraosseous findings on bone Scintigraphy using fusion SPECT/CT and correlative imaging. AJR Am J Roentgenol 2015;205(1):160–72.

60. Blake GM, Frost ML, Moore AEB, et al. The assessment of regional skeletal metabolism: studies of osteoporosis treatments using quantitative radionuclide imaging. J Clin Densitom 2011;14(3):263–71.

61. Ahuja K, Sotoudeh H, Galgano SJ, et al. 18F-Sodium fluoride PET: history, technical feasibility, mechanism of action, normal biodistribution, and diagnostic performance in bone metastasis detection compared with other imaging modalities. J Nucl Med Technol 2020;48(1):9–16.

62. Blake GM, Siddique M, Frost ML, et al. Radionuclide studies of bone metabolism: do bone uptake and bone plasma clearance provide equivalent measurements of bone turnover? Bone 2011; 49(3):537–42.

63. Frost ML, Moore AE, Siddique M, et al. ^{18}F-fluoride PET as a noninvasive imaging biomarker for determining treatment efficacy of bone active agents at the hip: a prospective, randomized, controlled clinical study. J Bone Miner Res 2013;28(6):1337–47.

64. Huang SCH. Pharmacokinetic modeling. Mol Imaging 2021;1625–31.

65. Carson RE. Tracer kinetic modeling in PET. In: Bailey DL, Townsend DW, Valk PE, et al, editors. Positron emission tomography: basic sciences. London: Springer; 2005. p. 127–59.

66. Puri T, Frost ML, Cook GJ, et al. [18F] sodium fluoride PET kinetic parameters in bone imaging. Tomography 2021;7(4):843–54.

67. Hawkins RA, Choi Y, Huang SC, et al. Evaluation of the skeletal kinetics of fluorine-18-fluoride ion with PET. J Nucl Med 1992;33(5):633–42. Available at: https://www.ncbi.nlm.nih.gov/pubmed/1569473.

68. Piert M, Zittel TT, Machulla HJ, et al. Blood flow measurements with [(15)O]H2O and [18F]fluoride ion PET in porcine vertebrae. J Bone Miner Res 1998;13(8):1328–36.

69. Griffith JF, Yeung DKW, Tsang PH, et al. Compromised bone marrow perfusion in osteoporosis. J Bone Miner Res 2008;23(7):1068–75.

70. Prisby RD, Ramsey MW, Behnke BJ, et al. Aging reduces skeletal blood flow, endothelium-dependent vasodilation, and NO bioavailability in rats. J Bone Miner Res 2007;22(8):1280–8.

71. Reeve J, Arlot M, Wootton R, et al. Skeletal blood flow, iliac histomorphometry, and strontium kinetics in osteoporosis: a relationship between blood flow and corrected apposition rate. J Clin Endocrinol Metab 1988;66(6):1124–31.

72. Cook GJR, Lodge MA, Blake GM, et al. Differences in skeletal kinetics between vertebral and humeral bone measured by 18F-fluoride positron emission tomography in postmenopausal women. J Bone Miner Res 2010;15(4):763–9.

73. Pantel AR, Viswanath V, Muzi M, et al. Principles of tracer kinetic analysis in oncology, Part I: principles and overview of methodology. J Nucl Med 2022; 63(3):342–52.

74. Aaltonen L, Koivuviita N, Seppänen M, et al. Correlation between 18F-Sodium Fluoride positron emission tomography and bone histomorphometry in dialysis patients. Bone 2020;134:115267.

75. Messa C. Bone metabolic activity measured with positron emission tomography and [18F]fluoride ion in renal osteodystrophy: correlation with bone histomorphometry. J Clin Endocrinol Metab 1993; 77(4):949–55.

76. Cook GJR, Blake GM, Marsden PK, et al. Quantification of skeletal kinetic indices in Paget's disease using Dynamic18F-fluoride positron emission tomography. J Bone Miner Res 2002;17(5):854–9.

77. Bloomfield SA, Hogan HA, Delp MD. Decreases in bone blood flow and bone material properties in aging Fischer-344 rats. Clin Orthop Relat Res 2002;396:248–57.

78. Vogt MT, Cauley JA, Kuller LH, et al. Bone mineral density and blood flow to the lower extremities: the

study of osteoporotic fractures. J Bone Miner Res 1997;12(2):283–9.

79. Nzeusseu Bol I. 18F-fluoride PET for monitoring therapeutic response in Paget's disease of bone. J Nucl Med 2005. Available at: https://jnm. snmjournals.org/content/46/10/1650.short.

80. Siddique A, Green T. Is response assessment of breast cancer bone metastases better with measurement of 18F-fluoride metabolic flux than with measurement of 18F-fluoride PET/CT SUV. J Nucl Med 2019. Available at. https://jnm.snmjournals. org/content/60/3/322.short.

81. Patlak CS, Blasberg RG, Fenstermacher JD. Graphical evaluation of blood-to-brain transfer constants from multiple-time uptake data. J Cereb Blood Flow Metab 1983;3(1):1–7.

82. Mathavan N, Koopman J, Raina DB, et al. 18F-fluoride as a prognostic indicator of bone regeneration. Acta Biomater 2019;90:403–11.

83. Puri T, Frost ML, Curran KM, et al. Differences in regional bone metabolism at the spine and hip: a quantitative study using 18F-fluoride positron emission tomography. Osteoporos Int 2013;24(2):633–9.

84. Morris MA, Lopez-Curto JA, Hughes SP, et al. Fluid spaces in canine bone and marrow. Microvasc Res 1982;23(2):188–200.

85. Schwartz AV. Marrow fat and bone: review of clinical findings. Front Endocrinol 2015;6:40.

86. Haddock B, Fan AP, Jørgensen NR, et al. Kinetic [18F]-Fluoride of the knee in normal volunteers. Clin Nucl Med 2019;44(5):377–85.

87. Assiri R, Knapp K, Fulford J, et al. Correlation of the quantitative methods for the measurement of bone uptake and plasma clearance of 18F-NaF using positron emission tomography. Systematic review and meta-analysis. Eur J Radiol 2022;146:110081.

88. Siddique B, Moore F. Quantitative PET imaging using 18F sodium fluoride in the assessment of metabolic bone diseases and the monitoring of their response to therapy. PET Clin 2012. Available at: https://www.pet.theclinics.com/article/S1556-8598(12)00060-0/abstract.

89. Vrist MH, Bech JN, Lauridsen TG, et al. Comparison of [18F] NaF PET/CT dynamic analysis methods and a static analysis method including derivation of a semi-population input function for site-specific measurements of bone formation in a population with chronic kidney disease-mineral and bone disorder. EJNMMI Res 2021;11(1):117.

90. Karakatsanis NA, Zhou Y, Lodge MA, et al. Generalized whole-body Patlak parametric imaging for enhanced quantification in clinical PET. Phys Med Biol 2015;60(22):8643–73.

91. Siddique M, Frost ML, Blake GM, et al. The precision and sensitivity of 18F-fluoride PET for measuring regional bone metabolism: a comparison of quantification methods. J Nucl Med 2011;52(11):1748–55.

92. Kurata S, Shizukuishi K, Tateishi U, et al. Age-related changes in pre- and postmenopausal women investigated with 18F-fluoride PET–a preliminary study. Skeletal Radiol 2012;41(8):947–53.

93. Ayubcha C, Zirakchian Zadeh M, Stochkendahl MJ, et al. Quantitative evaluation of normal spinal osseous metabolism with 18F-NaF PET/CT. Nucl Med Commun 2018;39(10):945–50.

94. Frost ML, Cook GJR, Blake GM, et al. A prospective study of risedronate on regional bone metabolism and blood flow at the lumbar spine measured by 18F-fluoride positron emission tomography. J Bone Miner Res 2003;18(12):2215–22.

95. Gnanasegaran G, Moore AE, Blake GM, et al. Atypical Paget's disease with quantitative assessment of tracer kinetics. Clin Nucl Med 2007;32(10):765–9.

96. Rhodes S, Batzdorf A, Sorci O, et al. Assessment of femoral neck bone metabolism using 18F-sodium fluoride PET/CT imaging. Bone 2020;136:115351.

97. Garnero P, Sornay-Rendu E, Chapuy MC, et al. Increased bone turnover in late postmenopausal women is a major determinant of osteoporosis. J Bone Miner Res 1996;11(3):337–49.

98. Clarke B. Normal bone anatomy and physiology. Clin J Am Soc Nephrol 2008;3(Suppl 3):S131–9.

99. Ceylan B, Özerdoğan N. Factors affecting age of onset of menopause and determination of quality of life in menopause. Turk J Obstet Gynecol 2015;12(1):43–9.

100. Siris ES, Chen YT, Abbott TA, et al. Bone mineral density thresholds for pharmacological intervention to prevent fractures. Arch Intern Med 2004;164(10):1108–12.

101. Stone KL, Seeley DG, Lui LY, et al. BMD at multiple sites and risk of fracture of multiple types: long-term results from the Study of Osteoporotic Fractures. J Bone Miner Res 2003;18(11):1947–54.

102. Marshall D, Johnell O, Wedel H. Meta-analysis of how well measures of bone mineral density predict occurrence of osteoporotic fractures. BMJ 1996;312(7041):1254–9.

103. Cranney A, Jamal SA, Tsang JF, et al. Low bone mineral density and fracture burden in postmenopausal women. CMAJ 2007;177(6):575–80.

104. Akkawi I, Zmerly H. Osteoporosis: Curr Concepts. Joints 2018;6(2):122–7.

105. Shetty S, Kapoor N, Bondu JD, et al. Bone turnover markers: emerging tool in the management of osteoporosis. Indian J Endocrinol Metab 2016;20(6):846–52.

106. Heaney RP. Is the paradigm shifting? Bone 2003; 33(4):457–65.

107. Garnero P, Hausherr E, Chapuy MC, et al. Markers of bone resorption predict hip fracture in elderly women: the EPIDOS Prospective Study. J Bone Miner Res 1996;11(10):1531–8.

108. Szulc P, Montella A, Delmas PD. High bone turnover is associated with acceated bone loss but not with increased fracture risk in men aged 50 and over: the prospective MINOS study. Ann Rheum Dis 2008;67(9):1249–55.

109. Grados Brazier, Kamel Mathieu. Prediction of bone mass density variation by bone remodeling markers in postmenopausal women with vitamin D insufficiency treated with calcium and vitamin D. J Clin Endocrinol Metab 2003;88(11):5175–9. Available at: https://academic.oup.com/jcem/article-abstract/88/11/5175/2656398.

110. Messa C, Goodman WG, Hoh CK, et al. Bone metabolic activity measured with positron emission tomography and [18F]fluoride ion in renal osteodystrophy: correlation with bone histomorphometry. J Clin Endocrinol Metab 1993;77(4):949–55.

111. Piert M, Zittel TT, Becker GA, et al. Assessment of porcine bone metabolism by dynamic. J Nucl Med 2001;42(7):1091–100. Available at: https://www.ncbi.nlm.nih.gov/pubmed/11438633.

112. Deal CL. Using bone densitometry to monitor therapy in treating osteoporosis: pros and cons. Curr Rheumatol Rep 2001;3(3):233–9.

113. Muncie HL Jr, LeBlanc LL. Monitoring osteoporosis treatment: DXA should not be routinely repeated. Am Fam Physician 2010;82(7):749–54. Available at: https://www.ncbi.nlm.nih.gov/pubmed/20879697.

114. Uchida K, Nakajima H, Miyazaki T, et al. Effects of alendronate on bone metabolism in glucocorticoid-induced osteoporosis measured by 18F-fluoride PET: a prospective study. J Nucl Med 2009; 50(11):1808–14.

115. Frost ML, Siddique M, Blake GM, et al. Regional bone metabolism at the lumbar spine and hip following discontinuation of alendronate and risedronate treatment in postmenopausal women. Osteoporos Int 2012;23(8):2107–16.

116. Borggrefe J, Graeff C, Nickelsen TN, et al. Quantitative computed tomographic assessment of the effects of 24 months of teriparatide treatment on 3D femoral neck bone distribution, geometry, and bone strength: results from the EUROFORS study. J Bone Miner Res 2010;25(3):472–81.

117. Sato M, Westmore M, Ma YL, et al. Teriparatide [PTH(1-34)] strengthens the proximal femur of ovariectomized nonhuman primates despite increasing porosity. J Bone Miner Res 2004;19(4):623–9.

118. Black DM, Greenspan SL, Ensrud KE, et al. The effects of parathyroid hormone and alendronate alone or in combination in postmenopausal osteoporosis. N Engl J Med 2003;349(13):1207–15.

119. Shi N, Foley K, Lenhart G, et al. Direct healthcare costs of hip, vertebral, and non-hip, non-vertebral fractures. Bone 2009;45(6):1084–90.

PET Imaging in Osteoarthritis

Mohamed Jarraya, MD[a],*, Frank W. Roemer, MD[b,c], Tobias Bäuerle, MD[c,d],
Feliks Kogan, PhD[e], Ali Guermazi, MD, PhD[f]

KEYWORDS

- Osteoarthritis • PET • MR imaging • CT

KEY POINTS

- Although PET is not routinely used in osteoarthritis, it can reveal early metabolic changes associated with early disease
- The combined use of PET and cross-sectional imaging, such as MRI, may increase sensitivity for detection of pain generator in osteoarthritis.

INTRODUCTION

Osteoarthritis (OA) is the single most common cause of disability in older adults, affecting at least more than 14 million Americans and resulting in joint pain, stiffness, and loss of mobility.[1,2] The high prevalence of OA results in high societal and personal costs, with a reported 140 billion dollars of arthritis-related medical expenditure in the United States in 2013 alone.[3] Although OA was traditionally considered a disease of "wear and tear" of cartilage, there is a growing consensus that OA is a complex condition involving different joint tissues. Although older age is a risk factor for OA, its pathogenesis remains poorly understood, with no disease-modifying treatments to date.

Radiological assessment of OA includes conventional radiography, computed tomography (CT), and MR imaging. Although CT and MR imaging provide information on the morphologic and functional aspects of OA, PET determines metabolic parameters depending on the administered radiopharmaceutical. ^{18}F-sodium fluoride (^{18}F-NaF) as a tracer has been established as a useful bone-seeking imaging tool, particularly when evaluating the local bone metabolism status.[4,5] Uptake of ^{18}F-fluorodeoxyglucose (^{18}F-FDG) in OA results from an increased glucose metabolism in bone or surrounding soft tissue due to processes like inflammation and infection.[6]

The advent of conventional MR imaging in OA research has led to the identification of biomarkers of disease progression such as bone marrow lesions and synovitis.[7,8] The importance of subchondral bone in OA pathogenesis is emphasized by the categorization of a separate subchondral bone phenotype in knee OA.[9] The use of PET/MR imaging in OA provides a useful addition to other imaging modalities assessment of bone turnover and represents a metabolic imaging of the subchondral bone. The purpose of this article is to review the use of PET in the imaging assessment of knee OA, with a focus on clinical research applications.

TECHNICAL CONSIDERATIONS
Hybrid Imaging (PET/Computed Tomography and PET/MR imaging)

There are several reports using hybrid PET/CT in imaging of OA. This is mainly due to the

[a] Department of Radiology, Massachusetts General Hospital, Harvard Medical School, 32 Fruit Street, YAW 6044, Boston, MA 02115, USA; [b] Department of Radiology, Boston University School of Medicine, 830 Harrison Avenue, 3rd Floor, Boston, MA 02118, USA; [c] Department of Radiology, Friedrich-Alexander University Erlangen-Nürnberg (FAU) and University Hospital Erlangen, Maximiliansplatz 391054, Erlangen, Germany; [d] Institute of Radiology, University Medical Center Erlangen, Maximiliansplatz 3, 91054 Erlangen, Germany; [e] Department of Radiology, Stanford university, 1201 Welch Rd, P266Stanford, CA 94305, USA; [f] Department of Radiology, VA Boston Healthcare System, 1400 VFW Parkway, 1B105, West Roxbury, MA 02132, USA
* Corresponding author.
E-mail address: mjarraya@mgh.harvard.edu

PET Clin 18 (2023) 21–29
https://doi.org/10.1016/j.cpet.2022.09.002
1556-8598/23/© 2022 Elsevier Inc. All rights reserved.

widespread use of PET/CT in clinical practice mainly for oncologic indications.[10,11] For instance, Nguyen and colleagues showed in a small clinical sample of 65 patients with oncologic indications that FDG uptake of the knee, shoulder, and hips correlated with pain and function[11] and demonstrated that standardized uptake value (SUV) was an independent predictor of progression of knee OA in these patients.[11] However, CT provides limited information about the presence of periarticular soft tissue and subchondral edema, both of which are important features in OA. For that reason, hybrid PET/MR imaging is particularly suited for the evaluation and clinical research of OA given the supplemental information on subchondral bone, synovium, and periarticular soft tissues. Obviously, the metabolic focus of hybrid OA imaging is defined by the administered radiophamaceutical (^{18}F-FDG or ^{18}F-NaF).

Attenuation Correction: Attenuation is by far the largest correction required for quantitative PET imaging with CT-based PET attenuation correction (AC) now widely accepted as the clinical standard.[12] AC for PET/MR imaging is more challenging as MR imaging signal results from proton density of tissues with its relaxation properties, therefore it does not provide direct information regarding PET AC as compared with CT where its linear AC is scaled to PET energy, that is, 511 keV, thus providing direct information of PET AC.[12,13] Instead, an MR imaging -based AC approach relies on a DIXON fat-water images to identifying four segments: soft tissue, fat, lung, and air. Each segment is then assigned an established AC coefficient.[13] However, with this method correction for bone which has no signal on conventional MR imaging is not possible. Therefore, more recent MR imaging methods based on zero echo time (ZTE) have helped providing patient-specific morphology of bone and estimate continuous-valued attenuation coefficients for bone.[13,14] Furthermore, novel methods for producing pseudo-CT attenuation coefficients maps from collected ZTE and Dixon images have been created using a deep learning-based technique. This approach allows capturing variability in bone density and improves SUV accuracy near bony anatomy significantly.[15]

Radiopharmaceuticals

^{18}F-fluorodeoxyoglucose: ^{18}F-FDG is a marker for rate of glucose metabolism, which integrates into the metabolic pathway of glucose resulting in FDG-6-phosphate. Because of its polar metabolic nature and inability to participate to Krebs cycle, the latter is entrapped into the intracellular space, which results in increased uptake within metabolically active cells. As a result, the metabolic activity can be measured using SUV.[16] In addition to its wide use for staging of malignancies, ^{18}F-FDG has proven its high sensitivity not only for inflammatory arthritis[17,18] but also for spinal[19] and peripheral OA.[20] Increased FDG uptake in OA knees was previously found in the intercondylar notch extending along the PCL, periosteophytic lesions, and subchondral bone marrow lesions.[6] Another study showed an increased ^{18}F-FDG uptake around the entire knee and in particular along the medial synovium.[21] Obviously, as ^{18}F-FDG records tissue changes like inflammation and infection resulting from mechanical aspects in OA, this technique is not specific, but relatively sensitive.

^{18}F-sodium fluoride: ^{18}F-NaF is a positron-emitting bone-seeking radiopharmaceutical tracer with an uptake mechanism similar to ^{99}mTc-HMDP and technetium 99m-methyl diphosphonate (^{99}mTc-MDP),[22] allowing quantification of calcium metabolism and is mainly used to evaluate skeletal metastases.[23,24] As analogue of the hydroxyl group found in the hydroxyapatite bone crystals, ^{18}F-NaF deposits in the bone compartment. The rapid bone clearance of ^{18}F-NaF as well as its minimum serum protein binding and fast renal clearance results in greater bone-to-background ratio and shorter time than conventional ^{99}mTc-based tracers.[25] In animal model, ^{18}F-NaF was shown to concentrate at freshly mineralizing bone sites,[26] explaining its use as a bone marker. Quantitative ^{18}F-NaF PET has been shown to be sensitive to variations in bone vascularization and metabolism in the healthy knee joint with significantly different uptake parameters between the cortical and trabecular bone.[27]

In addition, a recent study showing that exercise results in a significant increase of ^{18}F-NaF uptake in all bone tissue in both knees with up to 131% increase in $SUV_{(max)}$ in subchondral bone tissue.[28] These results show that bone loading induces an acute response in bone physiology as quantified by ^{18}F-NaF PET kinetics.

Last, several studies focused on the use of ^{18}F-NaF in OA showing its sensitivity in detecting early metabolic changes before structural changes are detected on conventional modalities.[29,30]

MORPHOLGIC AND COMPOSITIONAL MR IMAGING IN OSTEOARTHRITIS

Morphologic MR Imaging: One of the challenges of OA research is identifying risk factors of clinical and morphologic incidence and progression, especially among patients with normal radiographic findings. In this regard, MR imaging has been useful by demonstrating that MR imaging -detected bone marrow lesions[8] and synovitis[7] are independent predictors of OA progression.

Compositional MR Imaging: T1 rho and T2 relaxation times provide a measure of proteoglycan content and collagen orientation, respectively, reflecting the cartilage composition and biochemistry.[31,32] Elongated T1 rho and T2 relaxation times have been shown to predict cartilage damage progression in prior longitudinal study suggesting the role of compositional MR imaging as a biomarker of early hip OA.[33]

CLINICAL AND TRANSLATIONAL APPLICATIONS
Peripheral Joints

PET/MR imaging allows simultaneous evaluation of the metabolic activity of OA as well as structural and compositional biomarkers. PET/MR imaging also enables excellent spatial relationships between cartilage health and subchondral bone remodeling to be evaluated in a single examination with no added radiation from the MR imaging component of PET/MR imaging.[13]

Increased body mass index (BMI), which is considered a major risk factor in OA, was shown to correlate with increased ^{18}F-FDG and ^{18}F-NaF uptake in the knee[34] and sacroiliac and hips joints.[29] In addition, increased BMI was found to correlate with increased ^{18}F-NaF uptake, marker of subchondral bone formation in several joints including elbow, hands, knees, and feet.[35] Similar observation was also made in the cervicothoracic and lumbar spine which showed association between metabolic activity in the spine and increased BMI, but not age.[36]

The role of PET/MR imaging in early-stage OA has been demonstrated in several studies showing increased SUV$_{(max)}$ in the hip among patients with no radiographic joint space narrowing and those with severe pain.[37] The same investigators later showed in an overlapping cohort the role of PET SUV$_{(max)}$ as a predictor of OA progression, specifically, minimum joint space narrowing and pain worsening.[38]

Kobayashi and colleagues showed that although 18F-NaF PET positivity is found in 96% of joints with MR imaging-detected morphologic abnormality and increases with Kellgren–Lawrence grade and present in all cases with Kellgren–Lawrence grade 4, PET positivity was also found in a proportion of joint with no detected cartilage abnormalities, further emphasizing the potential role of PET/MR imaging as a predictor of disease.[39]

PET/MR imaging combines the high-resolution morphologic information on structural damage of the synovium, cartilage, subchondral bone (and meniscus in the knee), as well as advanced quantitative MR imaging measurement analyzing tissue microstructure (T2 or T1ρ relaxation times) and metabolic information on the subchondral bone brought by PET.

Watkins and colleagues found a correlation between tracer uptake rates calculated from ^{18}F-NaF

PET data and morphologic changes of knee OA using the MR imaging Osteoarthritis Knee Score scoring system. They found that abnormal bone metabolic biomarkers detected by PET correlated with regions of larger osteophytes, adjacent cartilage lesions, and bone marrow lesion (BML) relative to the bone that appeared to be normal on MR imaging [40] (**Fig. 1**). **Figs. 2** and **3** illustrate ^{18}F-FDG PET CT findings in the hand and knee, respectively, with MR imaging and CT correlates.

In a recent small study of 22 knees from 11 individuals, MacKay and colleagues found a positive correlation between SUV $_{(max)}$ of ^{18}F-NaF PET and synovitis quantified by dynamic contrast-enhanced MR imaging. The investigators found that areas of subchondral bone having high SUV$_{(max)}$ had more intense synovitis than the normal subchondral bone without ^{18}F-NaF uptake.[41] These results are in line with the hypothesis that synovitis may play some role in the formation of osteophytes.[42]

In a feasibility study involving 22 subjects Kogan and colleagues showed that SUV$_{(max)}$ in all subchondral bone marrow lesions was significantly higher than that of normal appearing subchondral bone on MR imaging, however, the investigators showed more than one-third of areas of high ^{18}F-NaF and ^{18}F-FDG uptake corresponded to normal appearing bone on MR imaging.[43] These findings suggest that increased metabolic activity detected by MR imaging can be an early sign of OA. These results were confirmed by Watkins and colleagues in 2021 showing altered bone metabolism using a 3T ^{18}F-NaF PET/MR imaging in OA knees within regions with and without structural findings, in comparison with healthy volunteers.[44] The role of bone physiology in OA instigation and progression may be quantified using kinetic characteristics in subchondral bone of ^{18}F-NaF uptake. The objective measurements of bone metabolism obtained from ^{18}F-NaF PET imaging can be used as supplementary information to MR imaging assessments of structural anomalies.[44]

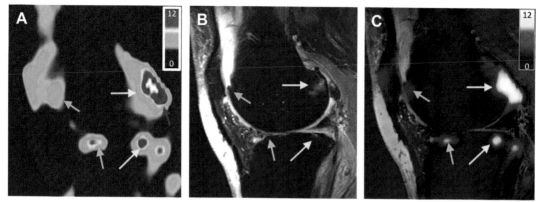

Fig. 1. (*A*) Sagittal ^{18}F-NaF PET, (*B*) sagittal T2-weighted (*W*) fat-suppressed (FS) fast spin echo (FSE), and (*C*) PET–MR imaging fusion in a 74-year-old woman with knee pain and known osteoarthritis (OA). ^{18}F-NaF PET shows increased uptake of the posterior lateral femoral condyle and tibial plateau at the site of bone marrow lesions (yellow *arrows*) with an SUV$_{max}$ of 17.9 and 8.4, respectively. There is also increased uptake of the anterior tibial plateau at the site of cartilage loss (green *arrow*) with an SUV$_{max}$ of 5.8, and mildly increased uptake at the site of small osteophyte formation in the lateral trochlea (SUV$_{max}$ of 3.4). Note also marked uptake of the fabella (red *arrow*, SUV$_{max}$ = 12).

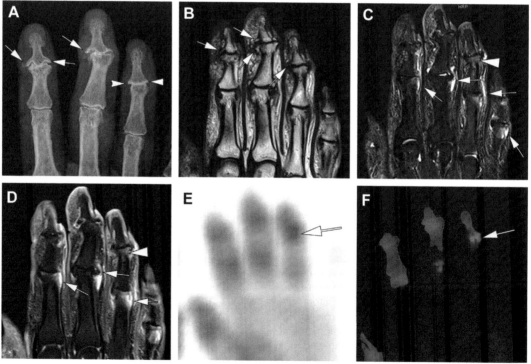

Fig. 2. Multimodality imaging of hand osteoarthritis (OA). (*A*) Frontal x-ray shows typical marginal osteophytes and gull-wing deformity of the articular surfaces of the index and long fingers distal interphalangeal (DIP) joints. There are minor osteoarthritis changes also in the ring finger DIP joint (*arrowheads*). (*B*) Corresponding coronal T1-weighted (*W*) image also exhibits osteophytes at the joint margins of multiple DIP joints (*arrows*). (*C*) Coronal T2w fat-suppressed image shows joint effusions in the index to little fingers proximal interphalangeal (PIP) joint depicted as intra-articular fluid-equivalent signal (*arrows*). In addition, there is an area of bone marrow edema (BME) at the distal epiphysis of the ring finger middle phalanx (*arrowhead*). (*D*) Coronal contrast-enhanced T1w fat-suppressed image shows synovial enhancement in the index to little fingers PIP joints. Area of BME of the ring finger middle phalanx distal epiphysis shows enhancement (*arrowhead*). (*E*) Corresponding PET image shows tracer accumulation in all DIP joints but particularly in the DIP joint of the ring finger (*arrow*). (*F*) The fusion PET/CT image shows that tracer uptake is particularly observed in the subchondral area of BME (*arrow*).

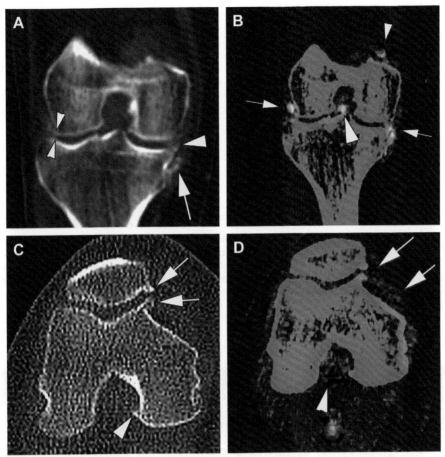

Fig. 3. ^{18}F-FDG PET/CT of advanced medial knee OA. (*A*) Coronal reformation of CT shows severe medial joint space narrowing (*arrows*) and osteophytes at the medial femur and the medial and lateral intercondylar notch (*arrowheads*). (*B*) Corresponding PET/CT fusion image shows perimeniscal tracer uptake corresponding to perimeniscal synovitis. Note also periligamentous synovitis around the PCL, the most common location of synovitis in knee OA (*arrowhead*). (*C*) Axial CT image shows patellofemoral OA with medial patellar and trochlea osteophytes (*arrows*). (*D*) Corresponding PET/CT fusion image shows medial patellofemoral synovitis (*arrows*). Periligamentous notch synovitis is seen around the PCL confirming finding on coronal images (*arrowhead*).

The interaction between subchondral bone and cartilage in early OA has been investigated by various studies using ^{18}F-NaF PET/MR imaging. In a limited sample of 10 individuals, a study focusing on the hip joint showed high correlation between SUV in the acetabulum with bone marrow lesions, which increased when corrected for age.[45] In some cases, elevated SUV was found in regions that did not show morphologic abnormality (cartilage or other joint tissue), however,

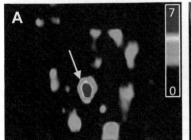
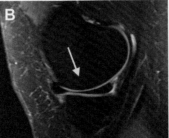
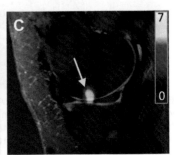

Fig. 4. (*A*) Sagittal ^{18}F-NaF PET, (*B*) sagittal T2-weighted FS FSE, and (*C*) PET–MR imaging fusion images in a healthy female individual. ^{18}F-NaF PET shows focal uptake in the central third of the medial femoral condyle (yellow *arrow*, $SUV_{max} = 5.0$) without MR-detected structural abnormality.

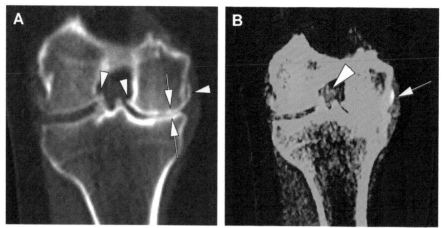

Fig. 5. ^{18}F-FDG PET/CT of knee OA with CPPD. (*A*) Coronal CT reformation shows definite joint space narrowing at the lateral joint space (small *arrowheads*). In addition, there is marked meniscal calcification (large *arrowhead*) and a calcification at the distal medial collateral ligament insertion (*arrow*) consistent with CPPD. (*B*) Corresponding coronal PET/CT fusion image shows marked perimeniscal tracer accumulation at the medial and lateral joint margins (*arrows*). In addition, there is tracer uptake in the intercondylar notch and superior-posterior at the medial femur (*arrows*).

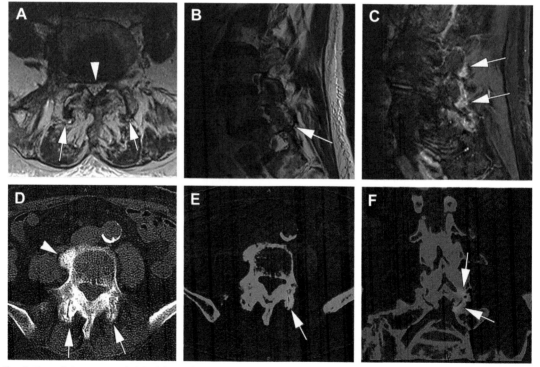

Fig. 6. Facet joint osteoarthritis. (*A*) Axial T2-weighted (*W*) MR image at the level L4/5 shows severe facet joint OA with severe osteophytes (*arrows*). In addition, there is a spinal canal stenosis due to disc bulging and ligament hypertrophy (*arrowhead*). (*B*) Sagittal T2w image shows hypertrophic facet OA on the left side of the level L4/5 (*arrow*). (*C*) Corresponding sagittal T1w fat-suppressed contrast-enhanced image shows marked synovial contrast enhancement at the levels L3/4 and L4/5 (*arrows*). (*D*) Corresponding axial CT shows hypertrophic OA of both facet joints at the level L4/5 (*arrows*). In addition, there is a large osteophyte anteriorly (*arrowhead*). (*E*) and (*F*) Axial and sagittal fusion images shows tracer accumulation only at the left facet joint. ^{18}F-FDG PET/CT enables visualization of inflammatory synovial activity complementary to non-enhanced MR imaging or CT.

these elevations were seen in regions of increased T1 rho and T2, further suggesting early changes in the bone-cartilage matrix.[45]

Savic and colleagues showed association between compositional MR imaging parameters including T1 rho and increased turnover in the adjoining bone in the knee but reduced turnover in the non-adjoining compartments.[46] This observation also emphasizes the complexity of the biochemical and biomechanical interactions between the subchondral bone and cartilage in OA joints and may pave the way to identify a target for the development of a disease-modifying OA drug.

In a cross-sectional study including 22 subjects with patellofemoral pain, the bone uptake on ^{18}F-NaF PET was found to not always correspond to MR imaging abnormalities suggesting that PET can provide additional information to MR imaging [47] (Fig. 4). Last, increased ^{18}F-FDG uptake can also be demonstrated in inflammatory arthropathies such as gouty arthropathy.[48] Fig. 5 illustrates ^{18}F-FDG PET CT findings in crystal pyrophosphate dihydrate (CPPD) arthropathy.

Spine

Current literature is limited; however, hybrid ^{18}F-NaF PET imaging was shown to correlate with sites of pain in the spine and sacroiliac joints by demonstrating increased ^{18}F-NaF uptake.[49] Specifically, this study showed that ^{18}F-NaF PET/CT identified the pain generator site in 37 (88%) out of 42 individuals with back pain and not history of surgery.[49] In addition, ^{18}F-NaF was reported to be only weakly correlated with CT morphologic changes suggesting that ^{18}F-NaF and CT can provide supplementary information for identification of pain-generating facet joints.[10] A different study showed a correlation between ^{18}F-NaF uptake and both MR imaging findings and clinical disability.[50] Fig. 6 illustrates a case of facet joint arthropathy with ^{18}F-FDG PET CT and MR imaging correlate.

Temporomandibular Joint

Although temporomandibular (TMJ) dysfunction may commonly be seen in young individuals, there is a large overlap between TMJ dysfunction and TMJ OA. Several studies focused on the role of ^{18}F-NaF PET/MR imaging in TMJ dysfunction showing a fair diagnostic performance of SUV(-max) for arthralgic TMJ and TMJ dysfunction.[51] ^{18}F-NaF PET was also shown to have superior diagnostic ability and suitable alternative to ^{99}Tc MDP bone scan.[52]

SUMMARY

The increase and widespread use of PET imaging with concomitant use of CT or MR imaging present new opportunities to understand pathogenesis of OA and hopefully identify therapeutic targets. The supplementary information provided by metabolic imaging often aids in localizing the pain-generating site. Hybrid PET imaging can also help identify early OA as demonstrated by increased uptake in areas with normal MR imaging morphologic findings. Metabolic information derived from dynamic ^{18}F-NaF PET imaging holds promise as a quantitative marker of bone metabolism. However, further large prospective studies are needed to better understand its role in OA management.

CLINICS CARE POINTS

- Hybrid PET imaging and especially PET/MR imaging increase sensitivity to detect pain generator sites in spinal osteoarthritis.
- PET can reveal early metabolic changes associated with compositional biomarkers of early osteoarthritis in the knee and hip joints.
- PET/MR imaging may pave the way to identify therapeutic targets for the development of disease-modifying osteoarthritis drugs.

DISCLOSURE

FWR: Shareholder Boston Imaging Core Lab (BICL), LLC. Consultant to Calibr, Grünenthal.FK: Receives research support from GE Healthcare.AG: Shareholder of BICL, LLC. Consultant for Pfizer, Regeneron, TissueGene, MerckSerono, AstraZeneca and Novartis.MJ and TB: None.

REFERENCES

1. Cisternas MG, Murphy L, Sacks JJ, et al. Alternative methods for defining osteoarthritis and the Impact on estimating prevalence in a US Population-based Survey. Arthritis Care Res 2016;68(5):574–80.
2. Deshpande BR, Katz JN, Solomon DH, et al. Number of Persons with symptomatic knee osteoarthritis in the US: Impact of Race and Ethnicity, age, Sex, and Obesity. Arthritis Care Res 2016;68(12):1743–50.
3. Murphy LB, Cisternas MG, Pasta DJ, et al. Medical expenditures and Earnings Losses among US adults with arthritis in 2013. Arthritis Care Res 2018;70(6):869–76.

4. Czernin J, Satyamurthy N, Schiepers C. Molecular mechanisms of bone 18F-NaF deposition. J Nucl Med Off Publ Soc Nucl Med 2010;51(12):1826–9.

5. Grant FD, Fahey FH, Packard AB, et al. Skeletal PET with 18F-fluoride: applying new technology to an old tracer. J Nucl Med Off Publ Soc Nucl Med 2008; 49(1):68–78.

6. Nakamura H, Masuko K, Yudoh K, et al. Positron emission tomography with 18F-FDG in osteoarthritic knee. Osteoarthritis Cartilage 2007;15(6):673–81.

7. Felson DT, Niu J, Neogi T, et al. Synovitis and the risk of knee osteoarthritis: the MOST Study. Osteoarthritis Cartilage 2016;24(3):458–64.

8. Roemer FW, Neogi T, Nevitt MC, et al. Subchondral bone marrow lesions are highly associated with, and predict subchondral bone attrition longitudinally: the MOST study. Osteoarthritis Cartilage 2010;18(1): 47–53.

9. Roemer FW, Collins J, Kwoh CK, et al. MRI-based screening for structural definition of eligibility in clinical DMOAD trials: rapid OsteoArthritis MRI Eligibility Score (ROAMES). Osteoarthritis Cartilage 2020; 28(1):71–81.

10. Mabray MC, Brus-Ramer M, Behr SC, et al. (18)F-sodium fluoride PET-CT hybrid imaging of the lumbar facet joints: tracer uptake and Degree of correlation to CT-graded arthropathy. World J Nucl Med 2016; 15(2):85–90.

11. Nguyen BJ, Burt A, Baldassarre RL, et al. The prognostic and diagnostic value of 18F-FDG PET/CT for assessment of symptomatic osteoarthritis. Nucl Med Commun 2018;39(7):699–706.

12. Chen Y, An H. Attenuation correction of PET/MR imaging. Magn Reson Imaging Clin N Am 2017;25(2): 245–55.

13. Jena A, Taneja S, Rana P, et al. Emerging role of integrated PET-MRI in osteoarthritis. Skeletal Radiol 2021;50(12):2349–63.

14. Leynes AP, Yang J, Shanbhag DD, et al. Hybrid ZTE/Dixon MR-based attenuation correction for quantitative uptake estimation of pelvic lesions in PET/MRI. Med Phys 2017;44(3):902–13.

15. Leynes AP, Yang J, Wiesinger F, et al. Zero-echo-time and Dixon deep pseudo-CT (ZeDD CT): direct generation of pseudo-CT images for pelvic PET/MRI attenuation correction using deep Convolutional Neural Networks with Multiparametric MRI. J Nucl Med Off Publ Soc Nucl Med 2018;59(5):852–8.

16. Lim MMD, Gnerre J, Gerard P. Mechanisms of uptake of common radiopharmaceuticals Radio-Graphics Fundamentals | online Presentation. Radiogr Rev Publ Radiol Soc N Am Inc 2018;38(5): 1550–1.

17. Palmer WE, Rosenthal DI, Schoenberg OI, et al. Quantification of inflammation in the wrist with gadolinium-enhanced MR imaging and PET with 2-[F-18]-fluoro-2-deoxy-D-glucose. Radiology 1995; 196(3):647–55.

18. Elzinga EH, van der Laken CJ, Comans EFI, et al. 2-Deoxy-2-[F-18]fluoro-D-glucose joint uptake on positron emission tomography images: rheumatoid arthritis versus osteoarthritis. Mol Imaging Biol 2007;9(6):357–60.

19. Rosen RS, Fayad L, Wahl RL. Increased 18F-FDG uptake in degenerative disease of the spine: Characterization with 18F-FDG PET/CT. J Nucl Med Off Publ Soc Nucl Med 2006;47(8):1274–80.

20. Parsons MA, Moghbel M, Saboury B, et al. Increased 18F-FDG uptake suggests synovial inflammatory reaction with osteoarthritis: preliminary in-vivo results in humans. Nucl Med Commun 2015;36(12):1215–9.

21. Shah J, Bural G, Houseni M, et al. The role of FDG-PET in assessing osteoarthritis. J Nucl Med 2007; 48(supplement 2):282P.

22. Ahuja K, Sotoudeh H, Galgano SJ, et al. 18F-Sodium fluoride PET: history, Technical feasibility, mechanism of action, normal Biodistribution, and diagnostic performance in bone Metastasis detection compared with other imaging modalities. J Nucl Med Technol 2020;48(1):9–16.

23. Iagaru A, Mittra E, Dick DW, et al. Prospective evaluation of (99m)Tc MDP scintigraphy, (18)F NaF PET/CT, and (18)F FDG PET/CT for detection of skeletal metastases. Mol Imaging Biol 2012;14(2):252–9.

24. Schmidkonz C, Ellmann S, Ritt P, et al. Hybrid imaging (PET-Computed tomography/PET-MR imaging) of bone metastases. PET Clin 2019;14(1):121–33.

25. Jadvar H, Desai B, Conti PS. Sodium 18F-fluoride PET/CT of bone, joint, and other disorders. Semin Nucl Med 2015;45(1):58–65.

26. Piert M, Zittel TT, Becker GA, et al. Assessment of porcine bone metabolism by dynamic. J Nucl Med Off Publ Soc Nucl Med 2001;42(7):1091–100.

27. Haddock B, Fan AP, Jørgensen NR, et al. Kinetic [18F]-Fluoride of the knee in normal Volunteers. Clin Nucl Med 2019;44(5):377–85.

28. Haddock B, Fan AP, Uhlrich SD, et al. Assessment of acute bone loading in humans using [18F]NaF PET/MRI. Eur J Nucl Med Mol Imaging 2019;46(12): 2452–63.

29. Al-Zaghal A, Yellanki DP, Kothekar E, et al. Sacroiliac joint Asymmetry regarding inflammation and bone turnover: assessment by FDG and NaF PET/CT. Asia Ocean J Nucl Med Biol 2019;7(2):108–14.

30. Raynor W, Houshmand S, Gholami S, et al. Evolving role of Molecular imaging with (18)F-sodium fluoride PET as a biomarker for calcium metabolism. Curr Osteoporos Rep 2016;14(4):115–25.

31. Li X, Majumdar S. Quantitative MRI of articular cartilage and its clinical applications. J Magn Reson Imaging JMRI 2013;38(5):991–1008.

32. Li X, Benjamin Ma C, Link TM, et al. In vivo T(1rho) and T(2) mapping of articular cartilage in osteoarthritis of the knee using 3 T MRI. Osteoarthritis Cartilage 2007;15(7):789–97.

33. Pedoia V, Gallo MC, Souza RB, et al. Longitudinal study using voxel-based relaxometry: association between cartilage T1ρ and T2 and patient reported outcome changes in hip osteoarthritis. J Magn Reson Imaging JMRI 2017;45(5):1523–33.

34. Al-Zaghal A, Yellanki DP, Ayubcha C, et al. CT-based tissue segmentation to assess knee joint inflammation and reactive bone formation assessed by 18F-FDG and 18F-NaF PET/CT: effects of age and BMI. Hell J Nucl Med 2018;21(2):102–7.

35. Khaw TH, Raynor WY, Borja AJ, et al. Assessing the effects of body weight on subchondral bone formation with quantitative 18F-sodium fluoride PET. Ann Nucl Med 2020;34(8):559–64.

36. Ayubcha C, Zirakchian Zadeh M, Stochkendahl MJ, et al. Quantitative evaluation of normal spinal osseous metabolism with 18F-NaF PET/CT. Nucl Med Commun 2018;39(10):945–50.

37. Kobayashi N, Inaba Y, Tateishi U, et al. New application of 18F-fluoride PET for the detection of bone remodeling in early-stage osteoarthritis of the hip. Clin Nucl Med 2013;38(10):e379–83.

38. Kobayashi N, Inaba Y, Yukizawa Y, et al. Use of 18F-fluoride positron emission tomography as a predictor of the hip osteoarthritis progression. Mod Rheumatol 2015;25(6):925–30.

39. Kobayashi N, Inaba Y, Tateishi U, et al. Comparison of 18F-fluoride positron emission tomography and magnetic resonance imaging in evaluating early-stage osteoarthritis of the hip. Nucl Med Commun 2015;36(1):84–9.

40. Watkins L, MacKay J, Haddock B, et al. Evaluating the relationship between dynamic Na[18F]F-uptake parameters and MRI knee osteoarthritic findings. J Nucl Med 2020;61(supplement 1):182.

41. MacKay JW, Watkins L, Gold G, et al. [18F]NaF PET-MRI provides direct in-vivo evidence of the association between bone metabolic activity and adjacent synovitis in knee osteoarthritis: a cross-sectional study. Osteoarthritis Cartilage 2021;29(8):1155–62.

42. Blom AB, van Lent PLEM, Holthuysen AEM, et al. Synovial lining macrophages mediate osteophyte formation during experimental osteoarthritis. Osteoarthritis Cartilage 2004;12(8):627–35.

43. Kogan F, Fan AP, McWalter EJ, et al. PET/MRI of metabolic activity in osteoarthritis: a feasibility study. J Magn Reson Imaging JMRI 2017;45(6):1736–45.

44. Watkins L, MacKay J, Haddock B, et al. Assessment of quantitative [18F]Sodium fluoride PET measures of knee subchondral bone perfusion and mineralization in osteoarthritic and healthy subjects. Osteoarthritis Cartilage 2021;29(6):849–58. https://doi.org/10.1016/j.joca.2021.02.563.

45. Tibrewala R, Bahroos E, Mehrabian H, et al. [18 F]-Sodium fluoride PET/MR imaging for bone-cartilage interactions in hip osteoarthritis: a feasibility study. J Orthop Res Off Publ Orthop Res Soc 2019;37(12):2671–80. https://doi.org/10.1002/jor.24443.

46. Savic D, Pedoia V, Seo Y, et al. Imaging bone-cartilage interactions in osteoarthritis using [18F]-NaF PET-MRI. Mol Imaging 2016;15:1–12.

47. Draper CE, Quon A, Fredericson M, et al. Comparison of MRI and 18F-NaF PET/CT in patients with patellofemoral pain. J Magn Reson Imaging JMRI 2012;36(4):928–32.

48. Shen G, Su M, Liu B, et al. A case of Tophaceous Pseudogout on 18F-FDG PET/CT imaging. Clin Nucl Med 2019;44(2):e98–100.

49. Gamie S, El-Maghraby T. The role of PET/CT in evaluation of Facet and Disc abnormalities in patients with low back pain using (18)F-Fluoride. Nucl Med Rev Cent East Eur 2008;11(1):17–21.

50. Jenkins NW, Talbott JF, Shah V, et al. [18F]-Sodium fluoride PET MR-based Localization and quantification of bone turnover as a biomarker for facet joint-Induced disability. AJNR Am J Neuroradiol 2017;38(10):2028–31.

51. Suh MS, Park SH, Kim YK, et al. 18F-NaF PET/CT for the evaluation of temporomandibular joint disorder. Clin Radiol 2018;73(4). 414.e7-414.e13.

52. Lee JW, Lee SM, Kim SJ, et al. Clinical utility of fluoride-18 positron emission tomography/CT in temporomandibular disorder with osteoarthritis: comparisons with 99mTc-MDP bone scan. Dento Maxillo Facial Radiol 2013;42(2):29292350.

Sarcopenia and Myositis Revisited
Emerging Role of Fluorine-18 Fluorodeoxyglucose PET in Muscle Imaging

Patrick Debs, MD[a], Abdullah Al-Zaghal, MD[a],*, Lilja B. Solnes, MD, MBA[a], Abass Alavi, MD, MD (Hon), PhD (Hon), DSc (Hon)[b]

KEYWORDS

- Myopathy • Sarcopenia • Myositis • FDG • PET/CT • PET/MRI

KEY POINTS

- The utility of fluorodeoxyglucose (FDG) PET/computed tomography (CT) in assessing age-related and malignancy-associated sarcopenia and its role in overall survival prediction.
- FDG PET, along with CT and MRI, can serve as an integral tool in quantifying clinically active myositis and myopathies.

INTRODUCTION

Fluorine-18 fluorodeoxyglucose (FDG) is a glucose analog and the most used PET radiopharmaceutical. Cellular uptake of FDG is determined by the expression of glucose transporter proteins in the targeted cells.[1] Given that this expression is increased in activated inflammatory cells and tumor cells, FDG PET has been established as a useful imaging modality in the diagnosis and management of patients with suspected inflammatory diseases.[2–4] Conventional cross-sectional imaging techniques; like computed tomography (CT) and MRI, have superior soft tissue contrast in comparison to PET. However, with the introduction of hybrid PET/CT and PET/MRI systems, we can not only have a better understanding of the structural and volumetric characteristics of a vast array of diseased and age-related changes, but also quantify its metabolic and functional behavior.[5]

Sarcopenia

Sarcopenia is characterized by progressive and generalized loss of skeletal muscle mass and strength and is strictly correlated with physical disability, poor quality of life, and mortality.[6,7] Although primarily considered a disease of the elderly, it can also develop in association with conditions that are not exclusively observed in the elderly population.[8] Its prevalence differs by age and increases from around 14% in individuals aged between 65 and 70 to around 53% in individuals above 80 years of age.[8] Even though its onset varies, evidence shows that loss of skeletal muscle mass begins as early as the fourth decade of life, with up to 50% of mass being lost by the eighth decade.[9] The consequences of sarcopenia are often severe in older adults, and the strength and functional declines associated with sarcopenia can contribute to several adverse health outcomes, including loss of function, disability, and

[a] The Russell H. Morgan Department of Radiology, The Johns Hopkins University School of Medicine, 601 North Caroline Street, Baltimore, MD 21205, USA; [b] Department of Radiology, Perelman School of Medicine at the University of Pennsylvania, 3400 Civic Center Boulevard, Philadelphia, PA 19104, USA
* Corresponding author.
E-mail address: aalzagh1@jhmi.edu
Twitter: @PatrickDebs (P.D.); @Abdullah_Zaghal (A.A.-Z.)

PET Clin 18 (2023) 31–38
https://doi.org/10.1016/j.cpet.2022.09.003
1556-8598/23/© 2022 Elsevier Inc. All rights reserved.

frailty.[10–12] Moreover, sarcopenia imposes a significant economic burden on health care services in the United States with a total estimated cost of approximately $18.4 billion in 2000.[13]

Sarcopenia is generally thought to be multifactorial; environmental causes, disease triggers, inflammatory pathway activation, mitochondrial abnormalities, loss of neuromuscular junctions, reduced satellite cell numbers, and hormonal changes are all thought to contribute to the overall decline in the size and number of skeletal muscle fibers as well as the fibrous and adipose tissue infiltration of muscles.[14] Age, gender, and level of physical activity are well-described risk factors, and resistance exercise is particularly effective at slowing the age-related loss of skeletal muscle.[8] Sarcopenia can be considered primary when no other cause is evident but aging itself and secondary when one or more other causes are evident.[15] Deficient intake of energy, protein, and vitamin D all contribute to muscle loss and low functionality in the elderly; acute and chronic co-morbidities can also play a role by leading to reduced physical activity and periods of bed rest on one hand and generating increased amounts of proinflammatory cytokines responsible for triggering muscle proteolysis on the other.[8] In addition, some drugs taken for common conditions can cause an imbalance between anabolic and catabolic muscle pathways and alter protein synthesis and degradation, ultimately leading to a form of drug-induced sarcopenia; common culprits include but are not limited to statins, sulfonylureas, and glinides.[16]

Sarcopenia is assessed using both imaging and nonimaging evaluation techniques, with nonimaging evaluation often involving clinical examinations, questionnaires for assessing physical function impairments and measurement of certain serum and urinary biomarkers.[17] The imaging technologies most used in evaluating sarcopenia include dual X-ray absorptiometry (DXA), MRI, CT, and ultrasound (US). These methods differ considerably in terms of reliability, radiation exposure, time taken to complete the examination and analyze the results, availability and complexity of the equipment involved and costs and applications.[17,18] DXA is the most frequently used modality to study body composition and can estimate bone mineral density, fat mass, and fat-free mass of the whole body or specific anatomic regions based on the attenuation of two X-ray beams with different energy levels. Low costs and a low radiation dose justify its widespread use in clinical practice; however, it cannot provide information on qualitative changes in muscle mass.[18–20] CT on the other hand is considered one of the more suitable methods for analyzing

quantitative and qualitative changes in body composition, investigating skeletal muscle mass, and distinguishing adipose tissue in different body compartments. The reliability of CT for the purpose of studying quantitative and qualitative changes in fat and fat-free mass with aging has been well documented; however, the high radiation levels associated with CT scans have limited its use to the field of research.[20,21] MRI can also evaluate skeletal muscle mass and distinguish it from fat as well as estimate fat mass and fat-free mass.[20,22] Even though MRI involves no radiation and is one of the most reliable techniques for studying body composition, its high cost, complexity and availability issues limit its use in clinical practice.[18,19,22] Finally, US scanning is a low-cost, non-invasive imaging technique used to study muscle damage or wasting diseases like sarcopenia and can be a good initial choice for assessing qualitative or quantitative changes in muscle mass. International guidelines recommend using other approaches to identify loss of muscle mass, but US can measure muscle thickness and provide an estimate of the reduction in lean body mass, and grayscale echogenicity analysis can provide a measure of qualitative changes such as adipose infiltration within the muscle.[18,23,24]

In recent years, several studies have attempted to study the emerging role that FDG PET/CT might play in the evaluation of sarcopenia, particularly in oncology. Given the utility of FDG PET/CT in the diagnosis and management of various oncologic diseases, these scans provide ample opportunities for studying any malignancy-associated sarcopenia and its implications. Bas and colleagues[25] studied the prevalence of sarcopenia in patients with Hodgkin's lymphoma using FDG PET/CT and found the modality to be useful not only for the evaluation of malignant lymphoid lesions, but also for the assessment of both muscle mass and metabolism. Albano and colleagues[26] compared the agreement of measurements of skeletal muscle area, visceral adipose tissue, subcutaneous adipose tissue and intramuscular adipose tissue between high-dose CT, considered to be the gold-standard imaging, and low-dose CT of FDG PET/CT in elderly patients affected by Hodgkin lymphoma. They found a strong correlation between all measurements and concluded that low-dose CT of PET/CT is a safe, accurate and precise method for the measurements of skeletal muscle area and visceral and subcutaneous adipose tissue. Zhou and colleagues[27] looked at the association between overall survival and body composition metrics derived from routine clinical FDG PET/CT examinations in patients with esophageal adenocarcinoma. They found that attenuation and SUVmax of the psoas muscle were significant independent predictors of survival, whereas cross-sectional area and SUVmean were not. Similarly, Mallet and used staging FDG PET/CT for assessment of sarcopenia and found it to be a prognostic factor for worse survival in patients with locally advanced esophageal cancer treated with chemoradiation. Anconina and colleagues looked at the prognostic value of sarcopenia measurements done on staging FDG PET/CT in surgically-treated patients with esophageal adenocarcinoma and found that combining skeletal mass index using CT-based segmentation with standard clinical data improved prediction for overall survival and relapse-free survival, whereas metabolic activity of the tumor on staging scan did not.[28,29] Umit and colleagues[30] evaluated sarcopenia in multiple myeloma patients using FDG PET/CT and concluded that PET/CT observations can be a useful surrogate for sarcopenia and possibly a promising option for evaluating muscle quality and quantity.

Finally, Kim and colleagues[31] analyzed FDG PET/CT of 288 patients who underwent surgical resection for invasive ductal carcinoma and found that higher SUVmax of the psoas muscle was associated with shorter disease-free survival (**Fig. 1**). They concluded that SUVmax of the psoas muscle has a strong potential as an independent prognostic factor for recurrence in patients with resectable breast cancer.

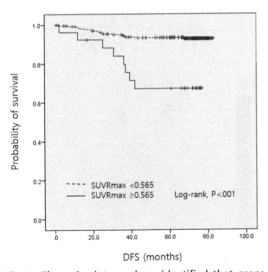

Fig. 1. The univariate analyses identified that psoas muscle of $SUVR_{max}$ greater than 0.565 is correlated with shorter DFS in patients with breast cancer. DFS, disease-free survival; $SUVR_{max}$, ratio of the maximum standard uptake value. (*From* Kim K, Kim IJ, Pak K, et al. Prognostic value of metabolic activity of the psoas muscle evaluated by preoperative 18F-FDG PET-CT in breast cancer: a retrospective cross-sectional study. BMC Cancer. 2021;21(1).)

Myositis and Myopathies

Myositis and myopathies are defined as inflammation of muscles and refer to a group of inflammatory disorders such as polymyositis, dermatomyositis, necrotizing myopathy, overlap syndrome with myositis or overlap myositis, and inclusion body myositis.[32] Inflammatory myopathies are rare and can affect several different organs apart from muscles, leading to severe impairment and diminishing the quality of life.[32,33] Clinical symptoms differ from one subtype to the other, but patients with myositis generally present with increasing difficulty with tasks requiring the use of proximal muscles, such as getting up from a chair, climbing steps, or lifting objects.[34] Patients also generally present with extra muscular manifestations such as skin and articular involvement, interstitial lung disease, and even malignancy.[34]

Myositis can have many different etiologies including infections, autoimmune conditions, genetic disorders, medication adverse events, electrolyte disturbances, and diseases of the endocrine system.[35] Infectious myositis, which is defined as infection of skeletal muscles, can be caused by a wide variety of pathogens such as bacteria, fungi, parasites, and viruses. The causes of inflammatory myopathies remain unknown, but autoimmune pathogenesis is strongly implicated. In dermatomyositis, early activation of complement C5b-9 membranolytic attack complex leads to infarction, necrosis and ultimately destruction of muscle fibers. In polymyositis and inclusion-body myositis, CD8+ cytotoxic T cells attack and destroy muscle fibers that aberrantly express MHC class I. The factors that trigger inflammatory muscle diseases also remain unknown, but genetic risk factors regulating immune responses against environmental agents have been proposed as possible etiologies.[34]

Diagnosis of myositis is typically based on a combination of clinical history and symptomatology, muscle enzyme levels, electromyographic findings and muscle biopsy results.[33,34] Conventional imaging had an ancillary role in diagnosing inflammatory muscle diseases in the past, but recent advances in imaging techniques have allowed some imaging modalities to occupy a more central role in the evaluation of myopathies.[36] MRI is a powerful modality capable of documenting the extent and intensity of muscle abnormalities and, depending on the disease stage, detecting certain muscle abnormalities such as edema, fatty replacement and atrophy.[37,38] Moreover, newer MRI techniques focusing not only on anatomy but also on muscle function provide a valuable tool for understanding the spectrum of muscle diseases.[36,39] US is also useful and can detect typical myositis features such as edema, calcifications, atrophy, fascial thickening, and degenerative processes.[40–42] In addition, US elastography can directly quantify tissue elasticity or stiffness that may be affected by structural alterations induced by disuse and pathologic processes.[43–45] Plain radiography plays a limited role in muscle imaging due to limitations in contrast resolution, but CT can evaluate muscle bulk, characterize soft tissue mineralization patterns and distinguish between bone, tendons and ligaments, muscles, fluid, and gas.[36,46,47]

Several studies have examined the rule of FDG PET/CT in detecting inflammatory muscle disorders (Fig. 2). Pipitone and colleagues[48] showed that the proximal muscle SUVmax was higher in patients with dermatomyositis and polymyositis than in normal controls, however, it did not correlate with disease duration or serum creatinine kinase. Matuszak and colleagues[49] showed that the SUVmax was increased in patients with inflammatory myopathies compared with controls and further allowed the differentiation between patients with high and low muscle disease activity, with good accuracy to detect changes in muscle disease activity on subsequent examination, with strong responsiveness and excellent interrater reliability. Sun and colleagues[50] showed that SUVmax in the paraspinal muscles correlated positively with serum creatinine-kinase and negatively with muscle strength in patient with polymyositis/dermatomyositis. Tanaka and colleagues[51] found significant correlations between metabolic activity of proximal muscles in 20 patients with polymyositis/dermatomyositis and histologic grading of inflammatory cell infiltration, as well as manual muscle test scores, serum creatinine kinase, and aldolase.

Several studies have also looked at the value of FDG PET/CT in detecting extra muscular manifestations of myositis. Inflammatory myopathies are often associated with malignant tumors and interstitial lung disease, which can be major causes of morbidity, and some patients are prone to developing life-threatening rapidly progressive

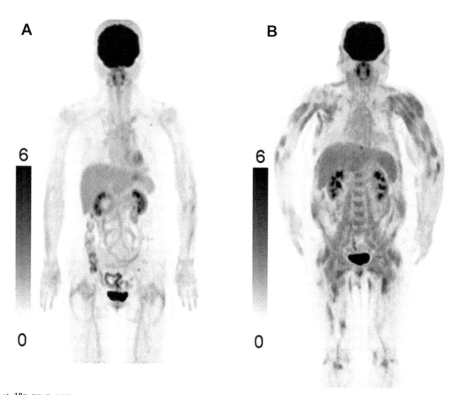

Fig. 2. (A) ^{18}F-FDG PET maximum intensity projection (MIP) image of a 58-year-old female as a control patient shows no increased uptake in the skeletal muscles. (B) ^{18}F-FDG PET MIP image of a 53-year-old female with dermatomyositis shows diffuse uptake in the proximal skeletal muscles.[67] (From Arai-Okuda H, Norikane T, Yamamoto Y, et al. 18F-FDG PET/CT in patients with polymyositis/dermatomyositis: correlation with serum muscle enzymes. European Journal of Hybrid Imaging. 2020;4(1).)

interstitial lung disease with risk of respiratory failure.[52–56] Li and colleagues[57] investigated use of FDG PET/CT in patients with idiopathic inflammatory myopathy; they analyzed a total of 38 patients and found that FDG PET/CT is helpful in identifying malignancies, observing the status of inflammatory myopathy, detecting interstitial lung disease and predicting the occurrence of rapidly progressive interstitial lung disease. Moreover, they found that an SUV_{max} threshold of ≥ 2.4 has a sensitivity of 100.0%, specificity of 87.0%, and accuracy of 90.0% in predicting rapidly progressive interstitial lung disease. Zhao and colleagues[58] investigated the use of FDG PET/CT in 67 patients with dermatomyositis and interstitial lung disease and found that patients with rapidly progressive interstitial lung disease had a significantly higher SUV in the lungs compared with patients with chronically progressed interstitial lung disease—a lung SUV cut off of 2.25 yielded a sensitivity of 77.8% and specificity of 72.8% in predicting disease progression. Cao and colleagues[59] analyzed FDG PET/CT characteristics of 26 patients with anti-melanoma differentiation-associated protein 5 antibody positive (anti-MDA5+) dermatomyositis and found the modality valuable in quantifying the pulmonary focal inflammation and potentially unveiling the distinctive characteristics and pathophysiological mechanisms of this disease subtype. Motegi and colleagues[60] studied the clinical value of FDG PET/CT for interstitial lung disease and myositis in 20 patients with dermatomyositis; they found a significant correlation between krebs von den lungen-6 (glycoprotein expressed by damaged type II alveolar cells) and SUVmax in each lung. A strong correlation was also noted between SUVmax in the muscles and serum cytokines.

Various case reports have also looked at the use of FDG PET/CT in identifying and evaluating rarer forms of myositis. Pereira and colleagues[61] highlighted the ability FDG PET/CT to detect two unusual cases of post-COVID-19 complications—diffuse panniculitis and inflammatory myositis. Suthar and colleagues[62] reported one case of myositis detected on FDG PET/CT and induced by Sunitinib, one of the most commonly used multi-kinase inhibitors for metastatic renal cell carcinoma. Spaas and colleagues[63] demonstrated the utility of FDG PET/CT in the early detection and monitoring of radiation myositis, an infrequent late adverse effect of radiotherapy, and Oueriagli and colleagues[64] reported FDG PET/CT findings of intense muscular hypermetabolism indicative of paraneoplastic polymyositis in a patient with lung epidermoid carcinoma.

FDG PET/CT is becoming a valuable tool with multiple advantages when evaluating myositis and myopathies but has its own limitations. Inflammatory diseases are characterized by a more diffuse and less pathognomonic pattern of FDG uptake than oncology FDG PET/CT, and patients referred to PET/CT with suspected infection or inflammation are rarely treatment naïve and may have received varying doses of antibiotics, corticosteroids or other immune-modulating drugs that could result in a higher rate of false positive FDG findings and in some cases lower sensitivity in detecting active disease.[65] One systematic review and meta-analysis by Kim and colleagues[66] concluded that, even though FDG PET/CT can be useful for the detection of active disease status in patients with inflammatory myopathies, more objective and updated criteria for the assessment of disease activity incorporated with FDG PET/CT should be introduced and validated, and further studies are necessary to determine if FDG PET/CT-based treatment of myositis can in fact improve disease outcomes.

SUMMARY

FDG PET/CT is a valuable diagnostic modality in the work-up of patients with suspected inflammatory myopathy. Sarcopenia and metabolic muscle activity on staging FDG PET/CT has been shown to correlate with overall survival in certain oncologic settings. However, most of the aforementioned studies are limited to retrospective analysis, and the available data and literature are still insufficient to establish a clear role for FDG PET in the management of inflammatory myopathies and sarcopenia. Moreover, knowledge of the physiologic FDG uptake in skeletal muscles and optimization of imaging protocols are key for proper image analysis. Further studies with prospective design and strict adherence to procedural protocols including fasting 6 to 8 h, optimizing serum glucose to physiologic levels, and total relaxation before image acquisition are needed to estimate the diagnostic accuracy and utility of FDG PET for muscle disorders.

DISCLOSURE

The authors have nothing to disclose.

REFERENCES

1. Kapoor V, McCook BM, Torok FS. An introduction to PET-CT imaging. Radiographics 2004;24(2). https://doi.org/10.1148/rg.242025724.
2. Love C, Tomas MB, Tronco GG, et al. FDG PET of infection and inflammation. Radiographics 2005;25(5). https://doi.org/10.1148/rg.255045122.

3. Zhuang H, Alavi A. 18-Fluorodeoxyglucose positron emission tomographic imaging in the detection and monitoring of infection and inflammation. Semin Nucl Med 2002;32(1). https://doi.org/10.1053/snuc.2002. 29278.

4. Boerman OC, Rennen H, Oyen WJG, et al. Radio-pharmaceuticals to image infection and inflammation. Semin Nucl Med 2001;31(4). https://doi.org/10.1053/snuc.2001.26189.

5. Kjaer A. Hybrid imaging with PET/CT and PET/MR. Cancer Imaging 2014;14(S1). https://doi.org/10.1186/1470-7330-14-s1-o32.

6. Goodpaster BH, Park SW, Harris TB, et al. The loss of skeletal muscle strength, mass, and quality in older adults: the Health, Aging and Body Composition Study. Journals Gerontol - Ser A Biol Sci Med Sci 2006;61(10). https://doi.org/10.1093/gerona/61.10.1059.

7. Delmonico MJ, Harris TB, Lee JS, et al. Alternative definitions of sarcopenia, lower extremity performance, and functional impairment with aging in older men and women. J Am Geriatr Soc 2007; 55(5). https://doi.org/10.1111/j.1532-5415.2007.01140.x.

8. Santilli V, Bernetti A, Mangone M, et al. Clinical definition of sarcopenia. Clin Cases Mineral Bone Metab 2014;11(3). https://doi.org/10.11138/ccmbm/2014.11.3.177.

9. Metter EJ, Conwit R, Tobin J, et al. Age-associated loss of power and strength in the upper extremities in women and men. Journals Gerontol - Ser A Biol Sci Med Sci 1997;52(5). https://doi.org/10.1093/gerona/52A.5.B267.

10. Dufour AB, Hannan MT, Murabito JM, et al. Sarcopenia definitions considering body size and fat mass are associated with mobility limitations: the framingham study. Journals Gerontol - Ser A Biol Sci Med Sci 2013;68(2). https://doi.org/10.1093/gerona/gls109.

11. Xue QL, Walston JD, Fried LP, et al. Prediction of risk of falling, physical disability, and frailty by rate of decline in grip strength: the women's health and aging study. Arch Intern Med 2011;171(12). https://doi.org/10.1001/archinternmed.2011.252.

12. Marsh AP, Rejeski WJ, Espeland MA, et al. Muscle strength and BMI as predictors of major mobility disability in the lifestyle interventions and independence for elders pilot (LIFE-P). Journals Gerontol - Ser A Biol Sci Med Sci 2011;66(12). https://doi.org/10.1093/gerona/glr158.

13. Janssen I, Shepard DS, Katzmarzyk PT, et al. The healthcare costs of sarcopenia in the United States. J Am Geriatr Soc 2004;52(1). https://doi.org/10.1111/j.1532-5415.2004.52014.x.

14. Walston JD. Sarcopenia in older adults. Curr Opin Rheumatol 2012;24(6):623–7.

15. Cruz-Jentoft AJ, Baeyens JP, Bauer JM, et al. Sarcopenia: European consensus on definition and diagnosis: report of the European working group on sarcopenia in older people. Age Ageing 2010; 39(4). https://doi.org/10.1093/ageing/afq034.

16. Campins L, Camps M, Riera A, et al. Oral drugs related with muscle wasting and sarcopenia. Annu Rev Pharmacol 2017;99(1–2). https://doi.org/10.1159/000448247.

17. Boutin RD, Yao L, Canter RJ, et al. Sarcopenia: current concepts and imaging implications. Am J Roentgenol 2015;205(3). https://doi.org/10.2214/AJR.15.14635.

18. Sergi G, Trevisan C, Veronese N, et al. Imaging of sarcopenia. Eur J Radiol 2016;85(8). https://doi.org/10.1016/j.ejrad.2016.04.009.

19. Rubbieri G, Mossello E, di Bari M. Techniques for the diagnosis of sarcopenia. Clin Cases Mineral Bone Metab 2014;11(3). https://doi.org/10.11138/ccmbm/2014.11.3.181.

20. Lustgarten MS, Fielding RA. Assessment of analytical methods used to measure changes in body composition in the elderly and recommendations for their use in phase II clinical trials. J Nutr Health Aging 2011;15(5). https://doi.org/10.1007/s12603-011-0049-x.

21. Woodrow G. Body composition analysis techniques in the aged adult: indications and limitations. Curr Opin Clin Nutr Metab Care 2009;12(1). https://doi.org/10.1097/MCO.0b013e32831b9c5b.

22. Selberg O, Burchert W, Graubner G, et al. Determination of anatomical skeletal muscle mass by whole body nuclear magnetic resonance. Basic Life Sci 1993;60. https://doi.org/10.1007/978-1-4899-1268-8_22.

23. Watanabe Y, Yamada Y, Fukumoto Y, et al. Echo intensity obtained from ultrasonography images reflecting muscle strength in elderly men. Clin Interventions Aging 2013;8. https://doi.org/10.2147/CIA.S47263.

24. Pillen S, van Alfen N. Skeletal muscle ultrasound. Neurol Res 2011;33(10). https://doi.org/10.1179/1743132811Y.0000000010.

25. Bas V, Umit EG, Korkmaz U, et al. Sarcopenia in Hodgkin's lymphoma evaluated with 18-FDG PET/CT, focus on age, performance, and treatment. Support Care Cancer 2021;29(5). https://doi.org/10.1007/s00520-020-05772-8.

26. Albano D, Camoni L, Rinaldi R, et al. Comparison between skeletal muscle and adipose tissue measurements with high-dose CT and low-dose attenuation correction CT of 18F-FDG PET/CT in elderly Hodgkin lymphoma patients: a two-centre validation. Br J Radiol 2021;94(1123):20200672.

27. Zhou C, Foster B, Hagge R, et al. Opportunistic body composition evaluation in patients with esophageal adenocarcinoma: association of survival with 18F-FDG PET/CT muscle metrics. Ann Nucl Med 2020;34(3). https://doi.org/10.1007/s12149-019-01429-7.

28. Anconina R, Ortega C, Metser U, et al. Influence of sarcopenia, clinical data, and 2-[18F] FDG PET/CT in outcome prediction of patients with early-stage adenocarcinoma esophageal cancer. Eur J Nucl Med Mol Imaging 2022;49(3). https://doi.org/10.1007/s00259-021-05514-w.

29. Mallet R, Modzelewski R, Lequesne J, et al. Prognostic value of sarcopenia in patients treated by Radiochemotherapy for locally advanced oesophageal cancer. Radiat Oncol 2020;15(1). https://doi.org/10.1186/s13014-020-01545-z.

30. Umit EG, Korkmaz U, Baysal M, et al. Evaluation of Sarcopenia with F-18 FDG PET/CT and relation with disease outcomes in patients with multiple myeloma. Eur J Cancer Care 2020;29(6). https://doi.org/10.1111/ecc.13318.

31. Kim K, Kim IJ, Pak K, et al. Prognostic value of metabolic activity of the psoas muscle evaluated by preoperative 18F-FDG PET-CT in breast cancer: a retrospective cross-sectional study. BMC Cancer 2021;21(1). https://doi.org/10.1186/s12885-021-08886-2.

32. Schmidt J. Current classification and management of inflammatory myopathies. J Neuromuscul Dis 2018;5(2). https://doi.org/10.3233/JND-180308.

33. Carstens PO, Schmidt J. Diagnosis, pathogenesis and treatment of myositis: recent advances. Clin Exp Immunol 2014;175(3). https://doi.org/10.1111/cei.12194.

34. Dalakas MC. Inflammatory muscle diseases. N Engl J Med 2015;372(18):1734–47.

35. Crum-Cianflone NF. Bacterial, fungal, parasitic, and viral myositis. Clin Microbiol Rev 2008;21(3). https://doi.org/10.1128/CMR.00001-08.

36. Kuo GP, Carrino JA. Skeletal muscle imaging and inflammatory myopathies. Curr Opin Rheumatol 2007;19(6). https://doi.org/10.1097/BOR.0b013e3282efdc66.

37. Schulze M, Kötter I, Ernemann U, et al. MRI findings in inflammatory muscle diseases and their noninflammatory mimics. Am J Roentgenol 2009;192(6). https://doi.org/10.2214/AJR.08.1764.

38. del Grande F, Carrino JA, del Grande M, et al. Magnetic resonance imaging of inflammatory myopathies. Top Magn Reson Imaging 2011;22(2). https://doi.org/10.1097/RMR.0b013e31825b2c35.

39. Malartre S, Bachasson D, Mercy G, et al. MRI and muscle imaging for idiopathic inflammatory myopathies. Brain Pathol 2021;31(3). https://doi.org/10.1111/bpa.12954.

40. Reimers CD, Fleckenstein JL, Witt TN, et al. Muscular ultrasound in idiopathic inflammatory myopathies of adults. J Neurol Sci 1993;116(1). https://doi.org/10.1016/0022-510X(93)90093-E.

41. Paramalingam S, Morgan K, Becce F, et al. Conventional ultrasound and elastography as imaging outcome tools in autoimmune myositis: a systematic review by the OMERACT ultrasound group. Semin Arthritis Rheum 2021;51(3). https://doi.org/10.1016/j.semarthrit.2020.11.001.

42. Bhansing KJ, van Rosmalen MH, van Engelen BG, et al. Increased fascial thickness of the deltoid muscle in dermatomyositis and polymyositis: an ultrasound study. Muscle Nerve 2015;52(4). https://doi.org/10.1002/mus.24595.

43. Wisdom KM, Delp SL, Kuhl E. Use it or lose it: multiscale skeletal muscle adaptation to mechanical stimuli. Biomech Model Mechanobiology 2015;14(2). https://doi.org/10.1007/s10237-014-0607-3.

44. Gennisson JL, Deffieux T, Fink M, et al. Ultrasound elastography: principles and techniques. Diagn Interv Imaging 2013;94(5). https://doi.org/10.1016/j.diii.2013.01.022.

45. Farrow M, Biglands J, Alfuraih AM, et al. Novel muscle imaging in inflammatory rheumatic diseases—a focus on ultrasound shear wave elastography and quantitative MRI. Front Med 2020;7. https://doi.org/10.3389/fmed.2020.00434.

46. Calò M, Crisi G, Martinelli C, et al. CT and the diagnosis of myopathies - preliminary findings in 42 cases. Neuroradiology 1986;28(1). https://doi.org/10.1007/BF00341766.

47. Swash M, Brown MM, Thakkar C. CT muscle imaging and the clinical assessment of neuromuscular disease. Muscle & Nerve 1995;18(7). https://doi.org/10.1002/mus.880180706.

48. Pipitone N, Versari A, Zuccoli G, et al. 18F-Fluorodeoxyglucose positron emission tomography for the assessment of myositis: a case series. Clin Exp Rheumatol 2012;30(4).

49. Matuszak J, Blondet C, Hubelé F, et al. Muscle fluorodeoxyglucose uptake assessed by positron emission tomography-computed tomography as a biomarker of inflammatory myopathies disease activity. Rheumatology (United Kingdom) 2019;58(8). https://doi.org/10.1093/rheumatology/kez040.

50. Sun L, Dong Y, Zhang N, et al. [18F]Fluorodeoxyglucose positron emission tomography/computed tomography for diagnosing polymyositis/dermatomyositis. Exp Ther Med 2018;15(6). https://doi.org/10.3892/etm.2018.6066.

51. Tanaka ahigeru, Ikeda K, Uchiyama K, et al. [18F]Fdg uptake in proximal muscles assessed by pet/ct reflects both global and local muscular inflammation and provides useful information in the management of patients with polymyositis/dermatomyositis. Rheumatology (United Kingdom) 2013;52(7). https://doi.org/10.1093/rheumatology/ket112.

52. Sontheimer RD, Miyagawa S. Potentially fatal interstitial lung disease can occur in clinically amyopathic dermatomyositis [3]. J Am Acad Dermatol 2003;48(5). https://doi.org/10.1067/mjd.2003.199.

53. Marie I, Hachulla E, Chérin P, et al. Interstitial lung disease in polymyositis and dermatomyositis.

Arthritis Care Res 2002;47(6). https://doi.org/10.1002/art.10794.

54. Yu KH, Wu YJJ, Kuo CF, et al. Survival analysis of patients with dermatomyositis and polymyositis: analysis of 192 Chinese cases. Clin Rheumatol 2011;30(12). https://doi.org/10.1007/s10067-011-1840-0.

55. Fathi M, Vikgren J, Boijsen M, et al. Interstitial lung disease in polymyositis and dermatomyositis: longitudinal evaluation by pulmonary function and radiology. Arthritis Rheum 2008;59(5):677–85.

56. Chen IJ, Jan Wu YJ, Lin CW, et al. Interstitial lung disease in polymyositis and dermatomyositis. Clin Rheumatol 2009;28(6). https://doi.org/10.1007/s10067-009-1110-6.

57. Li Y, Zhou Y, Wang Q. Multiple values of 18F-FDG PET/CT in idiopathic inflammatory myopathy. Clin Rheumatol 2017;36(10). https://doi.org/10.1007/s10067-017-3794-3.

58. Zhao Z, Li KP, Wang YY, et al. [The prediction of disease progression by 18Fluorodeoxyglucose-positron emission computed tomography/CT in patients with dermatomyositis and interstitial lung disease]. Zhonghua Nei Ke Za Zhi 2021;60(7):661–4.

59. Cao H, Liang J, Xu D, et al. Radiological characteristics of patients with anti-MDA5–antibody-positive dermatomyositis in 18F-FDG PET/CT: a pilot study. Front Med 2021;8. https://doi.org/10.3389/fmed.2021.779272.

60. ichiro Motegi S, Fujiwara C, Sekiguchi A, et al. Clinical value of 18F-fluorodeoxyglucose positron emission tomography/computed tomography for interstitial lung disease and myositis in patients with dermatomyositis. J Dermatol 2019;46(3). https://doi.org/10.1111/1346-8138.14758.

61. Pereira M, Shivdasani D, Roy D, et al. Post-COVID-19 unusual inflammatory syndromes detected on 18F-FDG PET/CT scan. Clin Nucl Med 2022;1. https://doi.org/10.1097/RLU.0000000000004088.

62. Suthar RR, Purandare N, Shah S, et al. Sunitinib-induced myositis detected on 18F-FDG PET/CT. Clin Nucl Med 2022;47(3):e311–2.

63. Spaas M, van den Broeck B, Creytens D, et al. Spatiotemporal evolution of radiation myositis on 18F-FDG PET/CT following hypofractionated radiotherapy of intramuscular melanoma metastases. Clin Nucl Med 2021;46(7). https://doi.org/10.1097/RLU.0000000000003596.

64. Oueriagli SN, Benameur Y, Sahel OA, et al. Unusual 18F-FDG PET-CT finding of paraneoplasic polymyositis in a patient with lung epidermoïd carcinoma. Nucl Med Rev 2020;23(2). https://doi.org/10.5603/NMR.2020.0022.

65. Pijl JP, Nienhuis PH, Kwee TC, et al. Limitations and pitfalls of FDG-PET/CT in infection and inflammation. Semin Nucl Med 2021;51(6). https://doi.org/10.1053/j.semnuclmed.2021.06.008.

66. Kim K, Kim SJ. 18F-FDG PET/CT for assessing of disease activity of idiopathic inflammatory myopathies. A systematic review and meta-analysis. Hell J Nucl Med 2021;24(2). https://doi.org/10.1967/s002449912353.

67. Arai-Okuda H, Norikane T, Yamamoto Y, et al. 18F-FDG PET/CT in patients with polymyositis/dermatomyositis: correlation with serum muscle enzymes. Eur J Hybrid Imaging 2020;4(1). https://doi.org/10.1186/s41824-020-00084-w.

Clinical Applications of PET in Evaluating the Aging Spine

Sanaz Katal, MD, MPH[a], Thomas G. Clifford, MD[b], George Matcuk, MD[c],
Liesl Eibschutz, MS[b], Ali Gholamrezanezhad, MD[b],*

KEYWORDS

- Positron emission tomography (PET) • Low back pain • Fluorine-18-fluorodeoxyglucose (FDG)
- NaF • Degenerative spine disorders • Osteoporosis • Vertebral compression fractures
- Spine infection

KEY POINTS

- Molecular imaging can potentially detect pathophysiology that precedes morphologic changes and therefore plays a useful role in the evaluation of back pain and age-related spinal disorders.
- PET/CT or PET/MR imaging (using NaF or FDG) can help early diagnose and characterize spine degeneration and/or osteoporotic changes in the elderly patients.
- FDG-PET can detect infectious spondylodiscitis with competitive diagnostic accuracy compared with MRI, and therefore, may be a good alternative or complementary modality in the appropriate clinical setting.

INTRODUCTION

The spine is a complex biomechanical system of vertebrae, intervertebral discs, and ligaments that provides protection and support to the spinal cord during movement and rest.[1–3] Each component of the spine tends to degenerate with age, contributing to disorders ranging from herniated discs to ligamentous weakening.[4] The complex process of degeneration changes the spinal morphology, shape, and structure, resulting in dysfunction and instability. which can manifest as low back pain (LBP) and other symptoms, such as radiculopathy.[5]

LBP is the most common musculoskeletal problem globally.[6] It is also the leading cause of disability worldwide, accounting for enormous medical and economic costs. It is therefore a significant global public health concern that is expected to account for even greater health care costs in the future.[7] Although most causes of LBP are nonspecific and self-limiting, age and other age-associated comorbidities are well-known risk factors for severe and chronic LBP.[8] In most cases, no specific structural abnormality is found to explain the symptoms of severe or chronic LBP, and its exact cause remains unknown. Understanding the underlying pathogenesis of age-related spine disorders may offer additional insight toward identifying high-risk patients and improving their symptom management.

Multiple imaging modalities provide information about the pathophysiology of the aging spine. They also play a crucial role in spine research and in diagnosing, risk-stratifying, and prognosticating spine disorders. However, spine imaging has limitations for both radiologists and clinicians. Traditional imaging methods, such as radiographs, computed tomography (CT), and magnetic resonance (MR) imaging, mostly reveal late, degenerative structural changes. They do not typically reveal early pathologic changes that precede

[a] Independent Researcher, Melbourne, Victoria, Australia; [b] Keck School of Medicine, University of Southern California (USC), Los Angeles, CA, USA; [c] Cedars-Sinai Medical Center, Los Angeles, CA, USA
* Corresponding authors. Department of Diagnostic Radiology, Keck School of Medicine, University of Southern California (USC), 1520 San Pablo Street, Los Angeles, CA.
E-mail addresses: A.gholamrezanezhad@yahoo.com; ali.gholamrezanezhad@med.usc.edu

PET Clin 18 (2023) 39–47
https://doi.org/10.1016/j.cpet.2022.08.001

pathologic, anatomic changes. Moreover, imaging findings of spine degeneration are seen in high proportions of asymptomatic individuals, increasing with age.[9] In fact, many imaging features of spine degeneration in elderly patients are likely related to normal aging rather than painful syndromes.

Nuclear medicine techniques can potentially detect pathophysiology that precedes morphologic changes and therefore play a useful role in the evaluation of back pain (**Fig. 1**). Several studies have evaluated the utility of PET tracers in investigating spine disorders. Studies have shown promise for the use of Fluorine-18-fluorodeoxyglucose–PET (FDG-PET) in detecting early inflammatory changes in the musculoskeletal system, including the spine. Of course, PET is already an established modality for differentiating benign from malignant diseases involving the aging spine. In addition, it is thought that other tracers, such as ^{18}F (Fluoride-18), may play a potential role in evaluating patients with back pain when, as is often the case, the exact pathologic condition is not identified by anatomic modalities. Herein, the authors briefly review potential applications of PET in the evaluation of spine disorders in the elderly population.

OSTEOARTHRITIS (DEGENERATIVE SPINE DISORDERS)

The incidence of spine degeneration, especially in the lumbar region, increases sharply with age and is a major source of LBP.[10] It has been suggested that various inflammatory mediators are linked to intervertebral disc degeneration and may play a role in its pathogenesis.

FDG-PET is a highly sensitive modality for early detection of inflammatory processes in many organs, including the musculoskeletal system. In 1 retrospective study, Parsons and colleagues[11] reported higher FDG uptake in the knee joints of symptomatic subjects than in controls, indicating an association between increased metabolic activity and knee pain in patients with osteoarthritis (OA). It is thought that FDG-PET may play a role in early diagnosis of arthritis response, in monitoring, and for prevention of further complications, such as joint damage, devastating pain, and the need for joint replacement.[12]

Saboury and colleagues[13] used FDG-PET to objectively quantify the degree of inflammation in various joint disorders by calculating the global knee inflammation, which has been shown to increase with age-related joint inflammation. Similar findings have shown increased ^{18}F-FDG uptake in the intervertebral discs and spinous processes with aging, likely reflecting the inflammatory component of age-related spine degeneration.[14] These findings suggest that inflammation may be implicated in the pathophysiology of age-related degenerative diseases and that PET may play a role in quantifying the burden of disease in OA.

In another study, Hong and Kong[15] found that ^{18}F-FDG uptake is increased in OA and such a metabolic alteration (represented by the change of mean standardized uptake value [SUVmean]) was consistent with the development of OA. Metabolic alterations in cartilage may be associated with vulnerability of the joint to stress in primary OA, and certain cellular changes that occur during aging may contribute to development of OA. Therefore, PET may be a valuable tool to predict early OA changes. They showed that clinically and radiologically diagnosed OA was consistently correlated with increased FDG uptake. More specifically, SUVs were shown to increase in association with aging and OA progression. Thus, ^{18}F-FDG uptake on PET/CT imaging may play a role in early detection of OA, which is critical to preventing progression to irreversible joint failure.

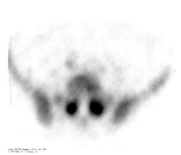 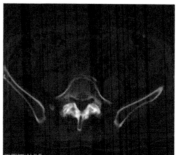 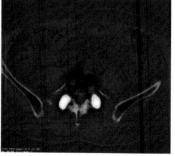

Fig. 1. Transaxial PET, CT, and fused PET/CT images of a 71-year-old woman showing focal hypermetabolic activity of ^{18}F-NaF at the facet joint in the lower back. Facet joint arthrosis is a common cause of LBP in the general population. (Figure reproduced with permission from Al-Zaghal A, Ayubcha C, Kothekar E, Alavi A. Clinical Applications of Positron Emission Tomography in the Evaluation of Spine and Joint Disorders. PET Clin. 2019 Jan;14(1):61-69.)

Lam and colleagues[16] studied the associations between FDG uptake on PET/CT and symptomatic MR imaging findings. They found that patients with symptomatic lumbar degenerative disease had increased ^{18}F-FDG metabolic activity corresponding to sites of disc and facet joint disease. However, there was no significant correlation between radiotracer uptake and the severity on MR imaging. There was also a moderate association between metabolic activity and levels of symptomatic spinal stenosis. Further studies are needed to evaluate the potential role of FDG-PET/CT in guiding epidural injections.

Rosen and colleagues[17] reported that incidental findings suggestive of degenerative spine disease are seen in 22% of patients on PET/CT, most commonly in the lumbosacral spine. Furthermore, the intensity of FDG uptake correlated with the severity of degenerative disc and facet disease as graded by CT. They also demonstrated that ^{18}F-FDG uptake is variable in patients with severe arthrosis owing to varying degrees of activity of inflammation.

At least 1 study has identified opportunity for ^{18}F-fluoride-PET/CT in identifying causes of persistent back pain following vertebral surgical interventions. Gamie and El-Maghraby[18] studied the role of ^{18}F-fluoride-PET/CT in the evaluation of facet and disc abnormalities in patients with LBP. They reported high sensitivity for identifying the source of pain in patients with or without previous surgical operations (76% and 88%, respectively).

Recently, PET/MRI has been introduced to detect and characterize osseous metabolic abnormalities seen in degenerative disorders. Simultaneous PET/MR imaging is a novel imaging technology that combines anatomic and metabolic data acquisition, proving an excellent soft tissue contrast and good spatial resolution, while significantly reducing radiation dose when compared with PET/CT.[19] PET/MR imaging may be a better diagnostic tool in evaluating both soft tissue structures (eg, cartilage morphology, intervertebral discs, major ligaments, and joint effusion) and osseous metabolic function. It has been suggested that by simultaneously assessing multiple early metabolic and morphologic markers of OA, PET/MR imaging may be able to detect early metabolic abnormalities of OA in normal-appearing joints on MR imaging. A study by Savic and colleagues[20] demonstrated that ^{18}F-NaF PET/MR depicts cartilage and bone interactions in knee OA, highlighting the complex biomechanical and biochemical interactions in knee OA and potentially better identifying therapeutic targets.

MR imaging provides excellent high-resolution anatomic delineation. In addition, delayed-contrast enhanced MR imaging can be used to assess synovitis.[21] MR imaging–based semiquantitative scoring systems that characterize pathologic features in osteoarthrosis have shown good reliability to predict OA disease progression.[22] However, structural degenerative changes seen on MR imaging likely reflect late-stage disease. Thus, by combining MR imaging findings with metabolic information from PET, PET/MR imaging better enables early thorough assessment of the whole joint, including soft tissues and bone.

PET/MR imaging can be performed with FDG or NaF, which provides different metabolic data about the degenerative process. For example, NaF can assess the activity of subchondral bone remodeling. Early PET/MR studies have suggested that different types of subchondral bony lesions on MR imaging have variable activity, indicating different stages of degeneration. Kogan and colleagues[23] used a novel technique of hybrid 3-T PET/MR imaging with ^{18}F-fluoride PET and semiquantitative methods. They found that maximum SUV values on PET were elevated in all subchondral bone lesions that appeared normal on MR imaging. Therefore, they suggested that metabolic abnormalities in subchondral bones might occur before structural changes can be seen on MR imaging, emphasizing the value of metabolic information provided by PET.

Finally, advanced imaging modalities play a role in the evaluation of spine degenerative diseases and their pathogenesis. PET imaging can depict active metabolism in articular and periarticular tissues while evaluating metabolic changes within the bone that occur with OA.[24] Thus, functional imaging with PET/CT or PET/MR imaging with (NaF or FDG) can help diagnose spine degeneration earlier, predict disease progression, and monitor treatment response.

OSTEOPOROSIS

Osteoporosis is a common systemic metabolic disease in the geriatric population that contributes significant morbidity, such as insufficiency fractures. Osteoporosis represents compromised bone strength, low bone mass, and microarchitectural deterioration of bone. Although not all elements of bone strength are represented by bone mineral density (BMD), BMD provides a useful estimate of fracture risk.[25,26] BMD normally decreases with aging. Beyond 50 years of age, the prevalence of osteopenia/osteoporosis is more than 50% in women and 30% in men.[27]

Conventional radiographs are notoriously unreliable for assessing BMD,[28] as it takes a long time before age-related structural changes are detectable. Currently, dual-energy x-ray absorptiometry (DXA) is the modality of choice for evaluating bone mineralization and diagnosing osteoporosis. Nevertheless, the DXA-derived BMD score has its own limitations, including its 2-dimensional nature and poor image quality. Moreover, the test needs to be repeated over long enough intervals to show significant BMD loss, which is inconvenient and sometimes impossible.[29] In addition, interindividual differences in age-related bone changes and therefore fracture risk may not be well represented by DXA.[30]

Other imaging modalities are available for BMD measurement, such as peripheral quantitative ultrasound and CT; however, to date they are primarily research tools. Recently, it has been proposed that molecular imaging methods may be superior in detecting the earliest changes in bone metabolism.[31] For example, studies of global bone metabolism using functional imaging techniques have shown that increased bone turnover is a feature of patients with osteoporosis. Israel and colleagues[29] found that cortical bone turnover (as depicted by quantitative ^{99m}Tc-methylene diphosphonate [^{99m}Tc-MDP] single-photon emission computed tomography [SPECT]) was significantly higher in women with osteoporosis. By providing imaging markers of bone turnover, SPECT and PET aid clinicians in identifying the populations at risk of bone loss and initiating appropriate prophylaxis.

In addition to MDP, NaF can also display increased bone turnover in osteoporotic patients and monitor the molecular effects of osteoporosis (**Fig. 2**).[32] Therefore, PET with ^{18}F-fluoride is a noninvasive tool for direct quantitative assessment of bone metabolism at certain sites in the skeleton, including the clinically important lumbar spine. Frost and colleagues[32] compared regional bone metabolism in the lumbar spine in women with and without osteoporosis using a dynamic ^{18}F-fluoride PET scan. They found significantly lower regional bone formation (manifested by lower K_i values) in patients with osteoporosis compared with women classified as osteopenic or normal. Surprisingly, they also reported higher values of bone-specific alkaline phosphatase (BSALP) in osteoporotic women. They stated that the K_i parameter is a regional measurement of bone formation, whereas BSALP is a measurement of global bone formation. These results suggest increased global bone turnover in women with postmenopausal osteoporosis despite relatively reduced regional

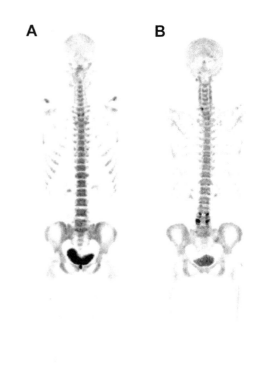

Fig. 2. Aging and ^{18}F-NaF uptake in the bone. Maximum intensity projection ^{18}F-NaF-PET images of 2 healthy subjects: (*A*) a 26-year-old woman and (*B*) a 62-year-old woman. The difference in ^{18}F-NaF uptake is visible particularly in the spine, pelvis, and proximal femur, which can be quantified in longitudinal studies to monitor disease progression and therapeutic response. Park, P.S.U.; Raynor, W.Y.; Sun, Y.; Werner, T.J.; Rajapakse, C.S.; Alavi, A. 18F-Sodium Fluoride PET as a Diagnostic Modality for Metabolic, Autoimmune, and Osteogenic Bone Disorders: Cellular Mechanisms and Clinical Applications. Int. J. Mol. Sci. 2021, 22, 6504. https://doi.org/10.3390/ijms22126504

bone formation at the predominantly trabecular lumbar spine.

Similarly, Uchida and colleagues[33] reported lower NaF activity in the lumbar spine in postmenopausal women with glucocorticoid-induced osteoporosis compared with healthy and osteopenic groups. They also reported that antiresorptive therapy with alendronate resulted in significant decreases in bone metabolism and turnover and an increase in lumbar BMD. Other studies have also investigated the usefulness of NaF PET in monitoring treatment response in patients with osteoporosis. Dynamic ^{18}F-fluoride PET scan has shown a significant increase in Ki and SUV from baseline following treatment, with larger increases in cortical bone than at trabecular sites.[34–36]

These findings suggest a promising role for molecular imaging methods (using NaF PET and

^{99m}mTc-MDP SPECT) to quantify bone turnover. Further studies are needed to establish the role of NaF in the management of osteoporosis.

COMPRESSION FRACTURES

Vertebral compression fractures are very common, especially in older adults. Differentiating between malignant and benign vertebral compression fractures can present a diagnostic dilemma, particularly in elderly patients who are potentially at risk of both.[37] Malignant and benign osteoporotic compression fractures have extremely different management and prognostic implications, highlighting the importance of making the correct diagnosis.

Advanced imaging plays a crucial role in distinguishing malignant and benign vertebral compression fractures. Although MR imaging and CT are widely used, they mainly provide anatomic data and on occasion do not yield a definitive diagnosis. Moreover, some patients are not good candidates for MR imaging owing to implanted devices, hardware, or other factors.

The metabolic information provided by ^{18}F-FDG-PET/CT may help in differentiating benign and malignant vertebral compression fractures.[38] Previous studies have evaluated the usefulness of FDG-PET in distinguishing benign and malignant acute vertebral compression fractures in patients with osteoporosis or preclinical osteoporosis.[39] Preliminary results indicated that unlike malignant pathologic fractures, acute osteoporotic vertebral fractures typically show no abnormally increased FDG uptake.[40]

Generally, fractures owing to tumors accumulate FDG, whereas benign fractures are not expected to accumulate FDG to a similar degree. It is thought that malignant pathologic fractures of various bones (pelvis, spine, rib, and long bones) demonstrate a significantly higher SUVmax compared with benign fractures.[41] Specifically, in the spine, the SUV should be significantly higher in malignant than benign compression fractures.[42] Most studies have applied a threshold SUV to classify the lesions, whereas others have used the mean liver SUV for comparison. An SUV cutoff between benign and malignant lesions of 3 to 4.7 has been proposed. Alternative criteria have suggested 2 standard deviations above (malignant) or below (benign) the liver SUV or direct comparison with the liver SUV in indeterminate (SUV 2–3) lesions.[38]

Nevertheless, ^{18}F-FDG-PET has its own limitations. There have been case reports of benign fractures demonstrating much higher than expected SUVs, even up to 9.3 in an acute pelvic fracture.[43] Therefore, acute fractures may be a source of false positives. In such scenarios, follow-up imaging is of value. It has been shown that FDG uptake is most intense in the acute phase and typically returns to normal by approximately 3 months.[44] Failure to return to a normal FDG uptake by 3 months raises concern for underlying malignancy or osteomyelitis.[45] Another limitation of ^{18}F-FDG-PET is false elevation of SUVmax values seen in patients on bone marrow–stimulating agents. To prevent incorrect interpretation, these factors should always be elicited and considered along with FDG uptake.[46]

In summary, ^{18}F-FDG-PET/CT may be able to differentiate malignant and benign fractures based on both SUVmax and ^{18}F-FDG uptake patterns.[47] It has high sensitivity and allows for semiquantitative assessment and thus provides additional information when evaluating vertebral compression fractures. It may provide the most benefit when CT or MR imaging findings are indeterminate. Again, further studies are needed to define the precise role of FDG-PET in the imaging of benign and malignant vertebral compression fractures.

SPINE INFECTION

The incidence of spine infections has been increasing owing to aging populations with substantial comorbidities and risk factors.[48] Spine infection accounts for 4% to 5% of all bone infections and represents the most frequent type of hematogenous osteomyelitis in patients older than 50 years.[49] Spine infections can be described as pyogenic, granulomatous (ie, tuberculous, brucella, fungal), and parasitic in cause. Hematogenic pyogenic spine infections can be thought of as a spectrum of disease that includes spondylodiscitis (a term encompassing vertebral osteomyelitis, spondylitis, and discitis), epidural abscess (which can be primary or secondary to spondylodiscitis), and facet joint arthropathy.[50] *Staphylococcus aureus* is the main pathogen, accounting for about half of nontuberculous cases. The average delay in diagnosis is about 2 to 4 months, which can contribute to permanent cord injury.[51] However, early diagnosis is difficult and often delayed or missed because of the nonspecific nature of its laboratory and radiographic findings. Infrequency of the disease coupled with the high frequency of LBP in the general population can make the diagnosis clinically challenging. Hence, the main problem in the management of spine infections is not treatment but early and accurate diagnosis.[52]

Unfortunately, it can take up to 6 weeks for bony erosive changes to become evident on plain

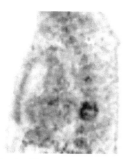 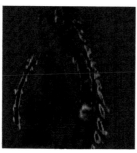 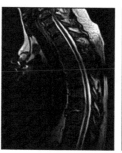 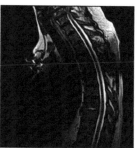

Fig. 3. ^{18}F-FDG-PET/CT and MR images of the spine in a 67-year-old man with *Streptococcus viridans* bacteremia. ^{18}F-FDG-PET/CT showed increased ^{18}F-FDG accumulation at the level Th8-Th9, correctly classified as spondylodiscitis. MR imaging correctly reported discitis with bulging into the spinal canal, suspect for an abscess. The patient received prolonged antibiotic treatment. (Figure reproduced with permission from Smids C, Kouijzer IJ, Vos FJ, Sprong T, Hosman AJ, de Rooy JW, Aarntzen EH, de Geus-Oei LF, Oyen WJ, Bleeker-Rovers CP. A comparison of the diagnostic value of MRI and 18F-FDG-PET/CT in suspected spondylodiscitis. Infection. 2017 Feb;45(1):41-49.)

radiographs. Thus, secondary imaging methods are of paramount importance in diagnosing spondylodiscitis. Contrast-enhanced MR imaging is the imaging modality of choice. When MR imaging is contradicted, a contrast-enhanced CT, PET, or combined gallium/Tc99m bone scan can assist in establishing the diagnosis.[53]

The usefulness of ^{18}F-FDG-PET/CT in the diagnosis and management of musculoskeletal infectious and inflammatory diseases has been widely debated in several publications to date.[54] Several meta-analyses have been performed to determine the diagnostic performance of ^{18}F-FDG-PET/CT in suspected musculoskeletal infections.[55,56] It has been suggested that ^{18}F-FDG-PET or PET/CT has excellent diagnostic ability in identifying infectious spondylodiscitis.[57] In a meta-analysis on ^{18}F-FDG-PET or PET/CT with suspicion of spondylodiscitis, the pooled sensitivity and specificity were reported to be 97% and 88%, respectively.[58] In addition, the diagnostic performance of ^{18}F-FDG-PET or PET/CT was higher compared with MR imaging. In a study by Yin and colleagues,[59] the diagnostic value of ^{18}F-FDG-PET or PET/CT for detecting spondylodiscitis was compared with MR imaging. Their findings demonstrated that the pooled sensitivity and specificity of ^{18}F-FDG-PET or PET/CT were higher compared with MR imaging (96% and 90% vs 76% and 62%, respectively). Other studies have reported similar results (95% and 88% vs 85% and 66%, respectively).[60] A recent study by Altini and colleagues[61] showed that ^{18}F-FDG-PET/CT is comparable to that of MR imaging for evaluation of spondylodiscitis in the entire spine (sensitivity, specificity, and accuracy of the MR imaging and ^{18}F-FDG-PET/CT were 100%, 60%, 97%, and 92%, 100%, 94%, respectively), indicating that ^{18}F-FDG-PET can be a complementary or alternative modality. Therefore, given its high diagnostic ability, ^{18}F-FDG-PET/CT should be considered for the diagnosis of spondylodiscitis, especially in cases with inconclusive clinical and/or MR imaging findings.[62] For example, it is often challenging to distinguish common Modic changes or sterile erosive osteochondritis from spinal infection by MR imaging. Adding ^{18}F-FDG-PET can improve the diagnosis of infectious spondylodiscitis (**Fig. 3**).[63,64] Moreover, FDG-PET/CT has been shown to predict treatment response in infectious spondylodiscitis with greater sensitivity and specificity than MR imaging.[65]

Other PET tracers have also been examined in the evaluation of infectious spondylodiscitis. Recently, Gallium-68-citrate PET/CT was used with promising results in patients with suspected bone infections, including 9 patients with spondylodiscitis.[66,67] Although preliminary, these results suggest a possible role for Gallium-68-citrate as a PET tracer in the diagnosis of spondylodiscitis.

In summary, nuclear medicine modalities can identify functional abnormalities that precede morphologic or anatomic changes, thereby playing an important role in the diagnosis of spinal infection. It has been suggested that ^{18}F-FDG-PET has equivalent if not better diagnostic accuracy compared with MR imaging in the detection of infectious spondylodiscitis. Therefore, it should be considered a useful alternative modality in the appropriate clinical setting. Finally, large multicenter studies are needed to validate the usefulness of other PET tracers (such as Gallium-68) in diagnosing spine infections.

SUMMARY

Previous studies have shown the ability of FDG-PET to demonstrate early inflammatory changes in the musculoskeletal system, including the spine. Complex inflammatory pathways may be implicated in the pathogenesis of age-related degenerative diseases, explaining the increased FDG uptake in the aging spine. Therefore, functional imaging with PET/CT or PET/MR imaging (using NaF or FDG) can help diagnose and characterize early spine degeneration, predict progression, and monitor treatment response.[68–75] In addition, as an imaging marker of bone turnover, NaF PET has a role in the diagnosis of osteoporosis and can help with earlier initiation of prophylactic therapies before a significant amount of bone loss occurs. In addition, ^{18}F-FDG-PET/CT may be able to differentiate between benign osteoporotic and malignant vertebral compression fractures. Last, ^{18}F-FDG-PET can detect infectious spondylodiscitis with competitive diagnostic accuracy compared with MR imaging, and therefore, may be a good alternative or complementary modality in the appropriate clinical setting.[76–78]

DISCLOSURE

The authors have nothing to disclose.

REFERENCES

1. Michelini G, Corridore A, Torlone S, et al. Dynamic MRI in the evaluation of the spine: state of the art. Acta Biomed 2018;89(1-S):89–101.
2. Prescher A. Anatomy and pathology of the aging spine. Eur J Radiol 1998;27(3):181–95.
3. Iorio JA, Jakoi AM, Singla A. Biomechanics of degenerative spinal disorders. Asian Spine J 2016; 10(2):377–84.
4. Benoist M. Natural history of the aging spine. Eur Spine J 2003;12(Suppl 2):S86–9.
5. Papadakis M, Sapkas G, Papadopoulos EC, et al. Pathophysiology and biomechanics of the aging spine. open orthopaedics J 2011;5:335.
6. Wu A, March L, Zheng X, et al. Global low back pain prevalence and years lived with disability from 1990 to 2017: estimates from the Global Burden of Disease Study 2017. Ann Transl Med 2020;8(6):299.
7. Cassidy JD, Cote P, Carroll LJ, et al. Incidence and course of low back pain episodes in the general population. Spine 2005;30(24):2817–23.
8. de Souza IMB, Sakaguchi TF, Yuan SLK, et al. Prevalence of low back pain in the elderly population: a systematic review. Clinics (Sao Paulo) 2019;74: e789.
9. Brinjikji W, Luetmer PH, Comstock B, et al. Systematic literature review of imaging features of spinal degeneration in asymptomatic populations. AJNR Am J Neuroradiol 2015;36(4):811–6.
10. Podichetty VK. The aging spine: the role of inflammatory mediators in intervertebral disc degeneration. Cell Mol Biol (Noisy-le-Grand, France) 2007;53(5):4–18.
11. Parsons MA, Moghbel M, Saboury B, et al. Increased 18F-FDG uptake suggests synovial inflammatory reaction with osteoarthritis: preliminary in-vivo results in humans. Nucl Med Commun 2015;36:1215–9.
12. Nguyen BJ, Burt A, Baldassarre RL, et al. The prognostic and diagnostic value of 18F-FDG PET/CT for assessment of symptomatic osteoarthritis. Nucl Med Commun 2018;39(7):699–706 [published correction appears in Nucl Med Commun. 2018; 39(10):960].
13. Saboury B, Parsons MA, Moghbel M, et al. Quantification of aging effects upon global knee inflammation by 18F-FDG-PET. Nucl Med Commun 2016; 37(3):254–8.
14. Aliyev A, Saboury B, Kwee TC, et al. Age-related inflammatory changes in the spine as demonstrated by (18)F-FDG-PET: observation and insight into degenerative spinal changes. Hell J Nucl Med 2012;15(3):197–201.
15. Hong YH, Kong EJ. 18F-Fluoro-deoxy-D-glucose uptake of knee joints in the aspect of age-related osteoarthritis: a case-control study. BMC Musculoskelet Disord 2013;22:14–141.
16. Lam M, Burke CJ, Walter WR. Correlation of 18F-FDG PET/CT uptake with severity of MRI findings and epidural steroid injection sites in patients with symptomatic degenerative disease of the lumbar spine: a retrospective study. Diagn Interv Radiol 2021;27(4):580.
17. Rosen RS, Fayad L, Wahl RL. Increased 18F-FDG uptake in degenerative disease of the spine: Characterization with 18F-FDG PET/CT. J Nucl Med 2006;47(8):1274–80.
18. Gamie S, El-Maghraby T. The role of PET/CT in evaluation of Facet and Disc abnormalities in patients with low back pain using (18)F-Fluoride. Nucl Med Rev Cent East Eur 2008;11(1):17–21.
19. Ramalho M, AlObaidy M, Catalano OA, et al. MR-PET of the body: early experience and insights. Eur J Radiol Open 2014;1:28–39.
20. Savic D, Pedoia V, Seo Y, et al. Imaging bone cartilage interactions in osteoarthritis using [18F]-NaF PET-MRI. Mol Imaging 2016;1:1–12.
21. Guermazi A, Roemer FW, Hayashi D, et al. Assessment of synovitis with contrast-enhanced MRI using a whole-joint semiquantitative scoring system in people with, or at high risk of, knee osteoarthritis: the MOST study. Ann Rheum Dis 2011;70(5): 805–11.
22. Hunter DJ, Guermazi A, Lo GH, et al. Evolution of semi-quantitative whole joint assessment of knee OA: MOAKS (MRI Osteoarthritis Knee Score). Osteoarthr Cartil 2011;19(8):990–1002.

23. Kogan F, Fan AP, McWalter EJ, et al. PET/MRI of metabolic activity in osteoarthritis: a feasibility study. J Magn Reson Imaging 2017;45:1736–45.

24. Roemer FW, Demehri S, Omoumi P, et al. State of the art: imaging of osteoarthritis—Revisited 2020. Radiology 2020;296(1):5–21.

25. Felsenberg D, Boonen S. The bone quality framework: determinants of bone strength and their interrelationships, and implications for osteoporosis management. Clin Ther 2005;27(1):1.

26. Lehouck A, Boonen S, Decramer M, et al. COPD, bone metabolism, and osteoporosis. Chest 2011; 139(3):648–57.

27. Zhang J, Morgan SL, Saag KG. Osteopenia: Debates and dilemmas. Curr Rheumatol Rep 2013; 15:384.

28. Taylor JA, Bussières A. Diagnostic imaging for spinal disorders in the elderly: a narrative review. Chiropractic Man Therapies 2012;20(1):1–9.

29. Israel O, Lubushitzky R, Frenkel A, et al. Bone turnover in cortical and trabecular bone in normal women and in women with osteoporosis. J Nucl Med 1994;35:1155–8.

30. Choksi P, Jepsen KJ, Clines GA. The challenges of diagnosing osteoporosis and the limitations of currently available tools. Clin Diabetes Endocrinol 2018;4(1):1–3.

31. Al-Zaghal A, Raynor W, Khosravi M, et al. Applications of PET imaging in the evaluation of musculoskeletal diseases among the geriatric population. InSeminars Nucl Med 2018;48(6):525–34.

32. Frost ML, Fogelman I, Blake GM, et al. Dissociation between global markers of bone formation and direct measurement of spinal bone formation in osteoporosis. J Bone Miner Res 2004;19(11):1797–804.

33. Uchida K, Nakajima H, Miyazaki T, et al. Effects of alendronate on bone metabolism in glucocorticoid-induced osteoporosis measured by 18F-fluoride PET: a prospective study. J Nucl Med 2009;50(11):1808–14.

34. Frost ML, Siddique M, Blake GM, et al. Differential effects of teriparatide on regional bone formation using (18)F-fluoride positron emission tomography. J Bone Miner Res 2011;26:1002–11.

35. Frost ML, Moore AE, Siddique M, et al. (18)F-fluoride PET as a noninvasive imaging biomarker for determining treatment efficacy of bone active agents at the hip: a prospective, randomized, controlled clinical study. J Bone Miner Res 2013;28:1337–47.

36. Moore AE, Blake GM, Taylor KA, et al. Assessment of regional changes in skeletal metabolism following 3 and 18 months of teriparatide treatment. J Bone Miner Res 2010;25:960–7.

37. Kubota T, Yamada K, Ito H, et al. High resolution imaging of the spine using multidetector-row computed tomography: differentiation between benign and malignant vertebral compression fractures. J Comput Assist Tomogr 2005;29(5):712–9.

38. Mauch JT, Carr CM, Cloft H, et al. Review of the imaging features of benign osteoporotic and malignant vertebral compression fractures. AJNR Am J Neuroradiol 2018;39(9):1584–92.

39. Schmitz A, Risse JH, Textor J, et al. FDG-PET findings of vertebral compression fractures in osteoporosis: preliminary results. Osteoporos Int 2002; 13(9):755–61.

40. Wan H, Xu T, Xiao J, et al. FDG-PET findings of vertebral compression fractures in osteoporosis. Bone 2008;43:S61.

41. Shin DS, Shon OJ, Byun SJ, et al. Differentiation between malignant and benign pathologic fractures with F-18-fluoro-2-deoxy-D-glucose positron emission tomography/computed tomography. Skeletal Radiol 2008;37:415–21.

42. Cho WI, Chang UK. Comparison of MR imaging and FDG-PET/CT in the differential diagnosis of benign and malignant vertebral compression fractures. J Neurosurg Spine 2011;14:177–83.

43. Ravenel JG, Gordon LL, Pope TL, et al. FDG-PET uptake in occult acute pelvic fracture. Skeletal Radiol 2004;33:99–101.

44. Shon IH, Fogelman I. F-18 FDG positron emission tomography and benign fractures. Clin Nucl Med 2003;28:171–5.

45. Zhuang H, Sam JW, Chacko TK, et al. Rapid normalization of osseous FDG uptake following traumatic or surgical fractures. Eur J Nucl Med Mol Imaging 2003;30(8):1096–103.

46. Bredella MA, Essary B, Torriani M, et al. Use of FDG-PET in differentiating benign from malignant compression fractures. Skeletal Radiol 2008;37:405–13.

47. He X, Zhao L, Guo X, et al. Differential diagnostic value of 18F-FDG PET/CT for benign and malignant vertebral compression fractures: comparison with magnetic resonance imaging. Cancer Management Res 2018;10:2105.

48. Babic M, Simpfendorfer CS. Infections of the spine. Infect Dis Clin North Am 2017;31(2):279–97.

49. Gouliouris T, Aliyu SH, Brown NM. Spondylodiscitis: update on diagnosis and management. J Antimicrob Chemother 2010;65(suppl_3):iii11–24.

50. Hadjipavlou AG, Mader JT, Necessary JT, et al. Hematogenous pyogenic spinal infections and their surgical management. Spine 2000;25(13):1668–79.

51. Gasbarrini AL, Bertoldi E, Mazzetti M, et al. Clinical features, diagnostic and therapeutic approaches to haematogenous vertebral osteomyelitis. Eur Rev Med Pharmacol Sci 2005;9(1):53–66.

52. Strohecker J, Grobovschek M. Spinal epidural abscess: an interdisciplinary emergency. Zentralblatt fur Neurochirurgie 1986;47(2):120–4.

53. Love C, Patel M, Lonner BS, et al. Diagnosing spinal osteomyelitis: a comparison of bone and Ga-67 scintigraphy and magnetic resonance imaging. Clin Nucl Med 2000;25(12):963–77.

54. Glaudemans AW, de Vries EF, Galli F, et al. The use of F-FDG-PET/CT for diagnosis and treatment monitoring of inflammatory and infectious diseases. Clin Developmental Immunol 2013;2013.

55. Wang GL, Zhao K, Liu ZF, et al. A meta-analysis of fluorodeoxyglucose-positron emission tomography versus scintigraphy in the evaluation of suspected osteomyelitis. Nucl Med Commun 2011;32(12): 1134–42.

56. Treglia G. Diagnostic performance of 18F-FDG PET/CT in infectious and inflammatory diseases according to Published meta-analyses. Contrast Media Mol Imaging 2019;2019:3018349.

57. Treglia G, Focacci C, Caldarella C, et al. The role of nuclear medicine in the diagnosis of spondylodiscitis. Eur Rev Med Pharmacol Sci 2012;16(Suppl 2): 20–5.

58. Prodromou ML, Ziakas PD, Poulou LS, et al. FDG PET is a robust tool for the diagnosis of spondylodiscitis: a meta-analysis of diagnostic data. Clin Nucl Med 2014;39(4):330–5.

59. Yin Y, Liu X, Yang X, et al. Diagnostic value of FDG-PET versus magnetic resonance imaging for detecting spondylitis: a systematic review and meta-analysis. Spine J 2018;18(12):2323–32.

60. Kim SJ, Pak K, Kim K, et al. Comparing the diagnostic accuracies of F-18 fluorodeoxyglucose positron emission tomography and magnetic resonance imaging for the detection of spondylodiscitis: a meta-analysis. Spine 2019;44(7):E414–22.

61. Altini C, Lavelli V, Niccoli-Asabella A, et al. Comparison of the diagnostic value of MRI and whole body 18F-FDG PET/CT in diagnosis of spondylodiscitis. J Clin Med 2020;9(5):1581.

62. Paez D, Sathekge MM, Douis H, et al. Comparison of MRI, [18F] FDG PET/CT, and 99mTc-UBI 29-41 scintigraphy for postoperative spondylodiscitis—a prospective multicenter study. Eur J Nucl Med Mol Imaging 2021;48(6):1864–75.

63. Ohtori S, Suzuki M, Koshi T, et al. 18F-fluorodeoxyglucose-PET for patients with suspected spondylitis showing Modic change. Spine (Phila Pa 1976) 2010; 35(26):E1599–603.

64. Fahnert J, Purz S, Jarvers JS, et al. Use of simultaneous 18F-FDG PET/MRI for the detection of Spondylodiskitis. J Nucl Med 2016;57(9):1396–401.

65. Righi E, Carnelutti A, Muser D, et al. Incremental value of FDG-PET/CT to monitor treatment response in infectious spondylodiscitis. Skeletal Radiol 2020; 49(6):903–12.

66. Nanni C, Errani C, Boriani L, et al. 68Ga-citrate PET/CT for evaluating patients with infections of the bone: preliminary results. J Nucl Med 2010;51(12): 1932–6.

67. Xu T, Chen Y. Research progress of [(68)Ga]citrate PET's utility in infection and inflammation imaging: a review. Mol Imaging Biol 2019;22(1):22–32.

68. Chaudhari AJ, Raynor WY, Gholamrezanezhad A, et al. Total-Body PET imaging of musculoskeletal disorders. PET Clin 2021;16(1):99–117.

69. Batouli A, Gholamrezanezhad A, Petrov D, et al. Management of primary osseous spinal tumors with PET. PET Clin 2019;14(1):91–101.

70. Behzadi AH, Raza SI, Carrino JA, et al. Applications of PET/CT and PET/MR imaging in primary bone Malignancies. PET Clin 2018;13(4):623–34.

71. Hancin EC, Borja AJ, Nikpanah M, et al. PET/MR imaging in musculoskeletal precision imaging - Third wave after X-ray and MR. PET Clin 2020;15(4): 521–34.

72. Katal S, Gholamrezanezhad A, Kessler M, et al. PET in the diagnostic management of soft tissue Sarcomas of musculoskeletal Origin. PET Clin 2018; 13(4):609–21.

73. Gholamrezanezhad A, Basques K, Batouli A, et al. Clinical Nononcologic applications of PET/CT and PET/MRI in musculoskeletal, Orthopedic, and Rheumatologic imaging. AJR Am J Roentgenol 2018; 210(6):W245–63.

74. Batouli A, Braun J, Singh K, et al. Diagnosis of non-osseous spinal metastatic disease: the role of PET/CT and PET/MRI. J Neurooncol 2018;138(2):221–30.

75. Manhas NS, Salehi S, Joyce P, et al. PET/Computed tomography scans and PET/MR imaging in the diagnosis and management of musculoskeletal diseases. PET Clin 2020;15(4):535–45.

76. Kooraki S, Assadi M, Gholamrezanezhad A. Hot Topics of research in musculoskeletal imaging: PET/MR imaging, MR Fingerprinting, dual-energy CT scan, Ultrashort Echo time. PET Clin 2019; 14(1):175–82.

77. Gholamrezanezhad A, Basques K, Batouli A, et al. Non-oncologic applications of PET/CT and PET/MR in musculoskeletal, Orthopedic, and Rheumatologic imaging: general Considerations, techniques, and Radiopharmaceuticals. J Nucl Med Technol 2017. jnmt.117.198663.

78. Gholamrezanejhad A, Mirpour S, Mariani G. Future of nuclear medicine: SPECT versus PET. J Nucl Med 2009;50(7):16N–8N.

PET-Computed Tomography in Bone and Joint Infections

Sarvesh Loharkar, MBBS, MD[a,b], Sandip Basu, MBBS, DRM, DNB, MNAMS[a,b],*

KEYWORDS

- PET • PET-CT • PET-MRI • FDG • Osteomyelitis • Diabetic foot • Prosthesis infection
- Aseptic loosening of prosthesis

KEY POINTS

- Hybrid imaging using fluorodeoxyglucose (FDG) PET/computed tomography (CT) is now considered a potentially useful imaging modality in the management of bone and joint infections, particularly for diagnosis and management of osteomyelitis, prosthetic joint infections, diabetic foot, and systemic infectious diseases with skeletal involvement (such as tuberculosis).
- FDG-PET/CT imaging aids in multiple aspects such as providing information on active disease extent in bones well of surrounding soft-tissue, identifying distant disease foci, and therapeutic response evaluation with great accuracy.
- FDG PET/CT imaging is not an alternative to other techniques like X-ray, MRI, and tissue diagnosis but to be used as complementary to them for best result.
- PET imaging using 18F sodium fluoride, gallium-68 citrate, 18F-fluorodeoxyglucose-labeled-white blood cells, and PET/MR imaging appears promising modalities in bone and joint infection. Their exact indications, protocol, and efficacy are yet to be established.

INTRODUCTION

Bone and joint infections form a major part of musculoskeletal ailments, and the spectrum of imaging techniques ranges from X-ray, computed tomography (CT) scan, and conventional Nuclear Medicine Scintigraphy to MRI scan in assisting clinical dilemmas in this specialty care. Over the last two decades, fluorodeoxyglucose (FDG)-PET and PET-CT imaging with its technological advances, has replaced many conventional Nuclear medicine scans in oncological practice. Recently, there is now growing evidence of the superiority of PET/CT imaging in non-oncological settings like infection-inflammation. Overall PET-CT hybrid imaging has multiple advantages when compared with other modalities, such as higher spatial resolution and accuracy, faster and single-day imaging protocols, one-stop-shop solution, simultaneous acquisition of both anatomic and functional data, whole-body imaging that aids in establishing other foci of infection and assesses whole-body disease extent, easy quantification of the degree of disease activity at the molecular level at both diagnosis and during response evaluation.

Elderly patients are more likely to have bone and joint infections because of preexisting conditions like diabetes mellitus, osteoarthritis rheumatoid arthritis, previous injuries/wounds, and reduced host immune response. In addition to native infections, prosthetic joint infections are quite peculiar in old age. Multiple imaging modalities are often used to delineate infection and to find infection coexistent with other conditions especially age-related degenerative changes and rheumatologic conditions. But many times, these additional

a Radiation Medicine Centre, Bhabha Atomic Research Centre, Tata Memorial Hospital Annexe, Jerbai Wadia Road, Parel, Mumbai 400 012, India; b Homi Bhabha National Institute, 2nd floor, BARC Training School Complex, Anushaktinagar, Mumbai, Maharashtra 400094, India
* Corresponding author. Radiation Medicine Centre, Bhabha Atomic Research Centre, Tata Memorial Hospital Annexe, Jerbai Wadia Road, Parel, Mumbai 400 012, India.
E-mail address: drsanb@yahoo.com

PET Clin 18 (2023) 49–69
https://doi.org/10.1016/j.cpet.2022.08.002
1556-8598/23/© 2022 Elsevier Inc. All rights reserved.

imaging adds to the complexity and further adds an inconvenience to patients, many of whom are elderly and debilitated. Here hybrid PET/CT evaluation is anticipated as one-stop solution in multiple clinical dilemmas.

18F-Fluorodeoxyglucose PET/Computed Tomography

The glucose analog FDG had been extensively studied in oncology imaging but soon it was observed that FDG uptake occurs in inflammatory cells owing to increased number and activity of glucose transporters during inflammation[1] and was considered an imaging pitfall because of false-positive findings in oncology practice in early years. Over time, this problem was turned into an opportunity, to image active infection-inflammation, especially in infections (eg, tuberculosis and bacterial abscess) and systemic inflammatory diseases like sarcoidosis. With this growing evidence joint European Association of Nuclear Medicine/Society of Nuclear Medicine and Molecular Imaging (EANM/SNMMI) guidelines for 18F-fluorodeoxyglucose (^{18}F-FDG) use in inflammation and infection were published in 2013[2] and advised few non-oncologic indications such as peripheral bone osteomyelitis (OM) and suspected spinal infection as major indications of FDG PET/CT with pooled accuracy of >85%, whereas few others like diabetic foot and prosthetic infections were listed as an unclear advantage over other scintigraphy methods.

Since then numerous heterogeneous studies and case series have been published worldwide and reported the role of FDG in these infective conditions and introduced a few new tracers in imaging armamentarium more specific than FDG. Though strong prospective trials and metanalysis are still sparse, this review provides a broad outline of present and possible future applications of mainly FDG-PET/CT and other explored novel PET tracers in the spectrum of infectious bone and joint diseases.

OM. It is defined as a spectrum of diseases where the bone is infected by microorganisms and varies as per the type and site of bone involved, the microorganism, and host immune response. It may be caused by contiguous spread, posttraumatic exposure of bone or by direct hematogenous route. Usually classified as per the period of occurrence, as acute (lasting <8 weeks), subacute or chronic OM. Acute OM is more commonly seen in children and immune-compromised adults and diagnosed using its clinical presentation.

The usual workup of bone infection is the physical examination, biochemical and pathologic tests, and imaging. The diagnosis requires the presence of at least two of the following four criteria:[3]

a. Purulent material draining from the site of OM,
b. Positive findings at bone tissue or blood culture,
c. Localized classical physical findings of bone tenderness and edema, and
d. Positive imaging findings

Imaging is a fast and noninvasive way of diagnosis, which primarily proves important in chronic OM. Imaging includes an X-ray which is usually done as a baseline evaluation, and has low sensitivity and specificities. CT and MRI scan comparatively provides high sensitivity and spatial resolution however these modalities have inherent drawbacks as their inability to diagnose pathology at very earlier stages where structural changes are not prominent, distinguish between acute and chronic disease and post-infection structural changes from chronic disease, and lower specificity in altered anatomic conditions like post-surgery/traumatic setting.[4]

In all these areas, the role of molecular imaging techniques has been emphasized, like 3-phase bone scan and technetium-99m (^{99m}Tc)-labeled leukocytes, which have superior performance in the aforementioned drawbacks and have been extensively used in low probability OM diagnosis.[5] Hybrid imaging with FDG-PET/CT gives added benefits and sensitivity and specificity of >90% in most studies[2] when compared with 78% and 84% for combined bone and leukocyte scintigraphy and 84%and 60% for MRI, respectively.[6,7] Recent metanalysis by Wang and colleagues[8] suggested the superior sensitivity and specificity of PET/CT of >90%, bone scintigraphy (83% and 45%), and labeled-white blood cell (WBC) scintigraphy (74% and 88%), respectively. Basu and colleagues[9] have reported higher sensitivity in acute-OM of 95% and specificity of 75% to 99%. Pawaskar and colleagues[10] concluded that MRI could be considered the primary imaging modality for uncomplicated unifocal cases of OM, whereas for multifocal disease or contraindications for MRI, FDG PET/CT is preferred. It also gives active disease sites to target biopsy in case of conspicuous clinical and imaging findings, multiple studies have shown a role of FDG PET/CT in response to antibiotic therapy in animal studies[11] and specific populations like children.[12,13] Larger studies with objective quantitative parameters in this arena are awaited to be established. It proves very useful in difficult scenarios like pediatric age group, and post-surgery/traumatic settings.

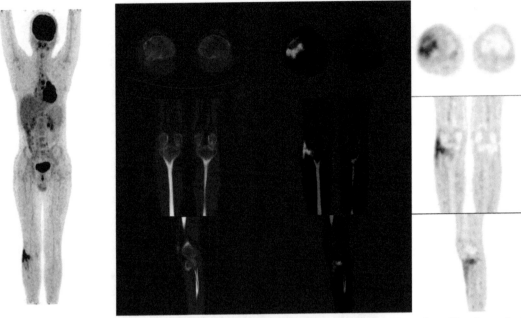

Fig. 1. A 19-year-old immunocompromised boy, past history of right-sided thigh pain and swelling 1 year back presented with nonhealing skin lesion, received empirical antibiotics for 3 months with partial symptomatic relief, was referred with suspicion for underlying bone and systemic involvement. FDG-PET/CT undertaken to map local disease and also other infective foci in the whole-body survey. FDG concentrating destructive lesion was noted at proximal end of right tibia with periosteal and subcutaneous soft-tissue edema and FDG concentrating sub centimetric left-sided axillary nodes (from left to right column wise MIP image, CT only, PET/CT fused, and PET-only images in transverse/coronal/sagittal sections at level of proximal tibia).

Overall, FDG PET/CT is a powerful tool in chronic OM where other modalities have failed to establish a diagnosis and in the assessment of response and complications (**Figs. 1** and **2**).

Osteomyelitis: Specific Subgroups

Spondylodiscitis

There are different types of infection described in the axial skeleton, and comprised of discitis (intervertebral disk infection), spondylodiscitis (SD) (infection of the intervertebral disk and adjacent vertebral body), and vertebral OM (infection of the vertebral body). Lumbar vertebrae are most common to get involved in SD but clinical diagnosis is difficult considering similar symptomatology of low back pain in many common skeletal diseases in the elderly. Early accurate diagnosis, assessment of disease extent, and complications considering the proximity of vital neurovascular structures are important considerations here for imaging and image-guided interventions. Routine radiological imaging such as X-ray and CT scans becomes useful when a significant part of cortical bone tissue is eroded; due to this and higher soft-tissue resolution, MRI has become an investigation of choice over these modalities where changes like marrow edema are also detected; but MRI suffers from higher false-positivity, especially in reactive marrow surrounding change, degenerative changes of disks, posttraumatic and post-intervention (eg, vertebral fixation procedures) and has shown poor correlation with clinical and microbiological response.

FDG-PET/CT has shown excellent accuracy and emerging as a promising tool in clinical decision-making. As per recent metanalysis[14] it has shown sensitivity and specificity of 97% and 88%, respectively, and<0.1% negative-likelihood ratio. This makes FDG-PET/CT imaging modality of choice to preclude infection in settings with equivocal/inconclusive MRI findings.

Meta-analysis by Kim and colleagues[15] comparing FDG-PET and MRI in spine infection comprising seven studies showed the sensitivity and specificity of FDG-PET/CT of 95% and 88%, respectively, whereas that of MRI at 85% and 65% highlighting diagnostic accuracy of FDG-PET over MRI. Meanwhile, FDG-PET/CT when used complimentarily with an MRI resulted in almost 100% detection of spinal infection as studied by Fuster and colleagues[16] Another additional benefit of FDG-PET/CT is its whole body screening and ability to image soft-tissue extent of disease;

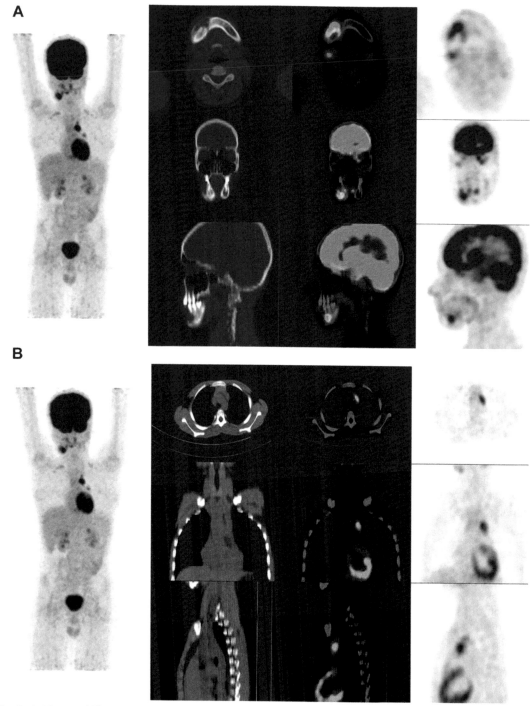

Fig. 2. A 14-year-old boy, case of mandibular osteomyelitis, presented with jaw swelling and gram-positive cocci on culture. (*A*) Focally FDG avid lytic lesion (SUVmax: 6.4) is noted right hemimandible. Mildly FDG avid (SUVmax: 3.2) tiny right-sided cervical level IB, II and bilateral level V nodes were noted (appears reactive) (from left to right column wise MIP image, CT only, PET/CT fused and PET-only images in transverse/coronal/sagittal sections at level of mandible). (B) FDG avid enlarged pre-vascular lymph node (SUVmax: 4.4) was noted measuring 2.0 cm × 1.5 cm, and also left-sided hilar node was noted (from left to right column wise MIP image, CT only, PET/CT fused, and PET-only images in transverse/coronal/sagittal sections at level of pre-vascular node).

thus, it has added benefits of distinguishing pyogenic vs. tubercular spine infection better than MRI.[17,18] However, for primary diagnosis, FDG-PET shows lower specificity owing to nonspecific uptake caused by several causes and diffuse uptake by inactive marrow in many common conditions like anemia.

A German study[19] on patterns of FDG-PET in SD established interpretation criteria based on the FDG uptake patterns, classified into different scores (from 0 to 4) related to different states of spine infection as:

- Score 0: normal findings and physiologic FDG distribution (consistent with no infection)
- Score 1: slightly enhanced uptake in the inter- or para-vertebral region (consistent with no infection)
- Score 2: clearly enhanced uptake with a linear or disciform pattern in the intervertebral space (consistent with discitis)
- Score 3: clearly enhanced uptake with a linear or disciform pattern in the intervertebral space and involvement of ground or cover plate or both plates of the adjacent vertebrae (consistent with SD)
- Score 4: clearly enhanced uptake with a linear or disciform pattern in the inter-vertebral space and involvement of ground or cover plate or both plates of the adjacent vertebrae + surrounding soft-tissue abscess (consistent with SD) (**Fig. 3**).

Response to therapy is another indication being successfully studied with FDG-PET. Several recent studies[20,21] have established that uptake and distribution of FDG is useful in assessing response and residual disease post 4 to 6 weeks of the therapy, however large prospective and comparison studies with quantitative parameters are awaited to establish this practice in guidelines (**Fig. 4**).

Overall owing to its high negative predictive value, the sensitivity FDG-PET/CT stands out over other modalities.

Skull-base osteomyelitis

This is a special form of OM comprised of face/skull base bones (temporal, sphenoid, or occipital) usually occurring as a complication of sino-nasal or ear infections and commonly noticed in diabetics. Though rare, it is potentially life-threatening. Infection usually passes through the Haversian system of compact bone and foramina of the cranial nerves (commonly jugular and facial). The complications include soft-tissue abscess in the cranial cavity, dural venous sinus thrombosis,

ischemic infections, meningitis, and cranial neuropathies depending on the nerve involved.[22]

The lack of underlying conditions like ear and nose infection, and conspicuous clinical findings like headache and neuropathy which is shared by multiple disorders (such as sinusitis, meningitis, and malignancy) makes diagnostic delay. Clinical examination and inflammatory markers are routinely used for diagnosis and response assessment but they do not elaborate on anatomy and extent and complications. High-resolution CT (HRCT) skull and MRI are commonly performed considering their legit spatial resolution, yielding detailed anatomic disease extent, marrow space involvement(by MRI), and information about complications; however they lack in specificity (especially in underlying disorders like fibrous dysplasia, Paget's) and functional information of disease activity in its chronic course.

A recent study by Kulkarni and colleagues[23] on 77 patients with clinically suspected skull-base osteomyelitis (SBO), FDG-PET/CT showed excellent accuracy with sensitivity, specificity, positive predictive value (PPV), negative predictive value (NPV), and accuracy of 96.7%, 93.3%, 98.3%, 87.5%, and 96.1%, respectively. In the same subset, 56 patients underwent an MRI scan in which soft-tissue involvement was corroborated with PET findings(83%), but MRI missed to show bone involvement in many cases (>30%) which were additionally shown by the PET study. Further, its role is response assessment where FDG-PET/CT was successful in detecting disease progression and regression and correlated well with other clinical and laboratory parameters.[23–25]

The overall experience of FDG-PET/CT in SBO is yet limited to a few discrete studies and case reports only. Though the initial experiences sound promising FDG PET/CT shows reduced accuracy in fungal infections, poorly controlled diabetes and false positivity in malignant disease (eg, nasopharyngeal carcinomas and metastatic secondaries). Recent reviews on imaging modalities of SBOs[26–30] concluded that CT shows bone erosion with a soft-tissue mass, whereas MRI is useful for evaluating the anatomic location and extent and shows an enhancing mass with an infiltrating pattern, bone marrow involvement, and adjacent soft-tissue edema. Nuclear imaging including FDG PET/CT scans is useful in confirmation of bone involvement in difficult cases and for follow-up response evaluation.

Infection of Prosthetic Joint Implants

In the last two to three decades, joint arthroplasty (commonly knee and hip) has become the

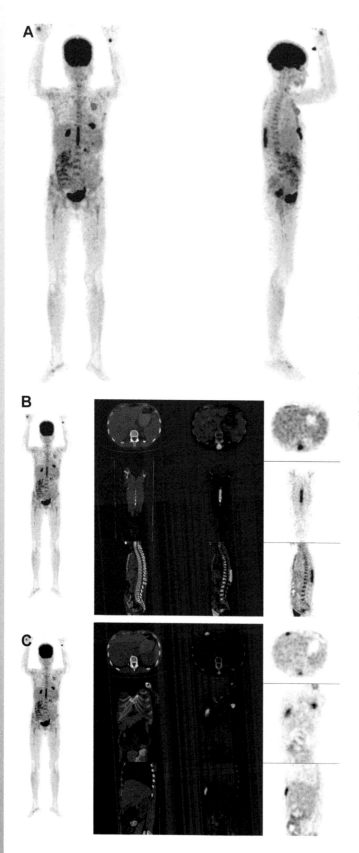

Fig. 3. 32-year-old woman, known case of right-sided carcinoma breast, post-mastectomy and post-adjuvant chemotherapy and radiotherapy, presented with back pain and swelling over back (thoracic region). (*A*) FDG-PET/CT was done for disease re-staging (MIP image in AP and right lateral view). (*B*) Linear FDG uptake is noted in soft-tissue density lesions with associated discrete destructive changes in spinous process of D9 to D12 with SUVmax 9.83. Soft-tissue lesion is seen extending into paraspinal muscles, subcutaneous tissues (from left to right column-wise MIP image, CT only, PET/CT fused, and PET-only images in transverse, coronal, and sagittal sections at level of D12 vertebra). (*C*) FDG uptake is noted in hypodense soft-tissue lesion in anterior part of sixth intercostal space on left sided and anterior part of seventh intercostal space on right side (from left to right MIP image, CT only, PET/CT fused, and PET-only images in transverse, coronal, and sagittal sections at level of 6th intercostal space). The destructive lesion on back was further evaluated by MRI and tissue diagnosis; this was proven to be of infective (bacterial), soft-tissue lesions in intercostal spaces region on both sides turned out to be abscess.

Baseline Post-antibiotic therapy

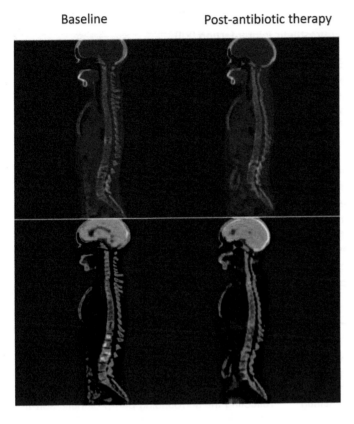

Fig. 4. Case of spondylodiscitis in a 55-year-old woman who presented with low back pain and tenderness, on tissue found to have gram-positive cocci, received IV antibiotics for 4 weeks; her baseline FDG-PET/CT (sagittal sections CT-only and fused PET/CT) showed multiple irregular FDG avid lytic lesions in lower dorsal and lumbar vertebrae, disk space narrowing, whereas posttreatment FDG-PET/CT scan showed resolution of FDG uptake in lesions.

standard of care in severe degenerative joint diseases and its incidence is exponentially increasing in all parts of the world. Although well tolerated, many of these land up into complications like loosening, dislocation, fracture, and infection. Infection of prosthesis is reported in approximately 2% of arthroplasties and increased up to 20% in revision surgeries. With the increase in the number of surgeries and follow-up years, the incidence of these complications is rising, whereas diagnosing them correctly clinically is demanding as they often share similar symptom complex of pain, movement difficulties, and swelling. As per the Musculoskeletal Infection Society (MSIS),[31] the recent definition for the adequate diagnosis of joint infection is given as (**Table 1**) score 1 of the 2 major criteria. OR for minor criteria joint infection is given as an aggregate score of >6, whereas score 2 to 5 is taken as possibly infected, whereas score of 0 to 1 does not reflect infection)

Many of the aforementioned criteria that are the backbone of the diagnostic workup are invasive and don't give an exact picture of the anatomic extent of the disease. The most important differential for joint infection is aseptic loosening which also shows some degree of peri-prosthetic inflammatory reactions and markers; as management

and prognosis of these two conditions differ significantly it is at most important to differentiate them in post-arthroplasty care. CT imaging is sensitive but it suffers from prostheses-related artifacts. MRI imaging provides an addition in addressing soft-tissue changes and complications it does suffer from metal artifacts. Routine bone scintigraphy shows degraded specificity of 50% to 60% because of reactive peri-prostheses tracer uptake and depends upon the time from surgery and type of prostheses used.[32]

A recent metanalysis by Verberne and colleagues showed[33] pooled sensitivity of FDG-PET/CT to be 70% and specificity of 84% for knee prostheses, whereas for hip prostheses[34] it was 86% and 93%, respectively. Another such review suggested similar results of pooled sensitivity of 87% and a pooled specificity of 87%. The recent joint consensus by European Association of Nuclear Medicine (EANM), European Bone and Joint Infection Society (EBJIS), and European Society of Radiology (ESR) on the diagnosis of prosthetic joint infections[35] which is based on recently available literature evidences such as randomized trials and observational studies in the topic compared accuracies of different modalities inprosthetic joint infection (PJIs). The group

Table 1
New scoring based MASIC criteria for periprosthetic joint infection (PJI)

A.	Major Criteria	Score
1.	Sinus tract communicating with the prosthesis	1
2.	pathogen is isolated by culture from at least two separate tissue or fluid samples obtained from affected prosthetic joint	1
Score ≥1 in major criteria—positive for infection		
B.	Minor Criteria	Score
1.	Serum elevated CRP or D-dimer	2
2.	Elevated ESR	1
3.	Synovial Elevated white blood cell count or leukocyte esterase	3
4.	Positive a-defensin	3
5.	Elevated polymorphonuclear cells	2
6.	Elevated CRP	1
Score ≥6 in minor criteria—positive for infection		

suggested that FDG-PET in patients with suspected prosthetic joint infection has high sensitivity (~90%) but lower specificity than WBC scintigraphy or anti-granulocyte antibody scintigraphy. Nonspecific synovial uptake or bone prostheses interface uptake is a major challenge before interpretation and excluding other differentials like aseptic loosening; only uptake of tracer results in poor specificity and to overcome this pattern of uptake has been studied by different groups with multiple criteria reported as elaborated by Thapa and colleagues.[36]

Visual assessment
In the study by Basu and colleagues,[37] the positivity criteria for infection in total hip arthroplasty (THA), was increased FDG uptake at the bone-prosthesis interface in the middle portion of the shaft of the hip prosthesis, whereas the negativity criteria adopted was FDG uptake limited to the soft-tissues, or adjacent only to the neck of the prosthesis. In total knee arthroplasty (TKR), only uptake at the bone/prosthesis interface was considered positive, whereas absent or minimal uptake was considered negative for infection. Many other groups also have suggested similar criteria and improving the accuracy of scan more than 90%.

Semiquantitative analysis
One of such method for evaluation of total knee prostheses is proposed by Gravius and colleagues,[38] which involves, Dividing the bone prosthesis interface into three segments (femoral prostheses is divided as anterior, posterior and stem region while tibial prostheses as medial lateral and stem region) and four other segments reflecting the surrounding peri-prosthetic soft-tissue (divided as upper inner, upper outer, lower inner and lower outer). FDG uptake in each of the segments is given a score compared with surrounding bone marrow uptake (0–3) as:

0: no uptake, 1: discrete uptake (intensity weaker than bone marrow), 2: moderate uptake (intensity analogous to bone marrow), 3: high uptake (intensity stronger than bone marrow). They further suggested 5 categories as per segment and FDG uptake score as (a) nNo Loosening or infection, (b) aseptic loosening of the tibial component, (c) aseptic loosening of the femoral component, (d) prosthesis infection, and (e) nonspecific synovitis. for example, as per above-mentioned criteria, femoral prostheses uptake can be labeled as infection [Category-d] if any one out of 3 the femoral segments shows a score of 3 FDG uptake.

FDG showed greater accuracy in the diagnosis of prosthetic joint infection when compared with most other imaging modalities but lesser specificity compared with labeled-WBC studies thus its routine clinical role is still in debate.,[39] elbow, ankle which are uncommonly performed, only discrete pilot studies are available and insufficient to comment on the exact role of FDG-PET/CT in these joints. Thus, considering the nonuniformity of multiple criteria in the diagnosis of infection from aseptic loosening as mentioned above, a multicenter evaluation is needed. In the review by

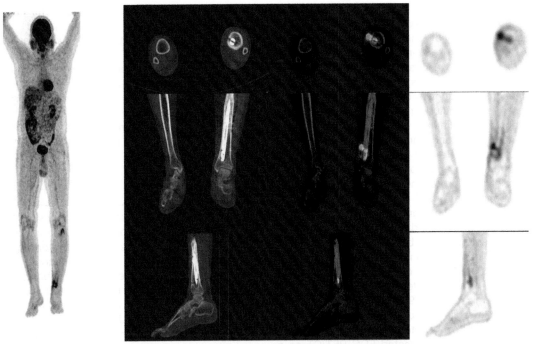

Fig. 5. A 56-year-old woman with history of traumatic fracture to left clavicle and tibia in 2018. Following open reduction and internal fixation of tibia 3 years back due to traumatic cause, now complained of pain and discharge at the postoperative site, FDG-PET/CT showed intense FDG uptake noted in ill-defined cutaneous soft-tissue thickening with surrounding fat stranding and edema involving the skin over the distal end of implant suggested soft-tissue infection with FDG uptake along the screw tracts at the distal end of implant with mild cortical lysis, suggestive of implant infection and patient was started with antibiotics as per culture (from left to right: MIP image, CT-only, PET/CT fused and PET-only images in transverse, coronal, and sagittal sections at level of distal end of tibia).

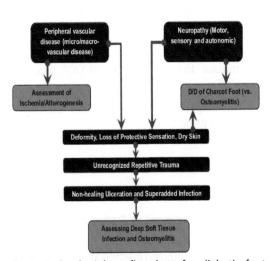

Fig. 6. Pathophysiology flowchart for diabetic foot where Primary pathogenetic factors (blue), the further complicating factors (brown), and diagnostic challenges where PET-CT/PET-MR imaging has a potential role (green). (*From* Basu S, Zhuang H, Alavi A. FDG PET and PET/CT Imaging in Complicated Diabetic Foot. PET Clin. 2012 Apr;7(2):151-60.)

Bhoil and colleagues FDG-PET/CT performs better than other clinical imaging modalities for implant-related infection; its limitations being in acute settings, differentiation of inflammation from infection, and in sterile infection (**Fig. 5**).[40]

Diabetic Foot

Diabetes mellitus is a modern-day pandemic with a high prevalence of 8.5% in adults worldwide. A diabetic foot is any pathology that results directly from peripheral arterial disease (PAD) and/or sensory neuropathy affecting the feet as a complication out of both macro-vascular and micro-vascular pathologies. Owing to loss of sensations and poor vascular conditions, the feet are prone to repeated trauma and infection. The estimated risk of a diabetic patient developing foot ulcer in his life is up to 25%[10] and it is noted that one-third of diabetic foot infections further lead to OM (**Fig. 6**).[41]

The main differential of bone involvement in diabetic foot is Charcot osteoarthropathy which leads to bone destruction and joint deformities because of repeated trauma precipitated by neuropathy. The clinical diagnosis of infection is guided by different criteria for example, Infectious Diseases Society of America (IDSA)[42] using signs like local warmth, tenderness, ulceration, temperature, heart rate, respiratory rate but clinical findings in the initial stages are quite similar as early infections in diabetics do not typically produce system signs (including leukocytosis), both conditions carry different management protocols and prognosis and early detection of infection enable the prevention of invasive and morbid treatments like an amputation. This is aided by different imaging techniques commonly an MRI and bone scan. MRI with its excellent soft-tissue spatial resolution, ability to detect early reactive changes, and surrounding soft-tissue involvement proves to be one of the most accurate methods to diagnose OM in the diabetic foot spectrum. But the dilemma of early OM and Charcot's remains unclear.

A systemic review of 9 studies and 299 patients derived by Treglia and colleagues[43] registered varied sensitivity of 60% to 85% and specificity of 85% to 96% and suggested FDG-PET/CT as a powerful tool when used combined with MRI. Another study by Nawaz and colleagues[44] compared FDG-PET and MRI and obtained assuring results with sensitivity, specificity, PPV, NPV, and accuracy of FDG PET as 81%, 93%, 78%, 94%, and 90%, respectively, whereas for MRI it was 91%, 78%, 56%, 97%, and 81%, respectively. In another such metanalysis of 27 papers by Laurie and colleagues,[45] FDG–PET showed sensitivity and specificity of 89% and 92%; for WBC scan with indium-111 (^{111}In)-oxine, it was 92% and 75%; whereas MRI showed 93% and 75%, respectively, highlighted similar sensitivity but higher specificity of FDG-PET/CT among other modalities.

Analysis of diagnostically difficult cases as in early Charcot's vs. infection the hybrid imagining with FDG PET/CT plays a vital role, as suggested by Basu and colleagues,[46] in their prospective study of 63 patients Charcot osteoarthropathy showed low-grade diffuse FDG uptake (SUV-max0.7–2.4) distinguishable from a normal joint (SUVmax0.2–0.7), whereas the group with superimposed OM had higher uptake (SUVmax6.5). Here overall accuracy of diagnosis Charcot's was >90% when compared with MRI in the range of 75% to 77%. In addition, using FDG PET for deeper etiopathological insights, Basu and colleagues[47] also studied atherosclerotic inflammation in the large vessels to evaluate the ischemic component of the disease in diabetic foot ulcers. The authors suggested the following indications of FDG-PET/CT in diabetic-foot in addition to MRI:

- Differentiation of Charcot's osteoarthropathy and OM
- Whole-body imaging to look for metastatic infective foci
- Response assessment in which clinical parameters are obscure
- Studying Ischemic and atherosclerotic changes
- Ruling out infection in areas of alerting or distorted anatomy (like previous surgical/orthopedic procedures)

Septic Arthritis

Septic arthritis is an infection of joint tissues and synovial fluid by a wide range of microorganisms; classified as per the type of causative organism, the onset of symptoms, and arthroscopic findings. Diagnosis is routinely done by nonspecific signs such as joint heat, redness, pain, swelling, movement restrictions, and fever. Apart from X-Ray which detects, USG is commonly performed imaging which provides high accuracy in establishing the initial diagnosis and guides invasive procedures to establish microbiological evidence. Further, an MRI scan with its ability to access bone marrow changes and great soft-tissue spatial resolution gives out high sensitivity and approximately 100% NPV, it also aids to diagnose complications like sinus track formation, abscess formation, and related destruction.[48] But it lags in specificity in an underlying inflammatory disorder, altered anatomy, and prostheses. Here procedures like labeled-WBCs scan and triple-phase ^{99m}Tc-MDP bone scan have been studied. The literature on FDG-PET/CT here is still limited due to its nonspecific uptake in inflammatory tissues. In practice, FDG-PET/CT has been used for

- Deciding the disease extent in destructive septic arthritis,
- Pinpointing of infective foci by whole-body survey,
- Response assessment in difficult and chronic cases.

Skeletal Involvement in Systemic Infectious Diseases

PET-CT hybrid imaging is empowered by its ability to scan the whole body to detect previously undiagnosed early bone involvement in a systemic infection. In such ways, PET/CT has become popular as a one-stop-shop imaging modality. A few of such applications are mentioned in the following section:

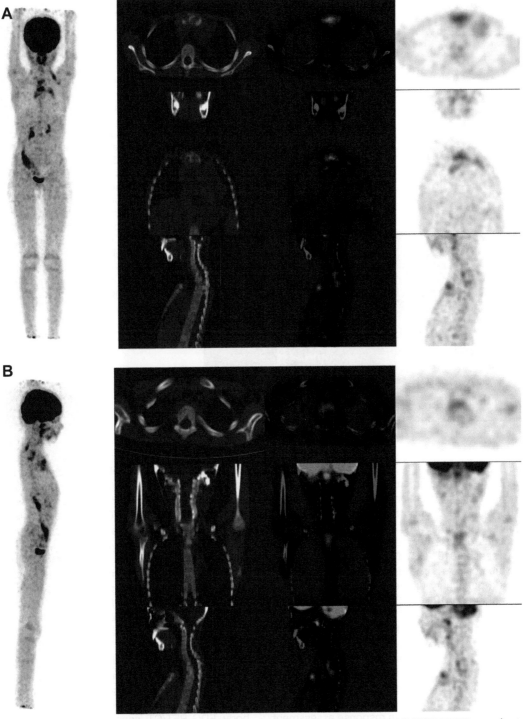

Fig. 7. An 8-year-old female patient who presented with central chest swelling, FNAC-GENE XPERT, mycobacterium tuberculosis detected very low and the patient was planned for AKT. She was referred for baseline evaluation of disease status. (*A*) FDG-PET/CT scan showed tracer concentrating destructive lytic lesion is noted at manubriosternal joint measuring ~3.0 cm in largest (transverse) dimension with SUVmax 3.2 (from left to right column wise MIP image in AP angle, CT-only, PET/CT fused, and PET-only images in transverse, coronal, and sagittal sections at level of manubrium). (*B*) Similar FDG concentrating destructive lytic changes were noted

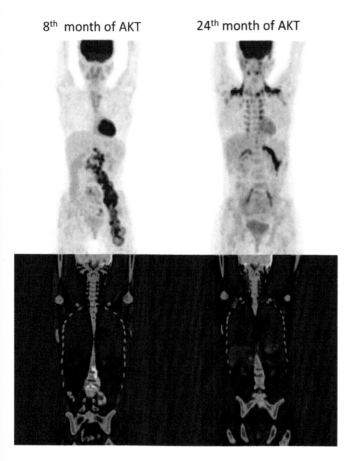

8th month of AKT   **24th month of AKT**

Fig. 8. A 26-year-old woman, known case of multidrug resistant Koch's disease with lumbar vertebral involvement; the baseline scan (MIP image and fused PET/CT image in coronal section) done at 8th month of anti-Koch's treatment showed abnormally increased FDG uptake (SUVmax: 8.3) in well-defined soft-tissue lesion in left para-vertebral region involving left psoas muscle extending from level of L3 vertebra to mid-thigh region. FDG uptake was also noted in D1 to D4 and D11-L3 vertebrae with lytic sclerotic changes and soft-tissue components. Around 24th month of the therapy response evaluation, FDG-PET/CT was performed, which showed (MIP and fused coronal images) nontracer concentrating destructive lytic lesions in multiple vertebrae. Mild FDG uptake in bilateral psoas muscles with normal anatomy, overall suggestive of metabolic response to therapy.

Tuberculosis

One of the most common systemic infectious disorders caused by infection due to mycobacteria, in 2020 itself it resulted in approximately 1.5million deaths being the second most common cause of infectious disease-related deaths after coronavirus disease-2019 (COVID-19). Skeletal infection with tuberculosis is one of the most common types of extra-pulmonary tuberculosis (EPTB), reported in as high as in10% to 30% of extra-pulmonary cases, most of them (~50%) are presented as spine infection known as Pott'sspine.[49] Identifying skeletal disease plays an important role in clinical judgment as they require different and longer anti-tubercular regimens. CT scan and MRI are being extensively used in studying bone destruction in tuberculosis but don't give input regarding the active disease, especially in response assessment scenarios (**Figs. 7** and **8**).

FDG uptake in tubercular infections has been notoriously affecting the accuracy of oncologic PET studies in multiple organ systems, however, this aspect of FDG-PET/CT in tuberculosis has been of considerable interest in recent times in the medical community. In the early stages of inflammation, FDG uptake is noted in the involving bone even if it is normal on CT images, especially before the occurrence of anatomic changes. Though sensitive, FDG-PET/CT lacks specificity in diagnosis, with tuberculosis and malignancies, sarcoidosis, and other inflammatory disorders being the major differentials, and tissue and microbiological diagnosis remain the gold standard. Multiple bone involvement is a common finding in tuberculosis: in one observational study, Dureja and colleagues[50] reported that baseline whole-body FDG-PET/CT scanning diagnosed 63.6% clinically occult noncontiguous multifocal skeletal

predominantly in body of vertebrae from D1 to D5 with SUVmax 2.8; there was also associated FDG concentrating para-vertebral soft-tissue component along D1 to D5 (left > right) with prominent bulge at left D4 level with SUVmax 2.5 (from left to right column wise MIP image in transvers angle, CT only, PET/CT fused, and PET-only images in transverse, coronal, and sagittal sections at level of third thoracic vertebra).

involvement. Recent expert opinion by Sharma and colleagues[51] suggested that modalities like FDG-PET/CT have facilitated precise anatomic localization of the lesions and mapping the extent of EPTB. Use of these image- and endoscopy-guided invasive diagnostic methods for diagnostic testing is now possible. Tubercular disease activity correlates with uptake on FDG-PET/CT, thus akin to its use in malignancies, it can be used to detect, stage, and assess response to therapy[52] in skeletal tuberculosis. FDG-PET/CT also gives insights and extent of surrounding soft-tissue involvement especially in the case of Pott's spine, para-spinal and psoas infection. Mittal and colleagues[53] studied 28 patients of spinal tuberculosis, using FDG-PET/CT and MRI in response assessment, PET/CT showed healed bone lesion in 100% compared with 68.42% in MRI. This is particularly relevant in the setting of extensive skeletal involvement where other imagining modalities cannot single-handedly map the whole-body disease.

Goyal and colleagues[54] studied FDG-PET/CT in assessing response to ATT and decision-making in 40 histologically proven joint tuberculosis patients, the time to complete response was correlated with metabolic volume and patients with CR in PET/CT maintained disease-free state during a mean follow-up of 271 days. The authors concluded FDG-PET/CT to be an excellent tool in estimating total disease burden, assessing response to ATT, and identification of treatment endpoint in joint tuberculosis.

Fungal infections including mucormycosis
Though uncommon and indolent, systemic invasive fungal diseases are a diagnostic and therapeutic challenges with high morbidity and mortality. Multiple types of fungi including coccidioidomycosis, blastomycosis, cryptococcosis, candidiasis, and sporotrichosis infest the bones. Diagnosis is often guided by clinical suspicion as these diseases may masquerade as other disorders.

Tissue biopsy and microbiological assay are labeled as gold standard diagnostic tools. Imaging is usually performed to assess the anatomic extent of disease and CT and MRI scans are routinely performed modalities. MRI with its high spatial resolution and ability to detect marrow changes is a current modality of choice but suffers from low specificity in early stages and underlying bony deformities. PET/CT has been recent of interest owing to the ability to detect active disease.

A recent study by Leroy-Freschini and colleagues[55] who evaluated FDG-PET/CT in 51 immunocompromised patients with invasive fungal disorders the sensitivity, specificity, positive and negative predictive values, and global accuracy noted were 93%, 81%, 95%, 72%, and 90%, respectively; as per their conclusion PET improved the primary staging workup of immune-compromised patients with invasive fungal infections and useful in assessing treatment effectiveness or disease relapse.

Mucormycosis has emerged as an important disorder in the post-COVID-19 pandemic area affecting vital structures on the face and skull including orbit; multiple modalities are being under evaluation to adequately diagnose the situation. As reported by Altini and colleagues[56] FDG-PET/CT can be used for initial staging in hand with an MRI and also it may be useful for the assessment of response to treatment.

Importantly these invasive infections are treated by toxic therapies for the long-term and often there is a dilemma for response assessment using clinical and conventional imaging due to severe postinfectious changes, here the role of PET with its advantage of molecular imaging to evaluate active disease is being considered by many groups,[57,58] but there is not yet any prospective study with large sample size available to define the role of PET in the management protocol of these diseases.

Other miscellaneous systemic infective disorders like melioidosis,[59] chikungunya virus infection,[60] and bone involvement because of these pathologies are also reported using FDG-PET/CT, with its utility in providing insights for pathology and active disease involvement in the whole body in a single go.

The authors suggest the following indications FDG-PET/CT in bone and joint infections in the elderly:

- For initial disease staging and extent assessment by whole-body survey
- To guide tissue diagnosis by pinpointing the active most disease
- To assess active disease involvement before and after invasive procedures
- To assess response to the therapy

Special Considerations for PET-CT Scan Acquisition and Interpretation for infectious disease in the elderly:

- Pre-imaging history should cover details of interfering factors, such as trauma, surgical, drug (antibiotics, immunosuppressants), known systemic conditions like diabetes, Koch's, and sarcoidosis with their duration.
- No stringent pre-imaging of blood glucose levels are advised (different from tumor imaging). Still as per the guideline statement[2] efforts should be made to decrease blood

glucose to the lowest possible level. Unstable or poorly controlled diabetes (often associated with infection), hyperglycemia should not be considered as an absolute contraindication for the imaging study.[61]

- Standard imaging protocol similar (to oncologic PET)[2]: post-injection 1-h imaging should be followed (many studies worldwide have followed dual time point imaging but the exact utility is not yet well established[2]).
- Imaging protocol should be modified as per disease and region under study.[62]

We suggest special local views, which provide excellent spatial resolution and give disease involvement with periosteal soft-tissue regions for example, regions of complicated anatomy as skull where regional acquisition with high dose HRCT (thin slice) provides better anatomic resolution. Viewer should always examine scans in triangulated views (eg, sagittal and coronal sections for the spine are more useful)

- Foreign bodies such as prostheses tend to interfere with CT acquisitions and this artifact produces errors in the form of excessive attenuation correction, thus it is always suggested to examine non-attenuation correlated PET only data.

As discussed above, FDG PET/CT has been extensively studied and established role in multiple scenarios in bone and joint infections, though it has some lacunae that can be mentioned as follows:

- Low specificity: FDG is not infection-specific agent, FDG uptake is seen in multiple conditions mainly malignancies and inflammatory conditions, and the same conditions are many times differentials to infection and/or co-existing with infections, which reduces the specificity.
- Drug interference: Multiple medications commonly given in infectious and inflammatory conditions as steroids and antibiotics significantly change FDG uptake.
- Difficult interpretation of images and physiologic uptake: Nonspecific marrow uptake, reactive marrow uptake, uptake in brown adipose tissue (BAT), and muscles overuse are common causes of increased physiologic FDG uptake which can significantly interfere with target bone uptake in the same vicinity.
- Radiation exposure: When compared with modalities like USG or MRI, PET/CT uses ionizing radiation which imposes radiation dose as high as 15 to 25 mSv per procedure, this defiantly becomes a concern in repeat imaging especially in pediatric age.

- Lack of systematized protocol for infection: No standardization of cutoff values and other parameters as in oncology.
- Poor availability and high cost: When compared with other modalities like CT scan/MRI/USG, PET-CT is still not widely available at peripheral locations.

Non-Fluorodeoxyglucose Tracers in Bone Infection Imaging

18F sodium fluoride (^{18}F-NaF) PET/CT

After FDG, NaF is the most extensively studied PET tracer in bone infection. The uptake of NaF is based on its chemisorption on hydroxyapatite.[63] Higher uptake in exposed bone surfaces and areas of remodeling in multiple benign and malignant conditions is the basis of its uptake mechanism. Owing to this nonspecificity of uptake in multiple bone etiologies,[64] the accuracy of the study is compromised, especially in unknown diagnoses. On the contrary, the benefits are its high sensitivity of accessing early bony change, well-defined tracer kinetics to study perfusion phase, and low background uptake especially in surrounding inflammatory infective or infective tissue and readily available CT features for correlation.

On the basis of triphasic-bone scintigraphy, the utility of ^{18}F-NaF has been studied in different skeletal conditions, Freesmeyer and colleagues[65] studied the strength of dynamic ^{18}F-NaF PET/CT in OM, where early 5 min dynamic scan was acquired in list mode. The study showed that in bone infection the 31 to 45 seconds frame had significantly higher SUVmax values compared with the healthy contralateral region similar to triphasic bone scan.

Lee and colleagues[66] studied 23 postoperative patients (non-oncology) under suspicion for surgical site infection of the bone using the dual-phase ^{18}F-NaF PET/CT acquisition, and showed encouraging sensitivity, specificity, and accuracy of 92.9%, 100.0%, and 95.7%, respectively, and highlighted high diagnostic ability in these scenarios where ^{18}F-FDG PET/CT reflects lower sensitivity.

The results in few prominent studies in PJIs are summarized in **Table 2**.

In conclusion, high sensitivity of ^{18}F-sodium fluoride for both benign and malignant lesions may pose a diagnostic dilemma. It may show higher specificity in specific conditions where FDG-PET findings are equivocal because of surrounding tissue inflammation. The exact role of NaF in bone and joint infections is still under

Table 2
Summary table for prominant studies (including their interpretation criteria, Results and inference) on NaF PET/CT in evaluation of PJIs

Study Sample	Interpretation Criteria	Results	Inference	Study Name and Ref No
65 hip joints	Significant uptake spreading through more than half of the bone-implant interface considered positive for infection	Sensitivity of 95% and Specificity 98%	NaF-PET/CT differentiates septic from aseptic loosening in considerable accuracy, quantifications using the SUVmax values can then provide objective evaluation.	Kobayashi et al,[67]
42 hip joints	Diffusely increased uptake in both early and delayed images along the femoral component of prostheses, and focal uptake on early images and diffusely increased uptake on delayed images along the femoral component considered positive for infection	Sensitivity of 75% and Specificity 96.1%	NaF PET/CT had shown slightly higher specificity but lesser sensitivity than FDG-PET/CT	Kumar et al,[68]
23 hip joints	Uptake region on the acetabular side more than 50% of the acetabular component with an SUVmax of > 5 and uptake region on the femoral more than 50% of the femoral component with an SUVmax of > 5considered positive for infection	Sensitivity of 75% Specificity 96%	NaF PET study in preoperative assessment before revision surgery improves the accuracy of tissue sampling, and aids in more definitive diagnosis of periprosthetic infection	Choi et al,[69]

(continued on next page)

Table 2
(continued)

Study Sample	Interpretation Criteria	Results	Inference	Study Name and Ref No
96 Hip joints + 14 Knee joints	Visual: uptake in the prosthesis/bone interface than in normal/bone/soft-tissue or contralateral asymptomatic prosthesis, the increased uptake included half the bone/metal interface in the femoral component or if the tibial stem in the tibial component was involved. Quantitative: average SUVmax values for septic loosening prostheses was10.5 ± 3.4, established threshold SUVmax cutoff of 6.9	Sensitivity of 97% Specificity 88%	Serial or single NaF-PET study is sensitive and specific tool for assessing joint prostheses.	Adesanya et al,[70]

evaluation, and less established compared with ^{18}F-FDG.

18F-Fluorodeoxyglucose-Labeled Leukocytes

As discussed, both of the above-mentioned tracers are not infection specific, which raises dilemmas in clinical practice, thus search for such exclusive infection-specific tracer has been undertaken in both preclinical and clinical studies worldwide. [111]In- and ^{99m}Tc-labeled WBC scintigraphy has been well studied and has provided the highest specificity in the spectrum of infection imaging including bones[71] and has given good accuracy in difficult situations like prosthetic infection and diabetic foot. But clinically this didn't get widely adopted because of high technical requirements that are not available in routine departments as well as the poor spatial resolution of the gamma camera. As per Rini and colleagues[72] FDG labeled-leucocytes gives comparable results compared with scintigraphy study but FDG-labeled leukocytes have further advantages are ease of availability, simpler labeling technique, a high spatial resolution of PET/CT, faster imaging time, and so on. Multiple groups have studied FDG-labeled leukocytes in infectious skeletal applications such as the use of FDG-labeled leukocytes in patients with diabetic foot OM with Charcot's neuropathy by Rastogi and colleagues[73] with MRI showed sensitivity and specificity of 83.3% and 100% compared with 83.3% and 63.6% for MRI, highlighting its role in early diagnosis and high accuracy. Akshoy and colleagues[74] studied the role of FDG-labeled leukocytes and FDG-PET/CT in 54 patients of suspicious prosthetic joint infection, where FDG uptake showed PPV only of 28%, whereas FDG-labeled Leukocytes showed strong sensitivity, specificity, and PPV of 93.3%, 97.4%, and 93.3%, respectively.

However, this method also comes with multiple issues and shortcomings such as (i) more preparation time and imaging time, (ii) higher cost (training, blood handling equipments, and procedures), (iii) nonuniform labeling yields, (iv) possible risk of infection to the patient as well as health care provider, and (v) propensity for homing in the reticuloendothelial system[75,76](physiologic process of clearing neutrophils through liver, spleen and marrow) causing more uptake and radiation exposure to these tissues. Few groups have also tried labeling leukocytes with other PET agent such as in vitro labeling of human leukocytes with longer half-life PET tracer copper-64(Cu) by Bhargava and colleagues.[77]Thus in conclusion, though being highly accurate it has multiple practice-related issues to answer well before its large-scale adoption worldwide.

Gallium-68 Citrate

[67]Ga has been historically studied in bone infections, however, suffered from multiple drawbacks such as high cost, unavailability of tracer, poor image quality, higher radiation dose, prolonged imaging time, and so on. For the last two decades, positron-emitting isotope of the same element viz. gallium-68 (^{68}Ga) is now routinely available in various Nuclear Medicine departments in a handy manner with the help of [68]Ge-^{68}Ga generator systems. It also provides a better spatial resolution of PET and a shorter procedure time. Considering this ^{68}Ga-citrate has been of recent interest in infection imaging.

The preclinical studies mainly explored the role of ^{68}Ga in Staphylococcus aureus infections, as noted by Mäkinen and colleagues,[78] who studied tibial OM in rats with both FDG and ^{68}Ga-citrate, both these tracers showed increased uptake (SUVratio); in addition, the intensity of ^{68}Ga uptake reflected pathologic changes of OM bones and does not show uptake in healing bone. Another similar preclinical study[79] by the same group using both ^{68}Ga-citrate and ^{68}Ga-chloride established that the SUVmax of ^{68}Ga-citrate was significantly higher than the uptake of ^{68}Ga-chloride, whereas both tracers accumulated in the infection.

The in vivo pilot study by Nanni and colleagues[80] studied 31 patients with suspected OM or discitis who underwent a total of 40 ^{68}Ga-citrate PET/CT scans along with other imaging such as MRI, WBC-scintigraphy, and biopsy and found to have sensitivity and NPV of 100% but reported specificity was76%. This could be contributed because of low-grade physiologic marrow uptake of gallium, especially in vertebrae. They also highlighted that SUVmax value in the infection region was between 2 and 4, not greatly above the background to clearly highlight an area in maximum intensity projection (MIP) images.

Another such study by Tseng and colleagues[81] studied ^{68}Ga-citrate-PET/CT in infected lower limb prostheses in 34 patients who also underwent FDG-PET/CT scans. The ^{68}Ga citrate showed sensitivity, specificity, and accuracy of 92%, 88%, and 91%, whereas for 18F-FDG the values were 100%, 38%, and 85%, respectively, highlighting its merit in differentiating inflammatory uptake.

Overall ^{68}Ga citrate appears a promising agent, whereas 18F-FDG has shown nonspecific uptake, especially in peripheral sites but needs larger clinical studies to incorporate into routine clinical practice.

Future Perspectives

PET/MR

Hybrid imaging with PET/MR has been introduced in the last two decades and with ongoing technological advances in PET detector technologies, it is being possible to image rapidly at many centers for routine clinical work. The amalgamation of (i) superior anatomic spatial resolution of MRI, (ii) features like dynamic contrast-enhanced MR, MR spectroscopy, and (iii) insights of pathophysiology using PET makes PET/MR a potential herculean imaging tool. After neurology, oncology, and cardiology, infection imaging is one of the potential grounds for its adequate harnessing. The ability and utility of MRI to assess bone-related soft-tissue, marrow changes, and occult bone changes has been discussed in this article which aids diagnosis in daily practice. PET-MRI could improve accuracy in detecting soft-tissue lesions in OM, by the symbiosis of the two impeccable modalities in bone infection imaging. Hybrid PET/MR imaging could solve many issues faced with PET/CT, and in addition, it could combine the quantification of the PET detectable functional changes with spectroscopy and measurable metabolites simultaneously in diabetic neuropathy.

Still, multiple challenges are yet to be answered pertaining to this modality, including MR sequence optimization, hybrid imaging protocols, artifacts, and related human resource training[82] which is beyond the limit of this article.

Newer tracers and machine learning

With advances in (i) molecular biology in identifying multiple infection-related targets mainly peptides and (ii) radiopharmaceutical developments with metal chelators, several infection-specific PET tracers are currently under active research, such as ^{68}Ga-Ciprofloxacin,[83] 68Ga-ubiquicidin,[84] ^{68}Ga-apo-transferrin,[85] N-cinnamoyl-phe-(d)-Leu-phe-(d)-Leu-phe-lys (^{64}Cu-labeled-cFLFLFK-PEG)[86] as an advanced form of leukocytes imaging; with this advancement in infection imaging, PET is expected to achieve higher accuracy and may cater to different types of infections in a specific way. Along with this, with advancements in machine learning and radiomics in medical imaging, the authors also foresee development in PET infection imaging similar to oncological imaging; especially in applications like diabetic foot, SD this will act as an aid in identifying and mapping disease more efficiently.

CLINICS CARE POINTS

- PET/CT imaging has multiple additional benefits over conventional modalities by providing information regarding disease extent in bone as well as whole body, gives an idea of active pathology at the molecular level, and response evaluation. Still it should not be used as first line alternative to routine methods like X-Ray.

- 18F-FDG PET/CT has distinguished role in deciding clinical management in multiple indications like osteomyelitis and PJIs, It has virtually replaced many scintigraphy tracers for these indications

- Both 18F-FDG PET/CT and 18F-NaF lacks specificity in infection imaging and it shows uptake in multiple inflammatory and degenerative conditions. It should never be used as alternative to tissue diagnosis/ microbiological-culture tests.

- FDG-labeled WBCs appears promising option which have resolution of PET imaging, ease of synthesising and better specificity; however its role is yet to be established in many routine infective conditions.

DISCLOSURE

The authors have nothing to disclose.

REFERENCES

1. Yamada S, KubotaK, Kubota R, et al. Highaccumulation of fluorine-18-fluorodeoxyglucose in turpentine-induced inflammatory tissue. J Nucl Med 1995;36(7):1301–6.

2. Jamar F, Buscombe J, Chiti A, et al. EANM/SNMMI guideline for 18F-FDG use in inflammation and infection. J Nucl Med 2013;54(4):647–58. Epub 2013 Jan 28. PMID: 23359660.

3. Shen CJ, Wu MS, Lin KH, et al. The use of procalcitonin in the diagnosis of bone and joint infection: a systemic review and meta-analysis. Eur J Clin Microbiol Infect Dis 2013;32(6):807–14.

4. Hartmann A, Eid K, Dora C, et al. Diagnostic value of (18)F-FDG PET/CT in trauma patients with suspected chronic osteomyelitis. Eur. J. Nucl. Med. Mol. Imaging 2006;34:704–14.

5. Weon YC, Yang SO, Choi YY, et al. Use of Tc-99m HMPAO leukocyte scans to evaluate bone infection: incremental value of additional SPECT images. Clin Nucl Med 2000;25(7):519–26.

6. Termaat MF, Raijmakers PG, Scholten HJ, et al. The accuracy of diagnostic imaging for the assessment

of chronic osteomyelitis: a systematic review and metaanalysis. J Bone Joint Surg Am 2005;87(11): 2464–71.

7. Palestro CJ. Radionuclide imaging of osteomyelitis. Semin Nucl Med 2015;45:32–46.

8. Wang GL, Zhao K, Liu ZF, et al. A meta-analysis of fluorodeoxyglucose-positron emission tomography versus scintigraphy in the evaluation of suspected osteomyelitis. Nucl Med Commun 2011;32(12): 1134–42.

9. Basu S, Kwee TC, Hess S, et al. FDG-PET/CT imaging of infected bones and prosthetic joints. Curr Mol Imaging 2014;3(3):225–9.

10. Basu S, Zhuang H, Alavi A. FDG PET and PET/CT Imaging in Complicated Diabetic Foot. PET Clin 2012;7(2):151–60.

11. Chatziioannou S, Papamichos O, Gamaletsou MN, et al. 18-Fluoro-2-deoxy-D-glucose positron emission tomography/computed tomography scan for monitoring the therapeutic response in experimental Staphylococcus aureus foreign-body osteomyelitis. J OrthopSurg Res 2015;10:132.

12. Warmann SW, Dittmann H, Seitz G, et al. Follow-up of acute osteomyelitis in children: the possible role of PET/CT in selected cases. J Pediatr Surg 2011; 46(8):1550–6.

13. Sahlmann CO, Siefker U, Lehmann K, et al. Dual time point 2-[18F] fluoro-2'-deoxyglucose positron emission tomography in chronic bacterial osteomyelitis. Nucl Med Commun 2004;25(8):819–23.

14. Prodromou ML, Ziakas PD, Poulou LS, et al. FDG PET is a robust tool for the diagnosis of spondylodiscitis: a meta-analysis of diagnostic data. Clin Nucl Med 2014;39(4):330–5.

15. Kim SJ, Pak K, Kim K, et al. Comparing the Diagnostic Accuracies of F-18 Fluorodeoxyglucose Positron Emission Tomography and Magnetic Resonance Imaging for the Detection of Spondylodiscitis: A Meta-analysis. Spine (Phila Pa 1976) 2019;44(7):E414–22.

16. Fuster D, Tomas X, Granados U, et al. Prospective comparison of whole-body 18F-FDG PET/CT and MRI of the spine in the diagnosis of haematogenous spondylodiscitis: response to comments by Soussan. Eur J Nucl Med Mol Imaging 2015; 42(2):356–7.

17. Lee IS, Lee JS, Kim SJ, et al. Fluorine-18-fluorodeoxyglucose positron emission tomography/computed tomography imaging in pyogenic and tuberculous spondylitis: preliminary study. J Comput Assist Tomogr 2009;33(4):587–92.

18. Rosen RS, Fayad L, Wahl RL. Increased 18F-FDG uptake in degenerative disease of the spine: characterization with 18F- FDG PET/CT. J Nucl Med 2006;47(8):1274–80.

19. Hungenbach S, Delank KS, Dietlein M, et al. 18F-fluorodeoxyglucose uptake pattern in patients with suspected spondylodiscitis. Nucl Med Commun 2013;34(11):1068–74.

20. Jeon I, Kong E, Kim SW, et al. Assessment of Therapeutic Response in Pyogenic Vertebral Osteomyelitis Using 18F-FDG-PET/MRI. Diagnostics (Basel) 2020;10(11):916.

21. Nanni C, Boriani L, Salvadori C, et al. FDG PET/CT is useful for the interim evaluation of response to therapy in patients affected by haematogenous spondylodiscitis. Eur J Nucl Med Mol Imaging 2012;39(10):1538–44.

22. Adams A, Offiah C. Central skull base osteomyelitis as a complication of necrotizing otitis externa: imaging findings, complications, and challenges of diagnosis. Clin Radiol 2012;67. e7–e16.

23. Kulkarni SC, Padma S, Shanmuga Sundaram P, et al. In the evaluation of patients with skull base osteomyelitis, does 18F-FDG PET CT have a role? Nucl Med Commun 2020;41(6):550–9.

24. Stern Shavit S, Bernstine H, et al. FDG-PET/ CT for diagnosis and follow-up of necrotizing (malignant) external otitis. Laryngoscope 2019;129:961–6.

25. Álvarez Jáñez F, Barriga LQ, Iñigo TR, et al. Diagnosis of Skull Base Osteomyelitis. Radiographics 2021;41(1):156–74.

26. Khan MA, Quadri SAQ, Kazmi AS, et al. A Comprehensive Review of Skull Base Osteomyelitis: Diagnostic and Therapeutic Challenges among Various Presentations. Asian J Neurosurg 2018; 13(4):959–70.

27. Chapman PR, Choudhary G, Singhal A, et al. Skull Base Osteomyelitis: A Comprehensive Imaging Review. AJNR Am J Neuroradiol 2021;42(3):404–13.

28. Blom AW, Brown J, Taylor AH, et al. Infection after total knee arthroplasty. J Bone JointSurg Br 2004; 86(5):688–91.

29. Kurtz S, Mowat F, Ong K, et al. Prevalence of primary and revision total hip and knee arthroplasty in the United States from 1990 through 2002. J Bone Joint Surg Am 2005;87(7):1487–97.

30. Zimmerli W, Trampuz A, Ochsner PE, et al. Prosthetic-joint infections. N Engl J Med 2004;351(16): 1645–54.

31. Parvizi J, Tan TL, Goswami K, et al. The 2018 Definition of Periprosthetic Hip and Knee Infection: An Evidence-Based and Validated Criteria. J. Arthroplast. 2018;33:1309–14. 31.

32. Seltzer A, Xiao R, Fernandez M, et al. Role of nuclear medicine imaging in evaluation of orthopedic infections, current concepts. J Clin Orthop Trauma 2019;10(4):721–32.

33. Verberne SJ, Sonnega RJ, Temmerman OP, et al. What is the accuracy of nuclear imaging in the assessment of periprosthetic knee infection? A meta-analysis. Clin OrthopRelat Res 2017;475:1395–410.

34. Verberne SJ, Raijmakers PG, Temmerman OP, et al. The accuracy of imaging techniques in the assessment of periprosthetic hip infection: a systematic

review and meta-analysis. J Bone Joint Surg Am 2016;98:1638–45.

35. Signore A, Sconfienza LM, Borens O, et al. Consensus document for the diagnosis of prosthetic joint infections: a joint paper by the EANM, EBJIS, and ESR (with ESCMID endorsement). European journal of nuclear medicine and molecular imaging 2019;46(4):971–88.

36. Thapa P, Kalshetty A, Basu S. FDG PET/CT in Assessment of Prosthetic Joint Infection. PET/CT in Infection and Inflammation 2018;43–54. https://doi.org/10.1007/978-3-319-90412-2_5.

37. Basu S, Kwee TC, Saboury B, et al. FDG PET for diagnosing infection in hip and knee prostheses: prospective study in 221 prostheses and subgroup comparison with combined (111)In-labeled leukocyte/(99m) Tc-sulfur colloid bone marrowimaging in 88 prostheses. Clin NuclMed 2014;39(7):609–15.

38. Gravius S, Gebhard M, Ackermann D, et al. Analysisof 18F-FDG uptake pattern in PET for diagnosis of aseptic looseningversusprosthesisinfection after total knee arthroplasty. A prospective pilotstudy. Nuklearmedizin 2010;49(3):115–23.

39. Falstie-Jensen T, Lange J, Daugaard H, et al, ROSA study-group. 18F FDG-PET/CT has poor diagnostic accuracy in diagnosing shoulder PJI. Eur J Nucl Med Mol Imaging 2019;46(10):2013–22.

40. Bhoil A, Caw H, Vinjamuri S, et al. Role of 18F-flurodeoxyglucose in orthopaedic implant-related infection: review of literature and experience. Nucl Med Commun 2019;40(9):875–87.

41. Marcus CD, Ladam-Marcus VJ, Leone J, et al. MR imaging of osteomyelitis and neuropathic osteoarthropathy in the feet of diabetics. Radiographics 1996;16:1337–48.

42. Lavery LA, Ryan EC, Ahn J, Crisologo PA, et al. The infected diabetic foot: re-evaluating the IDSA diabetic foot infection classification. Clin Infect Dis 2020;70(8):1573–9.

43. Treglia G, Sadeghi R, Annunziata S, et al. Diagnostic performance of fluorine-18-fluorodeoxyglucose positron emission tomography for the diagnosis of Osteomyelitis related to diabetic foot: a systematic review and a meta-analysis. Foot (Edinb) 2013;23:140–8.

44. Nawaz A, Torigian DA, Siegelman ES, et al. Diagnostic performance of FDG-PET, MRI, and plain film radiography (PFR) for the diagnosis of osteomyelitis in the diabetic foot. Mol Imaging Biol 2010;12:335–42.

45. Lauri Chiara, Tamminga Menno, Andor W, et al. Detection of Osteomyelitis in the Diabetic Foot by Imaging Techniques: A Systematic Review and Meta-analysis Comparing MRI, White Blood Cell Scintigraphy, and FDG-PET. Diabetes Care 2017;40(8):1111–20.

46. Basu S, Chryssikos T, Houseni M, et al. Potential role of FDG-PET in the setting of diabetic

neuroosteoarthropathy: can it differentiate uncomplicated Charcot's neuropathy from Osteomyelitis and soft tissue infection? Nucl Med Commun 2007;28:465–72.

47. Basu S, Zhuang H, Alavi A, et al. Imaging of lower extremity artery atherosclerosis in diabetic foot: FDG-PET imaging and histopathological correlates. Clin Nucl Med 2007;32(7):567–8.

48. Weber U, Østergaard M, Lambert RG, et al. The impact of MRI on the clinical management of inflammatory arthritis. SkeletRadiol 2011;40:1153–73.

49. spine Golden MP, Vikram HR. Extrapulmonary tuberculosis: an overview. Am Fam Physician 2005;72(9):1761–8.

50. Dureja S, Sen IB, Acharya S, et al. Potential role of F18 FDG PET-CT as an imaging biomarker for the noninvasive evaluation in uncomplicated skeletal tuberculosis: a prospective clinical observational study. Eur Spine J 2014;23:2449–54.

51. Sharma SK, Mohan A, Kohli M, et al. Extrapulmonary tuberculosis. Expert Rev Respir Med 2021;15(7):931–48. Epub 2021 Jul 14.

52. Ankrah AO, van der Werf TS, de Vries EF, et al. PET/CT imaging of mycobacterium tuberculosis infection. Clin Transl Imaging 2016;4:131–44.

53. Mittal S, Jain AK, Chakraborti KL, et al. Evaluation of Healed Status in Tuberculosis of Spine by Fluorodeoxyglucose-positron Emission Tomography/Computed Tomography and Contrast Magnetic Resonance Imaging. Indian J Orthop 2019;53(1):160–8. IJOrtho_224_18.

54. Goyal D, Shriwastav R, Mittal R, et al. Role of 18F-FDG PET/CT in the Assessment of Response to Antitubercular Chemotherapy and Identification of Treatment Endpoint in Patients with Tuberculosis of the Joints: A Pilot Study. Clin Nucl Med 2021;46(6):449–55.

55. Leroy-Freschini B, Treglia G, Argemi X, et al. 18F-FDG PET/CT for invasive fungal infection in immunocompromised patients. QJM 2018;111(9):613–22.

56. Altini C, NiccoliAsabella A, Ferrari C, et al. 18)F-FDG PET/CT contribution to diagnosis and treatment response of rhino-orbital-cerebral mucormycosis. Hell J Nucl Med 2015;18(1):68–70.

57. Dryden JR, Starsiak MD, Johnston MJ, et al. Bone Scan, PET-CT, and MRI in Disseminated Coccidioidomycosis. Clin Nucl Med 2017;42(4):319–22.

58. Emamian S, Fox MG, Boatman D, et al. Spinal blastomycosis: unusual musculoskeletal presentation with literature review. Skeletal Radiol 2019;48(12):2021–7.

59. Nair SS, Varsha N, Sunil HV, et al. Melidiosis presenting as septic arthritis: The role of 18F-FDG PET/CT in diagnosis and management. Indian J Nucl Med 2021;36:59–61.

60. Rose MV, Kjaer ASL, Markova E, et al. 18F-FDG PET/CT Findings in a Patient with Chikungunya Virus Infection. Diagnostics 2017;7(3):49.

61. Zhuang HM, Cortes-Blanco A, Pourdehnad M, et al. Do high glucose levels have differential effect on FDG uptake in inflammatory and malignant disorders? Nucl. Med. Commun. 2001;22:1123–8.

62. Signore A, Casali M, Lauri C. An easy and practical guide for imaging infection/inflammation by [18F] FDG PET/CT. Clin Transl Imaging 2021;9(4):283–97.

63. Hawkins RA, Choi Y, Huang SC, et al. Evaluation of the skeletal kinetics of fluorine-18-fluoride ion with PET. J Nucl Med. 1992;33(5):633-642.

64. Raynor WY, Borja AJ, Hancin EC, et al. Novel Musculoskeletal and Orthopedic Applications of 18F-Sodium Fluoride PET. PET Clin 2021;16(2):295–311.

65. Freesmeyer M, Stecker FF, Schierz JH, et al. First experience with early dynamic (18)F-NaF-PET/CT in patients with chronic osteomyelitis. Ann Nucl Med 2014;28(4):314–21.

66. Lee JW, Yu SN, Yoo ID, et al. Clinical application of dual-phase F-18 sodium-fluoride bone PET/CT for diagnosing surgical site infection following orthopedic surgery. Medicine (Baltimore) 2019;98(11):e14770.

67. Kobayashi N, Inaba Y, Choe H, et al. Use of F-18 Fluoride PET to differentiate septic from aseptic loosening in total hip arthroplasty patients. Clin Nucl Med 2011;36(11):e156–61.

68. Kumar R, Kumar R, Kumar V, et al. Potential clinical implication of (18) F-FDG PET/CT in diagnosis of periprosthetic infection and its comparison with (18) F-Fluoride PET/CT. J Med Imaging Radiat Oncol 2016;60(3):315–22.

69. Choe H, Inaba Y, Kobayashi N, et al. Use of 18F-fluoride PET to determine the appropriate tissuesampling region for improved sensitivity of tissue examinations in cases of suspected periprosthetic infection after total hip arthroplasty. Acta Orthop 2011;82(4):427–32.

70. Adesanya O, Sprowson A, Masters J, et al. Review of the role of dynamic 18F-NaF PET in diagnosing and distinguishing between septic and aseptic loosening in hip prosthesis. J OrthopSurg Res 2015;10(5).

71. Glaudemans AW, de Vries EF, Vermeulen LE, et al. A large retrospective single-centre study to define the best image acquisition protocols and interpretation criteria for white blood cell scintigraphy with 99mtc-HMPAO-labelled leucocytes in musculoskeletal infections. Eur J Nucl Med Mol Imaging 2013;40:1760–9.

72. Rini JN, Bhargava KK, Tronco GG, et al. PET with FDG-labeled leukocytes versus scintigraphy with 111In-oxine-labeled leukocytes for detection of infection. Radiology 2006;238(3):978–87.

73. Rastogi A, Bhattacharya A, Prakash M, et al. Utility of PET/CT with fluorine-18-fluorodeoxyglucose-labeled autologous leukocytes for diagnosing diabetic foot osteomyelitis in patients with Charcot's neuroarthropathy. Nucl Med Commun 2016;37(12):1253–9.

74. Aksoy SY, Asa S, Ozhan M, et al. FDG and FDG-labelled leucocyte PET/CT in the imaging of prosthetic joint infection. Eur J Nucl Med Mol Imaging 2014;41(3):556–64.

75. Dumarey N, Egrise D, Blocklet D, et al. Imaging infection with 18F-FDG-labeled leukocyte PET/CT: initial experience in 21 patients. J Nucl Med 2006;47(4):625–32. PMID: 16595496.

76. Hulsen DJW, Geurts J, Arts JJ, et al. Hybrid FDG-PET/MR imaging of chronic osteomyelitis: a prospective case series. Eur J Hybrid Imaging 2019;3(1):7.

77. Bhargava KK, Gupta RK, Nichols KJ, et al. In vitro human leukocyte labeling with (64) Cu: an intraindividual comparison with (111) In-oxine and (18)F-FDG. Nucl Med Biol 2009;36(5):545–9.

78. Mäkinen TJ, Lankinen P, Pöyhönen T, et al. Comparison of 18F-FDG and 68Ga PET imaging in the assessment of experimental osteomyelitis due to Staphylococcus aureus. Eur J Nucl Med Mol Imaging 2005;32(11):1259–68.

79. Lankinen P, Noponen T, Autio A, et al. A Comparative 68Ga-Citrate and 68Ga-Chloride PET/CT Imaging of Staphylococcus aureus Osteomyelitis in the Rat Tibia. Contrast Media Mol Imaging 2018;2018:9892604.

80. Nanni C, Errani C, Boriani L, et al. 68Ga-citrate PET/CT for evaluating patients with infections of the bone: preliminary results. J Nucl Med 2010;51(12):1932–6.

81. Tseng JR, Chang YH, Yang LY, et al. Potential usefulness of 68Ga-citrate PET/CT in detecting infected lower limb prostheses. EJNMMI Res 2019;9(1):2.

82. Sollini M, Berchiolli R, Kirienko M, et al. PET/MRI in Infection and Inflammation. Semin Nucl Med 2018;48(3):225–41.

83. oźmiński P, Gawęda W, Rzewuska M, et al. Physicochemical and Biological Study of 99mTc and 68Ga Radiolabelled Ciprofloxacin and Evaluation of [99mTc] Tc-CIP as Potential Diagnostic Radiopharmaceutical for Diabetic Foot Syndrome Imaging. Tomography 2021;7(4):829–42.

84. Bhusari P, Bhatt J, Sood A, et al. Evaluating the potential of kit-based 68Ga-ubiquicidin formulation in diagnosis of infection: a pilot study68Ga. Nucl Med Commun 2019;40(3):228–34.

85. Kumar V, Boddeti DK, Evans SG, et al. Potential use of 68Ga-apo-transferrin as a PET imaging agent for detecting Staphylococcus aureus infection. Nucl Med Biol 2011;38(3):393–8.

86. Locke LW, Chordia MD, Zhang Y, et al. A novel neutrophil-specific PET imaging agent: cFLFLFK-PEG-64Cu. J Nucl Med 2009;50(5):790–7.

Atherosclerosis Imaging
Positron Emission Tomography

Sze Jia Ng, MD[a], Hui Chong Lau, MD[a], Rizwan Naseer, MD[a], Simran Sandhu[b],
William Y. Raynor, MD[c,d], Thomas J. Werner, MS[c],
Abass Alavi, MD, MD (Hon), PhD (Hon), DSc (Hon)[c,*]

KEYWORDS

- PET/CT • FDG • NaF • Choline • Coronary artery disease • Peripheral arteries disease
- Alavi-Carlsen calcification score • Global assessment

KEY POINTS

- PET allows for earlier detection of atherosclerotic changes compared with anatomic modalities, facilitating early intervention with a higher chance of reversing disease progression.
- ^{18}F-fluorodeoxyglucose was the first PET tracer used for atherosclerosis imaging; however, its relatively weaker correlation with cardiovascular risk factor implies that its utility as such will be overshadowed by ^{18}F-sodium fluoride (NaF).
- NaF portrays active microcalcification, and its uptake in the arterial wall demonstrates excellent correlation with cardiovascular disease risk.
- Due to the influence of the partial volume effect, vascular uptake of PET tracers will be underestimated, underscoring the importance of global assessment.

INTRODUCTION

Atherosclerosis is a complex, multifactorial, and progressive process, which plays a significant role in the underlying mechanism of multiple life-threatening diseases, including coronary artery disease, stroke, and peripheral vascular disease.[1] According to the 2020 American Heart Association (AHA) statistical update, there were more than 1000 deaths caused by cardiovascular diseases (CVDs) every day in 2016 worldwide.[1] Therefore, atherosclerosis is considered one of the major contributing causes of morbidity and mortality worldwide; therefore, early detection of atherosclerosis is of utmost importance. Endothelial cell dysfunction caused by cardiovascular risk factors including hypertension, diabetes mellitus, aging,

or dyslipidemia is thought to be the beginning of the cascade of the development of atherosclerosis.[2] This is followed by recruitment of inflammatory cells, the development of fatty streaks, molecular microcalcification of atheromatous plaques, and gradually progressing to structural macrocalcification, leading to the risk of plaque rupture and eventually vessel occlusion.[2,3] Hence, it is crucial to develop diagnostic methods that can identify microcalcification of the vessels in the early stages. During the past few decades, multiple complementary imaging techniques has been used in identifying advanced macrocalcification of atherosclerosis, including computed tomography (CT) using the coronary artery calcium score, coronary CT angiography, and cardiac MR imaging[1,4] but these are of limited ability to visualize

Conflict of Interest: The authors have declared no conflicts of interest.
[a] Department of Medicine, Crozer-Chester Medical Center, 1 Medical Center Boulevard, Upland, PA 19013, USA; [b] College of Health and Human Development, Pennsylvania State University, 10 E College Avenue, University Park, PA 16802, USA; [c] Department of Radiology, Hospital of the University of Pennsylvania, 3400 Spruce Street, Philadelphia, PA 19104, USA; [d] Department of Radiology, Rutgers Robert Wood Johnson Medical School, 1 Robert Wood Johnson Place, MEB #404, New Brunswick, NJ 08901, USA
* Corresponding author. 3400 Spruce Street, Philadelphia, PA 19104.
E-mail address: abass.alavi@pennmedicine.upenn.edu

PET Clin 18 (2023) 71–80
https://doi.org/10.1016/j.cpet.2022.09.004
1556-8598/23/© 2022 Elsevier Inc. All rights reserved.

microcalcification in early stages of the disease. By contrast, PET molecular imaging is able to detect early-stage disease by identifying specific disease processes, such as glycolysis and microcalcification.[5] ^{18}F-fluorodeoxyglucose (FDG) and ^{18}F-sodium fluoride (NaF), markers of inflammation and microcalcification, respectively, are among the 2 most widely studied molecular tracers in the early detection of atherosclerosis.[6,7] This review will discuss the evolving role of PET in atherosclerosis imaging.

^{18}F-FLUORODEOXYGLUCOSE

FDG, the first molecular tracer being studied for the assessment of atherogenesis, is currently the most widely used PET radiotracer.[8,9] The study conducted by Yun and colleagues in 2001 first found the correlation between vascular uptake and the macrophages in atherosclerotic plaques,[8] being subsequently validated by multiple studies.[9,10] FDG serves as a glucose analog and tends to accumulate in macrophages due to increased glucose utilization.[11] According to Ogawa and colleagues,[11] there was a higher accumulation of FDG during the differentiation of macrophages to foam cells formation compared with the stage of completely differentiated foam cells, suggesting that FDG is useful in visualizing the disease in early stage.

In the past decades, multiple studies have been carried out to determine the vascular uptake of FDG in different arteries and aorta,[6,10,12–15] and they have been successfully established a strong correlation between FDG uptake and atherosclerotic plaque inflammation in these vessels.[12,13] When Rudd and colleagues advanced a further step to compare the FDG uptake in symptomatic and asymptomatic atherosclerotic plaques, they found that its accumulation rate was 27% higher in symptomatic lesions than in contralateral asymptomatic plaques, and no measurable uptake were detected in normal carotid arteries.[13] However, the data regarding the FDG uptake in the atherosclerotic plaques in peripheral arteries is limited. Myer and colleagues[15] discovered no significant correlation between FDG and the macrophage burden in peripheral arteries of the patients with symptomatic peripheral arteries disease (PAD). This can lead to devastating outcomes because PAD is known to affect around 8.5 million Americans.[16] Therefore, careful interpretation is needed when evaluating the focal vascular uptake of FDG in peripheral arteries.

In addition, studies have shown the clinical utility of FDG-PET imaging in assessing the risk of ischemic events.[17,18] According Figueroa and colleagues,[17] atherosclerotic plaques with one or more high-risk features including positive remodeling, luminal irregularity, and low attenuation, tend to have higher FDG accumulation and are associated with an increased risk of atherothrombosis. Although significant correlation was found between FDG and atherosclerotic process, discrepancy was noted between the accumulation of FDG and structural changes detected by the anatomic imaging modalities, especially CT imaging.[19–22] Tatsumi and colleagues[20] and Meirelles and colleagues[22] found no correlation between the accumulation of FDG and CT calcification. As disease progressed, the calcifications remained stable over time but there was less active inflammation, explaining why FDG uptake decreased in the advanced stage.[22] Multiple cardiovascular risk factors including age, dyslipidemia, smoking history, hypertension, diabetes, and so forth were known to play a vital role in the process of atherosclerosis.[2] However, the correlation between the cardiovascular risk factors and FDG uptake is poorly understood. To date, studies have only been able to prove the clear association between age and FDG avidity.[23,24]

Despite the promising evidence of FDG-PET in atherosclerosis imaging, there are still limitations in using FDG-PET to study atherosclerotic plaques. First, the physiologic uptake of FDG by myocardial tissues and combined cardiac and respiratory motion limit its utility in evaluating coronary vasculatures.[25] Although the physiologic myocardial uptake could be suppressed by adequate preparation before image acquisition including fasting and consuming a high-fat, low-carbohydrate diet,[26,27] the precise measurement is almost impossible due to the physiologic motion.[25] Besides, because atherosclerosis is a progressive disease, the questionable stability and "waxing and waning" features of FDG will yield a low sensitivity in detecting advanced, stable plaques, which can lead to misdiagnosis or underestimation of the disease.

^{18}F-SODIUM FLUORIDE

The second most common molecular radiotracer being studied in atherosclerosis imaging is ^{18}F-sodium fluoride (NaF). Unlike FDG, the uptake of which reflects macrophage activity, NaF shows microcalcification.[28] NaF-PET is a potential noninvasive imaging tool that can provide an invaluable insight regarding the activity of coronary plaque microcalcification. NaF differs from FDG by localizing specifically to areas of calcification; therefore, its uptake due to atherosclerotic changes is not obscured by physiological myocardial activity.[28] To now, stress testing and the gold standard coronary angiogram can only identify obstructive lesions but do not have the ability to detect high-risk plaques that could potentially cause acute thrombosis.

Unlike FDG, which is only able to prove the correlation between its uptake and age, studies have shown that NaF uptake has significant correlation with cardiovascular risk factors including age, hypertension, hyperlipidemia, diabetes, and so forth and with different cardiovascular scoring systems including Framingham Risk Score, atherosclerotic CVD risk scores, and CHADS-VASc score.[29–35] However, the correlation between the male and female gender has been demonstrated contradictory data. The study conducted by Derlin and colleagues[32] showed that male gender has significant correlation with increased NaF uptake, whereas Blomberg and colleagues[31] showed a significant correlation in female gender. Additionally, when Kwiecinski and colleagues followed up 203 patients with high coronary artery disease burden during 42 months, the authors found that increased coronary NaF activity is able to serve as an reliable prediction model of both fatal or nonfatal myocardial infarction, independently from age, sex, risk factors, segment involvement, coronary calcium scores, presence of coronary stents, coronary stenosis, REACH, SMART scores, the Duke coronary artery disease index, or recent myocardial infarction.[36] When compared with the high-risk plaque features on intravascular ultrasound (positive remodeling, microcalcification, and necrosis of the lipid core), Lee and colleagues demonstrated significant correlation with coronary plaques with high focal NaF uptake.[37] In another study, coronary NaF uptake was shown to have the ability to provide insight into the disease within the coronary circulation by identifying coronary segments with more rapid progression of coronary calcification.[38] In comparison to FDG, NaF was shown to be able to detect culprit lesions from nonculprit lesions among patient with acute coronary syndrome according to the prospective clinical trial by Joshi and colleagues.[39]

The accuracy of quantification of radiotracer activity in an atherosclerotic plaque on PET is questionable as most plaques are small with complex morphology. Maximum standardized uptake value (SUVmax) is the most commonly used parameter in measuring tracer activities. The use of the target-to-blood pool ratio in NaF imaging, a calculation derived by dividing the raw SUV by the venous blood pool SUV remains controversial.[12] This is mainly because of the variability in the measurement of venous blood pool SUV due to flow rate of venous blood.[40]

According to McKenney-Drake and colleagues,[41] the global NaF assessment of cardiovascular microcalcification has potential role risk stratification. These investigators also demonstrated that NaF has the ability to detect arterial calcifications earlier than CT, prompting the early identification of the disease. NaF could potentially overcome the difficulty in visualizing atherosclerotic plaque using PET due to the small size of coronary vessels and low spatial resolution from the cardiac contraction.[25] The use of NaF-PET in addition of the usual MR perfusion test or SPECT can be a monitoring tool of coronary calcification in patients requiring prolonged diagnostic intervention and monitoring. Nakahara and colleagues[42] and Strauss and colleagues[43] have proposed the theory regarding microcalcification as the initial biologic process for the development of atherosclerosis, suggesting that NaF might have better ability to detect disease in the early-stage compared with FDG (Fig. 1).

ALAVI-CARLSEN CALCIFICATION SCORE

According to PROSPECT (Providing Regional Observations to Study Predictors of Events in the Coronary Tree) study, the occurrence of major adverse cardiovascular events were equally attributable to culprit lesions and to nonculprit lesions in patients with acute coronary syndrome,[44] and similar findings were reported in VIVA (VH-IVUS in Vulnerable Atherosclerosis) Study.[45] Therefore, global assessment of plaque burden would provide more prognostic information compared with focal assessment of individual plaques. The Alavi–Carlsen Calcification Score (ACCS) was introduced based on the concept of global disease assessment as applied to atherosclerosis imaging (Fig. 2). The score is derived from measuring the total NaF uptake by segmenting the heart from the surrounding tissues and calculating the mean standardized uptake value (SUVmean).[46] Because the score is measured based on clearly delineated anatomic boundaries, it has less interrater variation. Furthermore, the implementation of artificial intelligence-based approaches in ACCS would ensure a fast and reliable method.[47] This can be integrated with developments in PET instrumentation; namely, total-body PET/CT, which allows the assessment of the whole body with greater sensitivity while administering less radiation (Fig. 3). Global assessment of atherosclerosis using ACCS has the potential to detect and quantify burden of disease by reliably detecting molecular changes not apparent by other means. This represents a landmark approach, with implications for

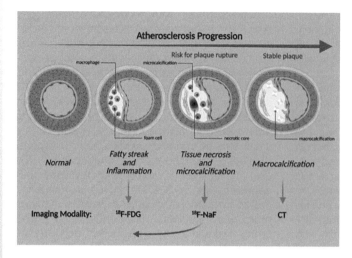

Fig. 1. Although inflammation has traditionally been thought to precede microcalcification in the course of atherosclerosis, new data suggest that microcalcification may be present earlier compared with previous expectations (*red arrow*). This observation supports the use of NaF (which is a specific marker of microcalcification) for the early detection of atherosclerosis. (*From* Raynor WY, Park PSU, Borja AJ, Sun Y, Werner TJ, Ng SJ, Lau HC, Høilund-Carlsen PF, Alavi A, Revheim ME. PET-Based Imaging with 18F-FDG and 18F-NaF to Assess Inflammation and Microcalcification in Atherosclerosis and Other Vascular and Thrombotic Disorders. Diagnostics (Basel). 2021 Nov 29;11(12):2234.[64])

both the diagnosis and treatment of atherosclerosis.

OTHER PET TRACERS IN ATHEROSCLEROSIS

Due to the nonspecific nature of FDG uptake, research has been directed toward tracer discovery with improved detectability, image quality, and ultimately clinical applicability.[48] Choline is a cation that exists as a phospholipid in cell membranes (as acetylcholine) and is required in the production of S-adenosylmethionine. It is also part of low-density lipoproteins. Humans do produce endogenous choline but the majority is obtained from dietary sources as a nutrient. Increased choline uptake in inflammatory tissue is established, and it has been used as a target molecule or tracer in atherosclerotic plaques in many studies. It is a water-soluble ion and passes through a fat-soluble cell membrane through 3 specific identifiable transport channels. It is metabolized to produce phosphatidylcholine, which becomes part of cell membranes. Both ^{18}F-choline and ^{11}C-choline have been successfully implemented in clinical and preclinical trials. Ex vivo mouse model studies by Laitinen and colleagues showed significantly higher ^{11}C-choline uptake in atherosclerotic aortic segments when compared with a healthy vessel.[49] In another mouse model study with comparative design by Matter and colleagues, ^{18}F-choline showed superiority in detecting atherosclerotic plaques when compared with FDG.[50] A retrospective analysis by Katsuhiko and colleagues demonstrated increased uptake of ^{11}C-choline in aortic and common carotid vessel segments in male patients aged 60 to 80 years.[51]

Somatostatin receptors are expressed by a wide range of human tissues and have 5 distinct human subtypes. Somatostatin type 2 receptors are found on the surface of activated macrophages and can be used to detect activated macrophages in unstable atherosclerotic plaques. ^{68}Ga-labeled somatostatin analogs collectively referred to as ^{68}Ga-DOTA peptides are currently in practice in PET imaging of somatostatin receptors on cancer cells.[52] The use of radiolabeled somatostatin receptor ligands demonstrated mixed results for the purpose of atherosclerosis imaging. A study by Rominger and colleagues showed differential uptake of ^{68}Ga-DOTA-TATE in the calcified plaque of coronary vessel and myocardium, highlighting its potential application in the identification of plaque and predicting clinical outcomes.[53] In a comparative analysis of the VISION trial, ^{68}Ga-DOTA-TATE showed superiority in certain aspects compared with FDG. It also showed the ability to identify the culprit versus nonculprit coronary vessels in acute coronary syndromes and transient ischemia attacks.[54]

The C-X-C chemokine receptor type 4, corresponding to a chemokine receptor overexpressed by leukocytes including macrophages and lymphocytes, can be assessed by the ^{68}Ga-pentixafor radioligand. C-type lectin CD206, commonly named the mannose receptor, is expressed by macrophages and has been used as well. Another small molecule ^{18}F-fluoro-3'-deoxy-3'-L-fluorothymidine is used to detect proliferating cells and to assess treatment response in patients with cancer and has shown an affinity for plaques with macrophages.[55]

The integrin alpha-V-beta-3 involved in inflammatory pathways can be detected using RGD sequence-derived PET probes such as ^{18}F-galacto-RGD and ^{68}Ga-NOTA-RGD.[56]

Fibroblast activation protein (FAP) is a serine protease whose expression is induced by

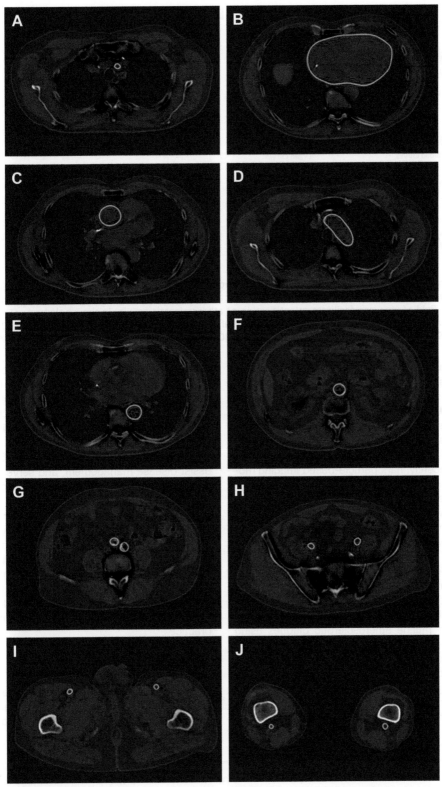

Fig. 2. NaF-PET/CT images of a 67-year-old patient with regions of interest used to quantify tracer uptake in the following vessels: left carotid artery (*A*), global coronary arteries (*B*), ascending aorta (*C*), aortic arch (*D*),

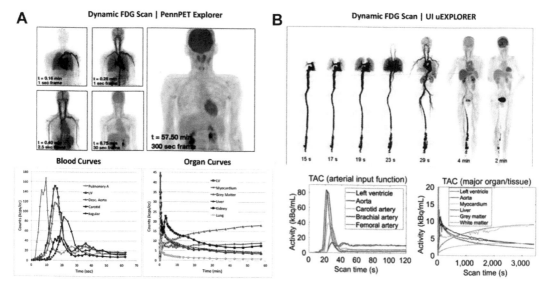

Fig. 3. Images acquired from PennPET Explorer (*A*) and UI uExplorer (*B*) showing the expanded field of view offered by total-body PET. Time activity curves (TACs) are provided for tissues captured by dynamic imaging. This larger field of view can facilitate quantification of atherosclerotic activity in the whole body. (This research was originally published in JNM. Ramsey D. Badawi et al. First Human Imaging Studies with the EXPLORER Total-Body PET Scanner*. J Nucl Med. Mar 2019, 60 (3) 299-303; DOI: 10.2967/jnumed.119.226498. © SNMMI.[66])

macrophage-derived tumor necrosis factor-alpha and is associated with thin-cap fibroatheromas through its contribution to type I collagen breakdown in fibrous caps. A study by Wu and colleagues showed its utilization as an imaging target using ^{68}Ga-conjugated quinoline-based FAP inhibitor ^{68}Ga-DOTA-FAPI-04.[57]

More recently, nanoparticle-based imaging modalities are being used to detect macrophages in atherosclerotic plaques. One of the first tested in humans was composed of an iron oxide core solubilized with hydrophilic polymers, such as dextran, with a mean diameter of 30 nm and called ultrasmall super paramagnetic particles of iron oxide (allowing for detection of contrast by MR imaging). Later, 13 nm dextran nanoparticles were developed and labeled with deferoxamine to allow radiolabeling with [89]Zr to detect inflammatory leukocytes in murine atherosclerotic plaques using PET. Woodard and colleagues tested Comb nanoparticle conjugating with C-type atrial natriuretic factor, known to bind the natriuretic peptide clearance receptor that has been demonstrated to be a biomarker for atherosclerosis in both animal models and human coronary arteries.[58] A 20-nm

spherical biocompatible nanoparticle composed of a macrophage sensor called Macrin was used by Nahrendorf and colleagues to image and quantify macrophage content using ^{64}Cu-Macrin PET to assess cardiovascular inflammation in animal studies. The authors concluded ^{64}Cu-Macrin PET imaging could stage inflammatory CVD activity, assist disease management, and serve as an imaging biomarker for emerging macrophage-targeted therapeutics.[59]

Although many new and novel agents have been described and used in preclinical and clinical studies, getting meaningful and applicable information from PET-based imaging of atherosclerosis remains a challenge. Although more data are needed to validate these experimental tracers, the focus of clinical trials should be on NaF, which has the highest likelihood of changing clinical practice.

LIMITATIONS OF PET

PET-based quantification of atherosclerotic disease burden comes with several limitations, the most significant of which involves nonspecific

descending aorta (*E*), abdominal aorta (*F*), bilateral common iliac arteries (*G*), external iliac arteries (*H*), femoral arteries (*I*), and popliteal arteries (*J*). The total body arterial uptake was calculated as 16.1. (*From* Raynor WY, Borja AJ, Rojulpote C, Høilund-Carlsen PF, Alavi A. 18F-sodium fluoride: An emerging tracer to assess active vascular microcalcification. J Nucl Cardiol. 2021 Dec;28(6):2706-2711.[65])

tracer uptake by surrounding tissues. FDG demonstrates diffuse uptake by highly metabolic tissues, such as myocardial tissue, obscuring visualization of atherosclerotic plaques within coronary vasculature. This decreases the available applications of FDG as an imaging modality for atherosclerosis.[41,60] In addition, blood pool activity of FDG has been found to affect the detection of vascular wall signal due to spatial blurring of PET images.[61] Finally, the retention of FDG in surrounding tissues and vessel walls leads to an overestimation of the inflammatory reaction seen in plaques.[41] In a study, Williams and Kolodny proposed a method to decrease average FDG uptake among subjects by imposing a high-fat, low-carbohydrate, protein-permitted diet before image acquisition.[26] Wykrzykowska and colleagues replicated this protocol and demonstrated "good" or "adequate" myocardial uptake suppression in 20 of the 32

patients, with the remaining cases of inadequate suppression secondary to self-reported nonadherence to the proposed diet.[62] Similarly, measurements of vascular NaF uptake may be confounded by uptake in adjacent structures such as bones or areas of soft tissue calcification. However, unlike FDG, NaF is rapidly cleared from circulation, greatly decreasing the degree of blood pool activity.[6]

Another unavoidable limitation of using PET as a probe of detecting atherosclerosis is its suboptimal spatial resolution. The resolution of PET is within the range of 5 to 8 mm, which is particularly relevant given the comparable size of atherosclerotic plaques. Thus, the partial volume effect is responsible for the underestimation of tracer uptake when measuring individual atheromas.[63] This particular limitation can be addressed by relying on methods of global assessment, such as ACCS (**Fig. 4**).

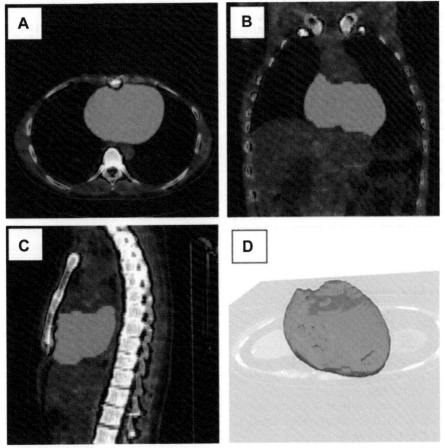

Fig. 4. Artificial intelligence-based cardiac segmentation of NaF-PET/CT images displayed with tomographic axial (*A*), coronal (*B*), and sagittal (*C*) images, as well as a 3D rendering (*D*). This region of interest can be used to calculate ACCS to determine the global cardiac atherosclerotic burden in this patient. (*From* Saboury B, Edenbrandt L, Piri R, Gerke O, Werner T, Arbab-Zadeh A, Alavi A, Høilund-Carlsen PF. Alavi-Carlsen Calcification Score (ACCS): A Simple Measure of Global Cardiac Atherosclerosis Burden. Diagnostics (Basel). 2021 Aug 5;11(8):1421.[67])

SUMMARY

In this review, we have discussed the clinical evidence of different molecular radiotracers in atherosclerosis imaging including FDG, NaF, choline, somatostatin receptor ligands, mannose receptors, and nanoparticles. FDG and NaF are the most studied radiotracers and have more evidence to support their clinical utility in PET imaging. In conclusion, the future of PET imaging in detecting atherosclerosis seems to be very promising. Compared with conventional CT or MR imaging, PET is able to detect disease in its early stage and allow early intervention and potential for prevention of an important cause of mortality.

CLINICS CARE POINTS

- Current data suggest that ^{18}F-sodium fluoride (NaF)-PET/computed tomography (CT) may become the leading modality for assessing atherogenic changes but larger prospective studies are needed.

- Due to the partial volume effect, the assessment of individual plaques (especially in small vessels such as the coronary arteries) is not feasible. Therefore, methods quantifying global uptake such as the Alavi-Carlsen Calcification Score are necessary for accurate interpretation.

- The introduction of total-body PET/CT offers the ability to assess atherosclerosis disease burden with higher sensitivity and lower radiation dose, which can be used for routine screening and monitoring.

DISCLOSURE

The authors have nothing to disclose.

REFERENCES

1. Virani SS, Alonso A, Benjamin EJ, et al. Heart disease and stroke statistics—2020 update: a report from the American heart association. Circulation 2020;141(9):e139–596.
2. Gimbrone MA, García-Cardeña G. Endothelial cell dysfunction and the pathobiology of atherosclerosis. Circ Res 2016;118(4):620–36.
3. Libby P. Inflammation in atherosclerosis. Nature 2002;420(6917):868–74.
4. Osborn EA, Jaffer FA. Imaging atherosclerosis and risk of plaque rupture. Curr Atheroscler Rep 2013; 15(10).
5. Syed MB, Fletcher AJ, Forsythe RO, et al. Emerging techniques in atherosclerosis imaging. Br J Radiol 2019;92(1103):20180309.
6. Mayer M, Borja AJ, Hancin EC, et al. Imaging atherosclerosis by PET, with emphasis on the role of FDG and NaF as potential biomarkers for this disorder. Front Physiol 2020;11:511391.
7. McKenney-Drake ML, Territo PR, Salavati A, et al. (18)F-NaF PET imaging of early coronary artery calcification. JACC Cardiovasc Imaging 2016;9(5): 627–8.
8. Yun M, Yeh D, Araujo LI, et al. F-18 FDG uptake in the large arteries: a new observation. Clin Nucl Med 2001;26(4):314–9.
9. Pasha AK, Moghbel M, Saboury B, et al. Effects of age and cardiovascular risk factors on (18)F-FDG PET/CT quantification of atherosclerosis in the aorta and peripheral arteries. Hell J Nucl Med 2015;18(1):5–10.
10. Davies JR, Rudd JHF, Fryer TD, et al. Identification of culprit lesions after transient ischemic attack by combined ^{18}F fluorodeoxyglucose positron-emission tomography and high-resolution magnetic resonance imaging. Stroke 2005;36(12):2642–7.
11. Ogawa M, Nakamura S, Saito Y, et al. What Can Be Seen by ^{18}F-FDG PET in Atherosclerosis Imaging? The Effect of Foam Cell Formation on ^{18}F-FDG Uptake to Macrophages In Vitro. J Nucl Med 2012; 53(1):55–8.
12. Tawakol A, Migrino RQ, Bashian GG, et al. In vivo 18F-fluorodeoxyglucose positron emission tomography imaging provides a noninvasive measure of carotid plaque inflammation in patients. J Am Coll Cardiol 2006;48(9):1818–24.
13. Rudd JHF, Warburton EA, Fryer TD, et al. Imaging atherosclerotic plaque inflammation with [^{18}F]-Fluorodeoxyglucose positron emission tomography. Circulation 2002;105(23):2708–11.
14. Graebe M, Pedersen SF, Borgwardt L, et al. Molecular pathology in vulnerable carotid plaques: correlation with [18]-fluorodeoxyglucose positron emission tomography (FDG-PET). Eur J Vasc Endovasc Surg 2009;37(6):714–21.
15. Myers KS, Rudd JH, Hailman EP, et al. Correlation between arterial FDG uptake and biomarkers in peripheral artery disease. JACC Cardiovasc Imaging 2012;5(1):38–45.
16. Allison MA, Ho E, Denenberg JO, et al. Ethnic-specific prevalence of peripheral arterial disease in the United States. Am J Prev Med 2007;32:328–33.
17. Figueroa AL, Subramanian SS, Cury RC, et al. Distribution of inflammation within carotid atherosclerotic plaques with high-risk morphological features. Circ Cardiovasc Imaging 2012;5(1):69–77.
18. Marnane M, Merwick A, Sheehan OC, et al. Carotid plaque inflammation on 18F-fluorodeoxyglucose positron emission tomography predicts early stroke recurrence. Ann Neurol 2012;71(5):709–18.

19. Dunphy MP, Freiman A, Larson SM, et al. Association of vascular 18F-FDG uptake with vascular calcification. J Nucl Med 2005;46(8):1278–84.

20. Tatsumi M, Cohade C, Nakamoto Y, et al. Fluorodeoxyglucose uptake in the aortic wall at PET/CT: possible finding for active atherosclerosis. Radiology 2003;229(3):831–7.

21. Ben-Haim S, Kupzov E, Tamir A, et al. Evaluation of 18F-FDG uptake and arterial wall calcifications using 18F-FDG PET/CT. J Nucl Med 2004;45(11): 1816–21.

22. Meirelles GS, Gonen M, Strauss HW. 18F-FDG uptake and calcifications in the thoracic aorta on positron emission tomography/computed tomography examinations: frequency and stability on serial scans. J Thorac Imaging 2011;26(1):54–62.

23. Yun M, Jang S, Cucchiara A, et al. 18F FDG uptake in the large arteries: a correlation study with the atherogenic risk factors. Semin Nucl Med 2002; 32(1):70–6.

24. Bural GG, Torigian DA, Chamroonrat W, et al. FDG-PET is an effective imaging modality to detect and quantify age-related atherosclerosis in large arteries. Eur J Nucl Med Mol Imaging 2008;35(3): 562–9.

25. Alavi A, Werner TJ, Høilund-Carlsen PF. What can be and what cannot be accomplished with PET to detect and characterize atherosclerotic plaques. J Nucl Cardiol 2018;25(6):2012–5.

26. Williams G, Kolodny GM. Suppression of myocardial 18F-FDG uptake by preparing patients with a high-fat, low-carbohydrate diet. AJR Am J Roentgenol 2008;190(2):W151–6.

27. Rogers IS, Nasir K, Figueroa AL, et al. Feasibility of FDG imaging of the coronary arteries: comparison between acute coronary syndrome and stable angina. JACC Cardiovasc Imaging 2010;3(4): 388–97.

28. Czernin J, Satyamurthy N, Schiepers C. Molecular mechanisms of bone 18F-NaF deposition. J Nucl Med 2010;51(12):1826–9.

29. Morbelli S, Fiz F, Piccardo A, et al. Divergent determinants of 18F-NaF uptake and visible calcium deposition in large arteries: relationship with Framingham risk score. Int J Cardiovasc Imaging 2014;30(2):439–47.

30. Gonuguntla K, Rojulpote C, Patil S, et al. Utilization of NaF-PET/CT in assessing global cardiovascular calcification using CHADS(2) and CHADS(2)-VASc scoring systems in high risk individuals for cardiovascular disease. Am J Nucl Med Mol Imaging 2020;10(6):293–300.

31. Blomberg BA, Thomassen A, de Jong PA, et al. Coronary fluorine-18-sodium fluoride uptake is increased in healthy adults with an unfavorable cardiovascular risk profile: results from the CAMONA study. Nucl Med Commun 2017;38(11):1007–14.

32. Derlin T, Wisotzki C, Richter U, et al. In vivo imaging of mineral deposition in carotid plaque using 18F-sodium fluoride PET/CT: correlation with atherogenic risk factors. J Nucl Med 2011;52(3):362–8.

33. Beheshti M, Saboury B, Mehta NN, et al. Detection and global quantification of cardiovascular molecular calcification by fluoro18-fluoride positron emission tomography/computed tomography–a novel concept. Hell J Nucl Med 2011;14(2):114–20.

34. Janssen T, Bannas P, Herrmann J, et al. Association of linear 18F-sodium fluoride accumulation in femoral arteries as a measure of diffuse calcification with cardiovascular risk factors: a PET/CT study. J Nucl Cardiol 2013;20(4):569–77.

35. Borja AJ, Bhattaru A, Rojulpote C, et al. Association between atherosclerotic cardiovascular disease risk score estimated by pooled cohort equation and coronary plaque burden as assessed by NaF-PET/CT. Am J Nucl Med Mol Imaging 2020;10(6):312–8.

36. Kwiecinski J, Tzolos E, Adamson PD, et al. Coronary (18)F-sodium fluoride uptake predicts outcomes in patients with coronary artery disease. J Am Coll Cardiol 2020;75(24):3061–74.

37. Lee JM, Bang JI, Koo BK, et al. Clinical relevance of 18 F-sodium fluoride positron-emission tomography in noninvasive identification of high-risk plaque in patients with coronary artery disease. Circ Cardiovasc Imaging 2017;10(11).

38. Doris MK, Meah MN, Moss AJ, et al. Coronary 18 F-fluoride uptake and progression of coronary artery calcification. Circ Cardiovasc Imaging 2020;13(12).

39. Joshi NV, Vesey AT, Williams MC, et al. 18F-fluoride positron emission tomography for identification of ruptured and high-risk coronary atherosclerotic plaques: a prospective clinical trial. Lancet 2014; 383(9918):705–13.

40. Chen W, Dilsizian V. PET assessment of vascular inflammation and atherosclerotic plaques: SUV or TBR? J Nucl Med 2015;56(4):503–4.

41. McKenney-Drake ML, Moghbel MC, Paydary K, et al. 18F-NaF and 18F-FDG as molecular probes in the evaluation of atherosclerosis. Eur J Nucl Med Mol Imaging 2018;45(12):2190–200.

42. Nakahara T, Strauss HW. From inflammation to calcification in atherosclerosis. Eur J Nucl Med Mol Imaging 2017;44(5):858–60.

43. Strauss HW, Narula J. 18 F-fluoride Imaging and other plaque-seeking diagnostic strategies. Circ Cardiovasc Imaging 2017;10(11).

44. Stone GW, Maehara A, Lansky AJ, et al. A prospective natural-history study of coronary atherosclerosis. N Engl J Med 2011;364(3):226–35.

45. Calvert PA, Obaid DR, O'Sullivan M, et al. Association between IVUS findings and adverse outcomes in patients with coronary artery disease: the VIVA (VH-IVUS in Vulnerable Atherosclerosis) Study. JACC: Cardiovasc Imaging 2011;4(8):894–901.

46. Høilund-Carlsen PF, Edenbrandt L, Alavi A. Global disease score (GDS) is the name of the game! Eur J Nucl Med Mol Imaging 2019;46(9):1768–72.

47. Trägårdh E, Borrelli P, Kaboteh R, et al. RECOMIA—a cloud-based platform for artificial intelligence research in nuclear medicine and radiology. EJNMMI Phys 2020;7(1).

48. Orbay H, Hong H, Zhang Y, et al. Positron emission tomography imaging of atherosclerosis. Theranostics 2013;3(11):894–902.

49. Laitinen IE, Luoto P, Nagren K, et al. Uptake of 11C-choline in mouse atherosclerotic plaques. J Nucl Med 2010;51(5):798–802.

50. Matter CM, Wyss MT, Meier P, et al. 18F-choline images murine atherosclerotic plaques ex vivo. Arterioscler Thromb Vasc Biol 2006;26(3):584–9.

51. Kato K, Schober O, Ikeda M, et al. Evaluation and comparison of 11C-choline uptake and calcification in aortic and common carotid arterial walls with combined PET/CT. Eur J Nucl Med Mol Imaging 2009; 36(10):1622–8.

52. Pauwels E, Cleeren F, Bormans G, et al. Somatostatin receptor PET ligands - the next generation for clinical practice. Am J Nucl Med Mol Imaging 2018;8(5):311–31.

53. Rominger A, Saam T, Vogl E, et al. In vivo imaging of macrophage activity in the coronary arteries using 68Ga-DOTATATE PET/CT: correlation with coronary calcium burden and risk factors. J Nucl Med 2010; 51(2):193–7.

54. Tarkin JM, Joshi FR, Evans NR, et al. Detection of atherosclerotic inflammation by (68)Ga-DOTATATE PET compared to [(18)F]FDG PET imaging. J Am Coll Cardiol 2017;69(14):1774–91.

55. Ye YX, Calcagno C, Binderup T, et al. Imaging macrophage and hematopoietic progenitor proliferation in atherosclerosis. Circ Res 2015;117(10):835–45.

56. Dietz M, Kamani CH, Deshayes E, et al. Imaging angiogenesis in atherosclerosis in large arteries with (68)Ga-NODAGA-RGD PET/CT: relationship with clinical atherosclerotic cardiovascular disease. EJNMMI Res 2021;11(1):71.

57. Wu M, Ning J, Li J, et al. Feasibility of in vivo imaging of fibroblast activation protein in human arterial walls. J Nucl Med 2022;63(6):948–51.

58. Liu Y, Abendschein D, Woodard GE, et al. Molecular imaging of atherosclerotic plaque with (64)Cu-labeled natriuretic peptide and PET. J Nucl Med 2010;51(1):85–91.

59. Nahrendorf M, Hoyer FF, Meerwaldt AE, et al. Imaging cardiovascular and lung macrophages with the positron emission tomography sensor (64)Cu-Macrin in mice, rabbits, and pigs. Circ Cardiovasc Imaging 2020;13(10):e010586.

60. Moghbel M, Al-Zaghal A, Werner TJ, et al. The role of PET in evaluating atherosclerosis: a critical review. Semin Nucl Med 2018;48(6):488–97.

61. Blomberg BA, Thomassen A, Takx RA, et al. Delayed (1)(8)F-fluorodeoxyglucose PET/CT imaging improves quantitation of atherosclerotic plaque inflammation: results from the CAMONA study. J Nucl Cardiol 2014;21(3):588–97.

62. Wykrzykowska J, Lehman S, Williams G, et al. Imaging of inflamed and vulnerable plaque in coronary arteries with 18F-FDG PET/CT in patients with suppression of myocardial uptake using a low-carbohydrate, high-fat preparation. J Nucl Med 2009;50(4):563–8.

63. Cal-Gonzalez J, Li X, Heber D, et al. Partial volume correction for improved PET quantification in (18)F-NaF imaging of atherosclerotic plaques. J Nucl Cardiol 2018;25(5):1742–56.

64. Raynor WY, Park PSU, Borja AJ, et al. PET-based imaging with (18)F-FDG and (18)F-NaF to assess inflammation and microcalcification in atherosclerosis and other vascular and thrombotic disorders. Diagnostics (Basel) 2021;11(12).

65. Raynor WY, Borja AJ, Rojulpote C, et al. 18F-sodium fluoride: an emerging tracer to assess active vascular microcalcification. J Nucl Cardiol 2021; 28(6):2706–11.

66. Badawi RD, Shi H, Hu P, et al. First human imaging studies with the EXPLORER total-body PET scanner. J Nucl Med 2019;60(3):299–303.

67. Saboury B, Edenbrandt L, Piri R, et al. Alavi-carlsen calcification score (ACCS): a Simple measure of global cardiac atherosclerosis burden. Diagnostics (Basel) 2021;11(8):1421.

Role of PET/Computed Tomography in Elderly Thyroid Cancer
Tumor Biology and Clinical Management

Sunita Nitin Sonavane, MBBS, DRM, DNB, MNAMS[a,b],
Sandip Basu, MBBS, DRM, DNB, MNAMS[a,b],*

KEYWORDS

- Thyroid carcinoma • Elderly • PET-CT • TENIS • FDG • ^{68}Ga-DOTATATE • ^{68}Ga-PSMA-11
- Tumor Biology

KEY POINTS

- An age cutoff of 55 years has been identified as an important predictive factor for disease prognosis in differentiated thyroid carcinoma (DTC).
- The elderly patients present with a higher incidence of aggressive histologic subtypes such as poorly differentiated and anaplastic cancer, tall/columnar cell variants of DTC, and Hurthle cell carcinoma. Even within well-differentiated DTCs, older patients have higher documentation of local invasiveness, lateral-sided lymph node involvement in the neck and vascular invasion.
- Metabolic imaging with fluorodeoxyglucose (FDG) PET-computed tomography (CT) has emerged as a valuable tool in disease evaluation, restaging, and treatment response assessment scenarios in aggressive variants of DTC and de-differentiated thyroid malignancies (including patients with thyroglobulin elevated negative iodine scintigraphy or thyroglobulin elevation with negative iodine scintigraphy [TENIS]).
- Exploring disease biology through FDG PET-CT plays a valuable complimentary role in assessing metastatic disease and directing appropriate therapeutic management on a case-to-case basis and prognostication.
- In addition to the important role of ^{68}Ga-DOTATATE/DOTANOC and ^{18}F-FDOPA PET-CT in medullary thyroid carcinoma (MTC), the other investigational PET-CT tracers that are being examined at this point include ^{18}F-tetrafluoroborate in DTC and Gallium-68 labeled somatostatin analogs, prostate-specific membrane antigen and RGD in patients with TENIS and other de-differentiated carcinomas of the thyroid.
- Primary thyroid lymphoma (PTL) primarily affects elderly females (age group: 50–80 years), and FDG-PET/CT plays a pivotal role in its treatment decisions.

INTRODUCTION

In the general population, the peak occurrence of thyroid cancer is between the ages of 51 and 60 years.[1] Papillary thyroid cancer (PTC) is one of the increasing cancers, and the incidence of PTC increases with age. It generally has a favorable prognosis but may behave more aggressively in older patients. Thyroid cancer is more common in women than men and among those with a family history of thyroid disease.[2] Histopathologically, differentiated thyroid cancer (DTC) that arises from thyroid follicular cells is further subclassified into papillary thyroid cancer (PTC), which is the

[a] Radiation Medicine Centre, Bhabha Atomic Research Centre, Tata Memorial Hospital Annexe, Parel; [b] Homi Bhabha National Institute, Mumbai, India
* Corresponding author. Radiation Medicine Centre (BARC), Tata Memorial Hospital Annexe Building, Jerbai Wadia Road, Parel, Mumbai 400012, India.
E-mail address: drsanb@yahoo.com

PET Clin 18 (2023) 81–101
https://doi.org/10.1016/j.cpet.2022.09.005
1556-8598/23/© 2022 Elsevier Inc. All rights reserved.

most common histologic type, follicular thyroid cancer (FTC), and Hürthle cell cancer (HTC). De-differentiated thyroid cancer evolves from poorly differentiated thyroid cancer (PDTC) to anaplastic thyroid cancer (ATC). Medullary thyroid cancer (MTC) arises from neuroendocrine parafollicular C cells that are derived from the neural crest.[3]

The analysis by Nixon and colleagues[4] led to the change in the age cutoff of prognosis in DTC, from 45 years to 55 years in the AJCC Cancer Staging Manual, 8th edition, describing the AJCC/UICC staging for well-differentiated thyroid cancer. Subsequently, this led to an international multi-institutional validation of the age of 55 years as a cutoff for risk stratification in the American Joint Committee on Cancer/Union for International Cancer Control (AJCC/UICC) staging system for well-differentiated thyroid cancer[5] In a study of low-risk PTC in older individuals of age ≥66 years with clinical T1N0M0 PTC, multivariate logistic regression to identify factors associated with extent of surgery (total thyroidectomy vs lobectomy) and radioactive iodine (RAI) administration concluded that most older adults with PTC underwent total thyroidectomy and a third received RAI; neither of the treatments improved disease-specific survival (DSS). It has been suggested that in the growing elderly population, less extensive interventions for low-risk PTC might reduce morbidity and improve quality of life while preserving an excellent prognosis.[6]

Variation in Histopathology, Disease Biology, and Extent of Disease in the Elderly

On histology, the elderly patients often present with aggressive histologic subtypes such as tall cell variant of papillary thyroid carcinoma and Hurthle cell carcinoma, poorly differentiated and anaplastic cancer. Even in presence of well-differentiated cancer, older patients had higher rates of local invasiveness, lateral lymph node involvement, and vascular invasion.[7] To evaluate the burden and risk of thyroid nodule evaluation in older patients, Angell and colleagues[8] recently analyzed a large cohort of elderly patients (age 70 years and older) who underwent thyroid nodule evaluation over a 20-year period. Thyroid cancer-specific mortality was observed in 8% of thyroid cancer patients in the age of 70 years with 2,527 nodules ≥1 cm. All such patients could be recognized during initial evaluation based on the presence of invasive tumor, extensive lymph node metastases, or distant metastases. The data suggested that although an identifiable group of older patients is at risk for mortality from thyroid cancer warranting aggressive treatment, many patients ≥70 year old derive little benefit by active intervention.[9]

Several studies have shown variance in histopathology distribution with rising age. Chereau and colleagues[10] evaluated histopathology and extent of disease at diagnosis in elderly (65–75 year old) and very elderly (>75 year old) patients compared with younger patients: the data were notable for significantly increased primary tumor size, tumor number, extra-capsular invasion, advanced TNM stage, and lymph node and distant metastasis in the very old group. Lin and colleagues[11] and Girardi and colleagues[1] highlighted a significant pattern of lower frequency of PTC and an increase in the frequency of FTC, poorly differentiated, and anaplastic thyroid carcinoma. Girardi and colleagues[1] demonstrated variability in other presenting features of thyroid cancer in elderly patients (age ≥ 65 years) compared with middle-aged cohorts (25–44 years or 45–64 years); specifically, there was a larger primary tumor size (median size being 2.1 cm for elderly vs 1.5 cm in 25–44 years and 1.1 cm in 45–64 years) and higher rates of extra-thyroidal disease (mean incidence 43% for elderly vs 25.3% in 25–44 years and 28.6% in 45–64 years).

Lymph node metastasis was greatest at the extremes of age (<24 years and >70 years). Payne and colleagues[12] showed that well-differentiated thyroid cancer (ie, PTC and FTC), and lymph node metastasis occurred more often in patients younger than 50 years, whereas micropapillary carcinoma was more common in patients 50 years or older. Collectively these studies reflected a pattern of more widespread disease at presentation in elderly patients and a relative increase in the frequency of more aggressive histologic sub-types. Diffuse intense immunostaining for a vascular endothelial growth factor (VEGF) in patients with papillary thyroid cancer has been associated with a high rate of local recurrence and distant metastases.[13] Expression of the tumor suppressor gene p53 has also been associated with an adverse prognosis for patients with thyroid cancer in the elderly.[14]

Incidence of mortality rate and recurrence risk in elderly thyroid cancer patients: comparison with other age groups.

Age has been incorporated into virtually all current clinical staging or prognostication systems for differentiated thyroid cancer, for example, the (i) American Joint Committee on Cancer (AJCC) 8th edition[15]; (ii) Metastasis, Age, Completeness of resection, Invasion, Size (MACIS) model[16]; (iii) Age, Grade, Extent, Size (AGES) score; and the (iv) Age, Metastasis, Extent, Size (AMES) score.[17] In all of these systems, advanced age is included as a risk factor predicting a worse prognosis. Age likely modifies prognosis in a continuous rather than dichotomous manner and that age itself may not be as relevant to thyroid cancer behavior, and likely the result of the multiple accompanying changes for example, accumulated cell mutations, immune senescence, and hormone changes that accompany aging.[18]

Ito and colleagues[19] in a study of 1,740 patients with PTC and by Sugino and colleagues[20] in 134 patients with FTC established a positive correlation between advanced age and worse prognosis in patients with DTC, as was shown in previously reported studies by Halnan[21] and Cady and colleagues.[22] Evaluation of over 30,000 patients in the Surveillance, Epidemiology, and End Result (SEER) database by Orosco and colleagues[23] demonstrated a linear association with age and thyroid cancer death. For elderly population (esp. patients ≥60 years of age) had worse DSS and DFS after a diagnosis of PTC, across all stages of the disease.[23] Given that patients over the age of 45 years have progressively worse survival as they age, the data support having three age groups, 18 to 44 years, 45 to 59 years, and ≥60 years as an independent predictor of survival and recurrence.

Kauffmann and colleagues[24] had shown that DSS and DFS are decreased in patients ≥60 years, after controlling for gender, race, comorbidities, stage, tumor size, extent of surgical treatment, RAI, insurance status, and hospital volume. They also confirmed the importance of age≥ 60 years on PTC-related survival in an American cohort. This has been ascribed to the biology of disease in elderly patients, which is inherently more aggressive than disease in younger individuals. Rukhman and colleagues[25] studied the influence of age and gender on morbidity and/or mortality in different groups of thyroid carcinoma patients. The PTC was the most common type, influenced by older age and male gender. Follicular carcinoma was the second most common type influenced by older age and male gender. The median age of diagnosis was 55 years and asymptomatic thyroid mass spreading mostly via the vascular system, associated with radiation exposure and iodine deficiency. Medullary thyroid cancer (MTC) constitutes 2% to 5% of thyroid malignancies, and is influenced by older age and male gender. In sporadic form(80% of cases), patients belong to a relatively older population, whereas the hereditary form (20% of cases) belong to younger age group. Anaplastic thyroid cancer (rare, bilateral and strongly related to older age) typically presents in the 7th decade of life. There are inconclusive reports on gender influence and the disease is frequently lethal with no effective systemic therapy. Primary thyroid lymphoma is relatively rare, presenting with a rapidly growing neck mass and related to older age and with increased risk in patients with Hashimoto's thyroiditis, with no specific influence by gender.

Numerous studies have demonstrated increased disease recurrence and mortality in thyroid cancer with rising age.[23,26] The recent data by Ylli and colleagues[18] suggest that thyroid cancer mortality and recurrence prediction is more robust when age is modeled as a continuous variable, with the suggestion on the elimination of a specific age cutoff from staging completely. Ganly and colleagues[26] found that disease-specific mortality increased progressively with advancing age, without a threshold age. Inferior outcome in older patients has been reported compared with younger patients with presence of lymph node involvement and extrathyroidal extension.[27] Extrathyroidal disease in older patients increased recurrence to 67% and death rates to 60% compared with those with an intrathyroidal disease, whereas in younger patients the relative increases were 12% and 4%, respectively. Similarly, the risk of death with distant metastasis is greater in older compared with younger patients (96% vs 63%).[22]

Recurrent/Metastatic Tumor Detection

At times, this is a challenge with anatomic imaging modalities, though they can be localized precisely including Ultrasonography (USG), computerized tomography (CT), and magnetic resonance (MR) imaging. USG of neck is useful for detecting small cervical adenopathy; however, it can be inconclusive in determining between malignant lesions and nonspecific tissue changes in neck, where, the role of fluorodeoxyglucose (FDG)-PET/CT can become useful in these scenarios.[28] Metabolic Imaging with PET/CT seems to be valuable complementary diagnostic tool in malignancy evaluation, staging, response assessment, and restaging scenarios in the elderly. The various radiopharmaceuticals of PET/CT that have been investigated for thyroid carcinoma have been ^{18}F-FDG, iodine-124 ([124]I), 18F-fluoride, ^{18}F-tetrafluoroborate, Gallium-68 labeled SSTR based PET agents, prostate-specific membrane antigen and RGD, and ^{18}F-dihydroxyphenylalanine (F-DOPA).

^{18}F-FDG could be useful in the initial staging of high-risk patients, and post-thyroidectomy assessment of DTC with aggressive histology. Nascimento and colleagues[29] in their study found FDG-PET/CT more sensitive than post-treatment radioiodine scan, thus suggesting routine uses in patients with aggressive histology. In a total of 38 consecutive patients with aggressive histology of DTC, FDG-PET/CT done within 3 months of the post-ablation scan, the metastases were found in 53% of patients.

Fluorodeoxyglucose Incidental Diffuse and Focal Fluorodeoxyglucose Uptake in Thyroid

Evaluation of FDG uptake in thyroid gland reveals that normal thyroid gland takes little or no FDG uptake; incidental increased FDG uptake in thyroid has been reported in 1.8% to 2.9% of all patients. Incidental focal thyroid uptake on PET/CT has a higher risk of malignancy (reported between 24%–36%), necessitating further diagnostic workup with ultrasound and fine-needle aspiration biopsy.

a. Focal FDG uptake in Thyroid

An incidental finding of focal unilateral uptake of FDG in the thyroid uptake corresponding to a nodule on the CT has a higher likelihood of malignancy[30] (Fig. 1). In such cases, further diagnostic workup with ultrasonography-guided fine-needle aspiration and cytology is recommended.[31] In one report, a nodule with a SUVmax $\geq$ 5 is highly suggestive of malignancy, regardless of its size.[32]

Higher SUV is reported in malignancy, with large overlap, SUV of benign nodule has been 4.8 (SD: 3.1) and SUV in malignancy being 6.9 (SD: 4.7).[33]

[18F]FDG-PET/CT texture analysis seems to be a promising approach to stratify the patients with thyroid incidentaloma identified on PET scans, with respect to the risk of the diagnosis of a malignant thyroid nodule and thus, could refine the selection of the patients to be referred for cytology.[34]

b. Diffuse, symmetric, bilateral FDG uptake in Thyroid:

Diffuse FDG uptake in the thyroid has an incidence of 0.1% to 4.5% (mean 1.9%), usually represents Hashimoto thyroiditis in ~85% (Fig. 2) and occasionally Graves' disease, with a low risk for malignancy.[33] Primary thyroid lymphoma usually presents in the form of an enlarging neck mass and a history of Hashimoto's thyroiditis. There have been significant advances in both diagnosis and treatment of patients with extranodal

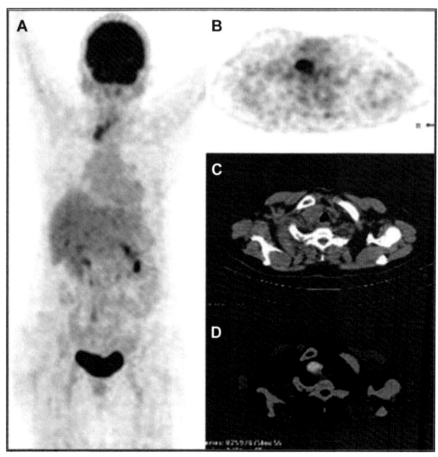

Fig. 1. Incidentaloma on FDG-PET/CT: the FNAC was positive suggestive of Hurthle cell carcinoma. A 60-year-old woman presented with pyrexia of unknown origin (A) anterior maximal intensity projection 18F-FDG PET image, (B–D) PET, CT, and fused PET/CT axial images showing metabolically active incidentaloma in right inferior pole thyroid nodule with SUVmax 4.6, FNAC was positive suggestive of Hurthle cell carcinoma.

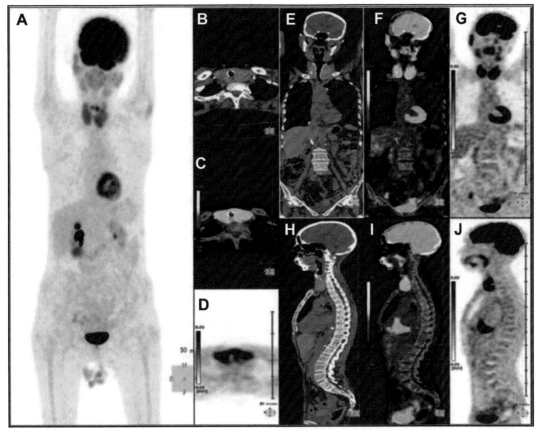

Fig. 2. Bilateral diffuse FDG uptake in thyroid suggestive of thyroiditis. A 69-year-old female patient case of carcinoma cervix presented with newly developed urethrovaginal fistula, referred to evaluate disease status, (*A*) Anterior maximal intensity projection 18F-FDG PET image; (*B–J*) CT, fused PET/CT, and PET images-axial (*B–D*), coronal (*E–G*) and sagittal (*H–J*) images showing only bilateral diffuse FDG uptake in thyroid, SUVmax: 9.36, suggestive of thyroiditis.

lymphoma (ENL), including primary thyroid lymphoma in recent years, with the increasing role of ^{18}F-FDG PET/CT in the diagnosis, staging, and assessment of therapy response and overall management of the disease.

Fluorodeoxyglucose-PET/Computed Tomography in Differentiated Thyroid Carcinoma

FDG-PET/CT has been investigated and used for different possible roles in the management of DTCs. One definitive indication for the PET scan included conventional indications, such as elevated thyroglobulin with non-iodine avid disease (**Figs. 3** and **4**), and more controversial uses, such as evaluation of the extent of disease or abnormalities on other imaging tests.[35] The American Thyroid Association recommends FDG PET and PET/CT for the evaluation of distant metastatic disease, especially bone lesions.[36] Poisson and colleagues[36] reported that patients with SUV greater than 18 on FDG PET/

CT had significantly worse 6-month survival rates than did those with SUV less than 18 (20% vs 80%), as did patients with FDG avid volume greater than 300 mL compared with patients with FDG uptake volume less than 300 mL (10% vs 90%). FDG-PET/CT can be used to evaluate response to systemic or local therapy in patients with the known persistent disease.[37] PET scan aided disease determination in patients with thyroglobulin elevated and radioiodine non-avid disease (thyroglobulin elevation with negative iodine scintigraphy [TENIS]), revealing the overall disease burden in such cases (see **Figs. 3** and **4**).

Top of Form

Bottom of form
Fluorodeoxyglucose PET-computed tomography in differentiated thyroid carcinoma patients with recurrent disease and/or high suspicion of recurrence In patients with a high risk of suspicion of disease recurrence or those in whom the basal

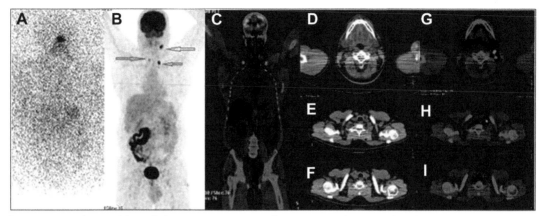

Fig. 3. TENIS with operable neck disease on FDG-PET/CT (see **Fig. 10** in the original PPT). A 63-year-old male post-total thyroidectomy and RAI therapy went in remission, subsequent radioiodine scan was negative despite serum Tg 77.5 ng/dL, (*A*) anterior whole-body planar ^{131}I scan showing no abnormal tracer concentration, (*B*) Anterior maximal intensity projection ^{18}F-FDG PET image, (*C*) fused coronal FDG-PET/CT image, (*D–F*) CT, and (*G–I*) fused PET/CT axial images showing metabolically active subcentimeter nodes (*arrows*) in left level IB (largest measuring 10 × 6 mm and SUVmax 4.2) and bilateral level V- FNAC proved metastatic nodal disease (*arrows*).

or stimulated Tg is ≥ 10 ng/mL, additional imaging studies to include whole-body FDG-PET/CT has been proposed: the patient-based sensitivity 84% specificity 84% and lesion-based sensitivity 92% specificity 78% in this subgroup.[30] Although high frequency of additional positive PET/CT lesions in patients with recurrent DTC (46%) (**Fig. 5**) and in patients with stage T3–T4N1 and tumor size > 2 cm (25%), only 3% to 6% of patients with stage T3–T4N0 or T1–T2N1 had additional PET/CT findings.[38] According to current European Guidelines, the application of PET or PET/CT using ^{18}F-FDG should only be considered for DTC patients with suspicion of disease recurrence (with rising thyroglobulin levels), and negative whole-body radioiodine scintigraphy.[39]

Fluorodeoxyglucose-PET in Aggressive Histologic Subtypes of Differentiated Thyroid Carcinoma and Other Characteristics of Aggressiveness

Grabellus and colleagues[40] reported increasing glucose transporter 1 expression with escalating de-differentiation and aggressiveness of thyroid cancer cells and PDTCs. Aggressive histologic subtypes of DTC include patients with tall cell, diffuse sclerosing,[41] solid/trabecular[42] and insular variants.[43] FDG-PET or PET/CT has been proposed as a useful imaging tool for the staging and restaging of such tumors and also aid in prognostication and treatment approach. DTCs presenting with high FDG uptake on PET scan and histologic features of necrosis have been considered aggressive differentiated cancers and the FDG uptake in these tumors is highly prognostic for survival.[44] Similarly, Treglia and colleagues[45]

showed that DTCs with radioiodine refractory disease and FDG-PET positive should be considered aggressive tumors with poor prognosis, indicating the potential usefulness of FDG-PET or PET/CT in patients with aggressive histologic subtypes of DTC (**Figs. 6** and **7**).

Fluorodeoxyglucose-PET in Hurthle Cell Thyroid Carcinoma

The role of FDG-PET or PET/CT has been emphasized in patients with Hurthle cell thyroid carcinoma (HCTC) in initial staging and/or follow-up of invasive and metastatic tumors.[45] Approximately 3.6% of thyroid cancers, HCTC was initially included in the FTC group, but has been found to have a different oncogenic expression and is now considered as a different histologic and clinical disease. HCTC has a 10-year disease-free survival of 40%, associated with a high risk of distant and lymph nodal metastases, having a worse prognosis compared with DTC. HCTC seems to demonstrate poor radioiodine accumulation, and is reported to be FDG-avid tumor. Only few studies about the role of FDG-PET/CT in HCTC have been published in the literature. Overall, FDG-PET demonstrated high sensitivity and specificity in HCTC(sensitivity: 92%, specificity: 80%, PPV: 92%, NPV: 80%, and an accuracy of 89%), and also provides prognostic information in patients with Hurthle cell thyroid carcinoma.[30] **Fig. 6**.

Fluorodeoxyglucose-PET in Poorly Differentiated Thyroid Carcinoma

Poorly differentiated thyroid carcinoma is often low RAI avid or radioiodine-negative. In a negative

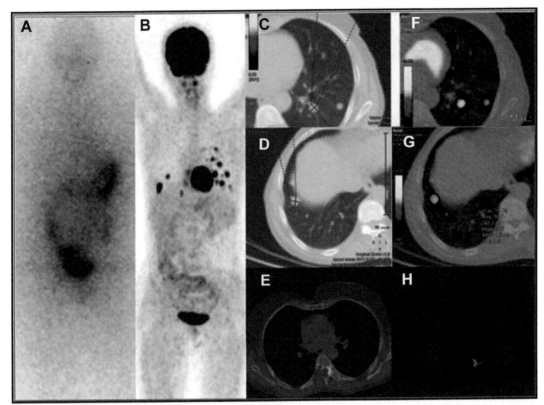

Fig. 4. TENIS with elevated Tg: role of FDG-PET/CT in whole body disease evaluation. A 61-year-old womanpresented with back pain with inability to walk since 2 months and swelling in anterior neck, underwent total thyroidectomy with histopathology pT size 6.2 × 5.6 cm, follicular carcinoma (Hurthle cell carcinoma) of right lobe. No Vascular and capsular invasion or nodal metastasis. Patient developed paraparesis with bony tenderness along spine. Tg > 300 ng/ml patient was treated thrice with RAI therapy cumulative 724 mCi, fourth LDS (A) Anterior whole body planar 131I-Iodine scan revealed no abnormal tracer concentration despite Tg 147; (B) Anterior maximal intensity projection 18F-FDG PET image in TENIS, (C–E) CT and (F–H) Fused FDG PET/CT axial images, (C–G) showing metabolically active multiple bilateral micro and macro lung nodules (left > right), largest in right lower lobe measuring 1.2 cm × 1.1 cm (SUVmax 18.39), largest in left lobe measuring 1.1 cm × 1 cm (SUVmax 14.66). (E,H) Minimal FDG uptake noted in lytic lesion involving D8 vertebra and right 8th rib with soft tissue component invading the spinal canal, measuring 2.5 cm × 2.9 cm (SUVmax: 2.8).

RAI scenario, there are cases that show multiple metastasis on 18F-FDG PET/CT. FDG-PET/CT is often considered for initial staging and disease evaluation in the subsequent stages of poorly differentiated thyroid cancer[46] (see **Fig. 7**).

Complementary Role of Fluorodeoxyglucose-PET in Radio-Iodine Concentrating Metastases of Differentiated Thyroid Carcinoma

FDG-PET has been investigated for its complementary role to iodine-131 (131-I) scanning in metastatic DTC.[47] 18F-FDG PET/CT undertaken concurrently with ^{131}I therapy detected additional lesions in 14% of DTC patients and was particularly helpful for detecting additional lesions in patients undergoing ^{131}I therapy after resection of recurrent tumor or in stage T3–T4N1 disease with

tumor size > 2.0 cm.[48] FDG-PET may fail to localize the tumor sites in some patients with well-differentiated thyroid cancer that retain good radioiodine avidity. This is a well-described phenomenon, known as "flip-flop", that depends on the differentiation of the thyroid cancer. Multiple studies have documented higher accuracy of FDG-PET, compared with other imaging modalities in the evaluation of patients with recurrent or metastatic differentiated thyroid cancer.[49]

Fluorodeoxyglucose-PET in Non-Radioiodine Concentrating Metastases of Differentiated Thyroid Carcinoma

In Tg elevated non-radioiodine concentrating tumors that is, TENIS, there is 'NIS downregulation and GLUT receptor upregulation' forming the

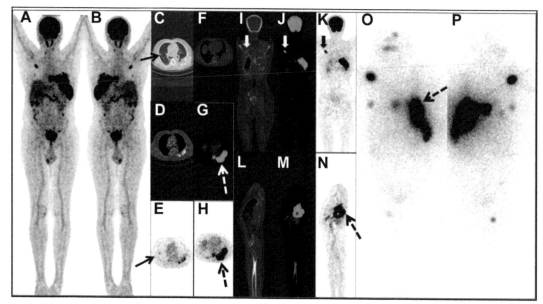

Fig. 5. DTC with suspicion of recurrence & metastatic disease). A 57-year-old man post-total thyroidectomy, FVPCT of right lobe, post-radioiodine therapy(56 mCi) defaulted for 3 years, presented with Tg 300 ng/ml, maximal intensity projection anterior (A) and posterior (B) ^{18}F-FDG PET images showing metabolically active metastatic lung and bone disease, (C–E) lung window CT, fused PET/CT and PET axial images showing metabolically active multiple bilateral lung nodules, largest measures 1.5 cm (SUVmax 3.39) at right lung upper lobe (*thin arrow*); bone window CT, fused PET/CT and PET axial (F–H), sagittal (L–N) images showing hypermetabolic destructive large soft tissue mass involving left posterolateral chest wall muscles and left sided 6th to 9th ribs (dotted *arrow*), measuring 8.8x9x6.4 cm (SUVmax 10.85), D7 and D8 vertebra (SUVmax 11.35); (I–K) bone window CT, fused PET/CT and PET coronal images reveal additional lytic lesion (*bold arrow*) with soft tissue component in spine of right scapula (SUVmax: 11.35). Anterior (O) and posterior (P) whole body planar 131I-Iodine scan showing iodine avid all metastatic bone sites, treated with high dose RAI and palliative EBRT.

basis behind FDG-PET molecular imaging that helps in evaluating the disease burden. DTCs in the course of time, including recurrent or metastatic settings often exhibit negative ^{131}I uptake and positive findings on ^{18}F-FDG PET/CT due to cell de-differentiation.[50,51] In a study of 239 patients with metastases and high Tg, the sensitivity of FDG-PET was 49%, the sensitivity of 131-I was 50%, and the combined sensitivity was 90%. It was also observed that FDG-PET was more likely to be positive in 131-I negative patients.[52]

From a prognostic viewpoint, radioactive iodine-refractory (RAIR), and FDG-PET positive thyroid carcinomas represent the major cause of deaths from thyroid carcinomas and are therefore the main focus of novel targeted therapies. Although most of the RAIR, FDG-PET positive metastatic diseases belong to PDTCs, DTC can also present as RAIR disease. In one study, histologic characterization of metastases/recurrence in 70 RAIR, FDG-PET positive thyroid carcinoma patients, 47.1% had PDTCs, 20% had tall-cell variant of PTC, 22.9% had well-differentiated PTCs (including classic and follicular variants), 8.6% had HCTC, and 1.4% had ATC.[53]

Fluorodeoxyglucose-PET for Prognostic Information: Irrespective of Radioiodine Scan Results

Robbins and colleagues[54] demonstrated that patients with a positive FDG-PET had a 7-fold increased risk of mortality compared with thyroid cancer survivors who had a negative FDG study. Robbins and colleagues[54] demonstrated only age and PET results continued to be strong predictors of survival under multivariate analysis. There were significant inverse relationships between survival and (i) the glycolytic rate of the most active lesion and (ii) the number of FDG-avid lesions.

Fluorodeoxyglucose-Positron Emission Tomography/Computed Tomography in Anaplastic Thyroid Carcinoma

FDG-PET or PET/CT is recommended for staging, follow-up, and post-treatment restaging of ATC, especially in metastatic disease, as published in ATA guidelines.[45] ATC demonstrates a higher incidence in elderly and patients with anaplastic cancer who are older than those with differentiated cancer; the mean age at diagnosis is 65 years,

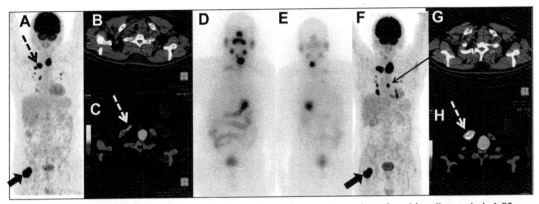

Fig. 6. FDG-PET/CT in Hurthle cell with anaplastic carcinoma (aggressive variant thyroid malignancies). A 59-year-old man post-total thyroidectomy status, serum Tg 2929 ng/mL, ATA negative (*A*) anterior maximal intensity projection of baseline ^{18}F-FDG PET image showing metabolically active left thyroid bed, subcm bilateral lung metastasis, lytic bone metastases-right anterior end of clavicle (*dotted arrow*) and right proximal femur (*bold arrow*), (*B,C*) CT and fused FDG PET/CT axial images showing metabolically active left thyroid bed, lytic right anterior end of clavicle (*dotted arrow*). Patient was treated with high dose ^{131}iodine therapy 252 mCi; post-radioiodine therapy scan (*D*) anterior and (*E*) posterior whole body planar ^{131}iodine scan showed uptake only in thyroid neck remnant. On adequate thyroid suppression, Follow-up at 6 months, Tg-2463 ng/mL (*F*) Anterior maximal intensity projection 18F-FDG PET image showing progression-new metabolically active sub-carinal node measuring 1.3 × 1.2 cm (SUVmax 32.73- *long thin arrow*); increase in size, metabolic activity and number of subcentimetric multiple bilateral lungs nodules, largest being 7.6 mm (SUVmax 13.98), persistent lytic bone lesions with soft tissue component in the medial end of right clavicle (*dotted arrow*) and proximal right femur (*bold arrow*). (*G,H*) CT and fused FDG PET/CT axial images showing increase in size and metabolic activity of left thyroid bed soft tissue, abutting and displacing trachea and esophagus posteriomedially; anteriorly fat planes with strap muscles are lost suggestive of disease infiltration and lytic bone lesion with soft tissue component in the medial end of right clavicle. subcm, subcentimeter.

and fewer than 10% are younger than 50 years. Thyroid gland involvement is multifocal and bilateral with short duration history of symptoms. Sixty to 70% of tumors occur in women,[55,56] clinically presenting with rapidly expanding thyroid mass with hoarseness, dyspnea, dysphagia, cervical pain, tracheal obstruction, and metastasis. Histologically 3 predominant features include spindle cell, giant cell and squamoid cell types. The treatment remains controversial. In over 70% of the

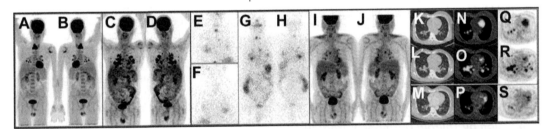

Fig. 7. FDG-PET/CT in Anaplastic thyroid carcinoma arising on a background of poorly differentiated thyroid carcinoma and columnar cell variant of papillary thyroid carcinoma (aggressive variants of thyroid carcinoma). A 66-year-old male, PREOPERATIVE anterior (*A*) and posterior (*B*) maximal intensity projection ^{18}F-FDG PET images; post-total thyroidectomy (Tg 417.2 ng/mL) Anterior (*C*) and posterior (*D*) maximal intensity projection 18F-FDG PET images showed a significant increase in number and FDG avidity of bilateral multiple lung nodules; diagnostic ^{131}I neck and chest anterior (*E*) posterior (*F*) images show neck remnant and faint lung uptake; treated with 200 mCi of radioiodine therapy subsequent ^{131}iodine post-therapy anterior (*G*) and posterior (*H*) whole body images confirm concentration in neck remnant and bilateral lung nodules; post-RAI therapy (Tg 19.26 ng/mL). On follow-up at 6 months- Anterior (*I*) and posterior (*J*) maximal intensity projection ^{18}F-FDG PET images showed a significant decrease in number and FDG avidity of residual (*K,L,M*) CT, (*N,O,P*) fused FDG PET/CT and (*Q,R,S*) FDG PET axial images, (*K,N,Q*) preoperative showing FDG avid few right lower lobe nodules; (*L,O,R*) postoperative increase in number, size, and avidity of multiple bilateral lung nodules; (*M,P,S*) post radioiodine showing significantly reduced number, size and avidity of lung nodules suggesting good response to RAI therapy.

patients, the tumor infiltrates surrounding tissues & median survival time is about 6 to 8 months.

This aggressive thyroid tumor does not demonstrate uptake of radioiodine and/or produce Tg.[57] Conversely, ATC whether primary or metastatic, consistently show high FDG uptake.[58] PET/CT with FDG is very sensitive and also useful for evaluation for metastases (especially skeletal) for specific treatment planning surgical vs radiation therapy planning and also for evaluation of treatment response. Bogsrud and colleagues[35,59] reported that PET findings had a direct impact on the management of approximately 50% of patients diagnosed with ATC (n = 16). Both SUV_{max} and FDG avid volume were found to be of prognostic value for survival of patients with ATC. **Figs. 6 and 7.**

Disease-specific treatment approach aided by FDG, 68Ga-DOTATATE and 68Ga-PSMA correlation in TENIS and de-differentiated malignancies

Different patterns of lesional uptakes have been documented on ^{18}F-FDG, ^{68}Ga-DOTATATE, and ^{68}Ga-PSMA-11 PET/CT, as a demonstration of tumor heterogeneity.[60] The TENIS has been investigated as a potential indication of peptide receptor radionuclide therapy (PRRT) in patients who demonstrate substantial tracer avidity on ^{68}Ga-DOTATATE-positive scan.[61] Abundant PSMA expression in tumor vasculature with relative sparing of normal tissue makes it a potential agent for targeted imaging and radionuclide therapy for solid tumors.[62] Depending upon the FDG-PET lesions and correlation with ^{68}Ga-DOTATATE, or ^{68}Ga-PSMA-11, whichever tracer shows equivalent lesions with SUVmax uptake more than liver uptake could be further planned for targeted radionuclide therapies (Lu-177 DOTATATE/PSMA-617), when patients cannot tolerate or resistant to the tyrosine kinase inhibitor therapies (**Figs. 8 and 9**).

Role of Thyroid Stimulating Hormone Stimulation by Thyroid Hormone Withdrawal/ Recombinant Thyroid Stimulating Hormone

(rhTSH) use with fluorodeoxyglucose-PET/ computed tomography in differentiated thyroid carcinoma patients

A number of studies have examined the effect of thyroid hormone withdrawal or recombinant TSH (rhTSH) use on FDG-PET/CT performance. Iwano and colleagues[63] performed ^{18}F-FDG PET/CT with serum TSH stimulation 3 to 4 days before ^{131}I ablation in 54 patients with DTC. ^{18}F-FDG PET/CT findings were positive in 33% of enrolled patients, and most of the positive lesions were located in the thyroid bed and cervical lymph nodes.[63] rhTSH primed FDG-PET examined in Tg positive radioiodine negative patients, demonstrated more lesions in post-rh-TSH PET/CT scans (odds ratio: 4.9), more patients with true positive lesions (OR: 2.5), and better target-to-background and change of management in 9% of patients. rhTSH was found to be more sensitive for lesion detection (95 vs 81%), more sensitive for detection of involved organs (94 vs 79%), and not significantly different in the detection of patients (with any lesions). It is proposed that this approach is most useful when there is a normal neck & chest CT scan & normal neck US & elevated, but not very high Tg. Although T4 therapy is generally not withdrawn before FDG-PET, in one small study, more lesions were identified when T4 therapy was withdrawn.[64] In another study, the use of rhTSH before an FDG-PET scan significantly increased the number of lesions detected, but patient-wise treatment changes due to true positive lesions were uncommon (6% in one study of 63 patients).[65]

Non-Fluorodeoxyglucose PET/Computed Tomography Radiopharmaceuticals in Thyroid Cancer Management

The value of non-FDG PET/CT tracers in thyroid cancer management is evolving. Beyond ^{18}F-FDG, the other tracers used for PET imaging of thyroid malignancies include iodine-124 ([124]I), ^{18}F-fluoride, ^{18}F-tetrafluoroborate, and gallium-68-based SSTR-PET, prostate-specific membrane antigen and RGD.

Iodine-124

I-124 a positron-emitting radioiodine. Some facts regarding this PET radioisotope for consideration are: (i) better resolution of PET (4–5 mm) vs. SPECT (8–10 mm); and (ii) high energy of positrons (2.1 MeV; 23% abundance), mean range in the tissue of about 3.5 mm (compared with 0.6 mm for F-18); (iii) I-124 allows for lesion dosimetry, better quantitation of uptake with PET with half-life of 4.2 days. I-124 can be produced in cyclotron, but is volatile and contaminates cyclotron.

PET with [124]I has been investigated as a valuable diagnostic tool for the detection of recurrent or residual DTC. The imaging can be performed as early as 24 hours after the administration of the radio-tracer without sacrificing diagnostic accuracy compared with high-dose ^{131}I-WBS.[66] PET with [124]I has greater spatial resolution than planar ^{131}I-WBS, even at lower radioiodine activities and therefore gives considerably low radiation exposure. [124]I PET can provide specific dosimetric information, allowing quantification of the volume

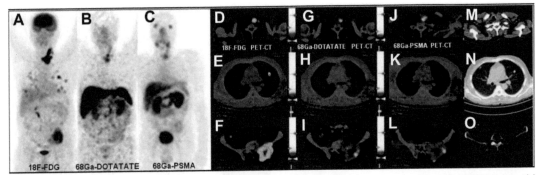

Fig. 8. Comparison of investigational PET tracers (^{68}Ga-DOTATATE & ^{68}Ga-PSMA-11) with FDG-PET/CT in Hurthle cell Ca. Anterior maximal intensity projection PET images (*A*) 18F-FDG PET, (*B*) ^{68}Ga-DOTATATE, (*C*) 68Ga-PSMA-11; fused PET/CT axial images (*D–F*) 18F-FDG, (*G–I*) ^{68}Ga-DOTATATE, (*J–L*) ^{68}Ga-PSMA-11 PET, (*M-O*) CT transaxial images [Window: (*M*)- soft tissue, (*N*)- lung, (*O*)- bone]; (*D,G,J,M*) showing left level III nodes largest measuring 27 × 27.5 mm with SUVmax: 18F-FDG 27.81, ^{68}Ga-DOTATATE 1.8 (Krennings score 2), ^{68}Ga-PSMA 8.3 (miPSMA score 1); (*E,H,K,N*) showing multiple (>10) tiny bilateral pulmonary nodules, largest left lower lobe measuring 11.5 × 9.7 mm, with SUVmax: 18F-FDG 25.63, ^{68}Ga-DOTATATE 9.0 (Krennings score 1), ^{68}Ga-PSMA-11 1.6 (single 13 mm left lung with miPSMA score 0); (*F,I,L,O*) showing lytic lesion with soft tissue component in left iliac bone 88 × 80.7 mm with SUVmax: [68]F-FDG 58.5, ^{68}Ga-DOTATATE 9.9 (Krennings score 2), ^{68}Ga-PSMA-11 7.4 (miPSMA score 1) (**Table 1**).

of the thyroid tumor, and can be used as a surrogate marker before therapeutic intervention with [131]I. Simultaneous administration of the therapeutic dose of ^{131}I and a tracer dose of [124]I allows accurate measurement of iodine uptake during therapy.[67] The localization of metastasis is also improved with the use of [124]I-PET/CT compared with conventional imaging.

[68]Ga-Labeled PET/Computed Tomography Radiopharmaceuticals

[68]Ga-labeled somatostatin receptor PET/computed tomography
[68]Ga-somatostatin receptor PET/CT has been used to determine the somatostatin receptor density in the residual tumor/metastatic lesions for PRRT in refractory thyroid cancer and to assess the treatment response.[68] The lesions in TENIS show variable expression of somatostatin receptors (SSTR-2) on their cell surface.[69–71] ^{68}Ga-DOTATOC/TATE-PET/CT can be used for

visualization of SSTR-2 expressing lesions and can be used as a potential indication of PRRT in patients who demonstrate substantial tracer avidity on ^{68}Ga-DOTATATE PET-CT. However, not all patients with TENIS lesions express SSTR-2(in our experience, this constitute only 15%–20% of cases).[61,69–71] PET-based tracers such as ^{68}Ga-DOTA-NOC/TATE, compared with SRS or somatostatin receptor scintigraphy, offer the advantages of better resolution and quantification, and hence have been useful for treatment response evaluation.

Angiogenesis Imaging in Thyroid Cancer

[68]Ga-prostate-specific membrane antigen
Prostate-specific membrane antigen (PSMA) overexpression secondary to tumor neovasculature has been reported in a variety of cancers.[72] Abundant PSMA expression in tumor vasculature with relative sparing of normal tissue makes it a potential agent for targeted imaging and radionuclide

Table 1			
Comparison of investigational PET tracers (^{68}Ga-DOTATATE & ^{68}Ga-PSMA-11) with FDG-PET/CT in Hurthle cell Ca			
Lesions	^{68}Ga-DOTATATE	^{68}Ga-PSMA-11	FDG
Left level III lymph node, 27 × 27.5 mm	1.8	8.3	27.81
Bilateral multiple pulmonary nodules, largest left lower lobe, 11.5 × 9.7 mm,	9.0	1.6 (single 13 mm left lung)	25.63
Lytic lesion with soft tissue component in left iliac bone 88 × 80.7 mm, SUV max	9.9	7.4	58.5

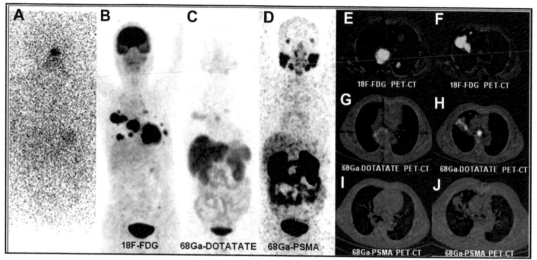

Fig. 9. Comparison of investigational PET tracers (^{68}Ga-DOTATATE & ^{68}Ga-PSMA-11) with FDG-PET/CT in TENIS. A 56-year-old male, k/c/o TENIS, serum thyroglobulin 330.21, ATA negative, (*A*) anterior whole-body planar ^{131}I-Iodine scan showing no abnormal tracer concentration; Anterior maximal intensity projection (MIP) PET images (*B*) ^{18}F-FDG PET showing uptake in right hilar, subcarinal nodes, Multiple small >10 nodules in both lungs (*C*) ^{68}Ga-DOTATATE, (*D*) ^{68}Ga-PSMA-11; (*E–J*) Fused PET/CT transaxial images; (*E,F*) ^{18}F-FDG, (*G,H*) 68Ga-DOTATATE, (*I,J*) 68Ga-PSMA; (*E,G,I*) showing right parahilar large nodal mass, SUVmax: ^{18}F-FDG 36.7, ^{68}Ga-DOTATATE 8.9 (Krennings score 2), ^{68}Ga-PSMA-11 1.2 (miPSMA score 0); (*F,H,J*) lung window fused PET/CT transaxial images showing largest lung nodule in right middle lobe, measuring 44.2 × 42 mm, SUVmax: ^{18}F-FDG 40.1, ^{68}Ga-DOTATATE 5.7 (Krennings score 2), ^{68}Ga-PSMA-11 1.92 (miPSMA score: 0), all other lung nodules non PSMA concentrating (**Table 2**).

therapy for solid tumors and their metastases.[62] ^{68}Ga-PSMA-PET/CT thus can be considered as a beneficial adjunct to the well-established ^{18}F-FDG-PET/CT for a few individually selected patients of ATC, PDTC, and TENIS to detect lesions that are not evident on ^{18}F-FDG-PET/CT and to determine patients' eligibility for a radioligand therapy.

It is postulated that both radiolabeled PSMA-ligands in the future may represent a promising theragnostic approach with only minor side effects for selected individual patients with ATC and PDTC who need alternative treatment options in case of progression and when established therapies are no longer effective.[73] PSMA representing a marker of neovasculature formation also has the potential to contribute in the prediction of tumor aggressiveness and patient outcome.[74]

^{68}Ga-DOTA-RGD$_2$ and [^{18}F]Tetrafluoroborate PET

Neovascularization in the cancer microenvironment is a multistep process that is necessary during the progression of solid tumors.[75–77] As in other solid and hematological tumors, the microvessel density (MVD) has been shown to correlate with disease-free survival in thyroid cancers, particularly in PTC and in follicular thyroid carcinoma (FTC).[78,79] Differences have been demonstrated amongst tumor types in the patterns of spread and metastasis, probably due to the influence of tumor metastasis route by phenotype,

Table 2
Comparison of investigational PET tracers (^{68}Ga-DOTATATE & ^{68}Ga-PSMA-11) with FDG-PET/CT in TENIS

Lesions	^{68}Ga-DOTATATE	^{68}Ga-PSMA-11	FDG
Right parahilar large nodal mass and	8.9	1.2	36.7
Subcarinal carinal node (11 mm)	7.6	1.1	2.5
Multiple small >10 nodules in both lung, left hilar 15.2 × 14.33 mm nodule shows	no	No	12
Largest lung nodule in RML 44.2 × 42 mm	5.7	1.92	40.1

angiogenesis or their interactions determining a more aggressive behavior.[80,81] Angiogenesis imaging can prove useful in RAI-refractory DTC (RAIR-DTC), especially in patients with negative/suspicious ^{18}F-FDG PET/CT. In one study, most of the patients (82.1%) positive on ^{68}Ga-DOTA-RGD$_2$ PET/CT showed radiotracer avidity toward the higher end of the spectrum (grade IV and grade V); it was postulated that novel ^{177}Lu-based theranostics can be a potential treatment for these patients.[82] The targeted therapies for RAIR-DTC, in particular, act primarily through two mechanisms of action, by inhibition of angiogenesis and inhibition of cell proliferation and survival.

^{18}F-TFB shows a biodistribution similar to ^{99m}Tc-pertechnetate, a known non-organified hNIS tracer, and is pharmacologically and radiobiologically safe in humans. Imaging using ^{18}F-TFB imparts a radiation exposure similar in magnitude to many other ^{18}F-labeled radiotracers.[83,84] Recently, [^{18}F]tetrafluoroborate ([^{18}F]TFB or [^{18}F]BF$_4^-$) and other fluorine-18 labeled iodide analogs have emerged as a promising iodide analog for PET imaging. These fluorine-18 labeled probes have biochemical properties that allow them to closely mimic iodide transport by NIS in thyroid, as well as in other NIS-expressing tissues. Unlike radioiodides, they do not undergo organification in thyroid cells, which results in an advantage of relatively lower uptake in normal thyroid tissue. Initial clinical trials of [^{18}F]TFB have been completed in healthy human subjects and thyroid cancer patients. The excellent imaging properties of [^{18}F]TFB for the evaluation of NIS-expressing tissues indicate its bright future in PET NIS imaging.[83] In a reported study, [^{18}F]TFB-PET was not inferior to [I]NaI-PET for detecting thyroid cancer and its metastases and was able to detect [I]NaI-PET-negative viable differentiated thyroid cancer metastases,[85] with an indication that [^{18}F]TFB-PET shows higher sensitivity and accuracy than [^{131}I]iodine WBS and SPECT-CT in detecting recurrent DTC. The combination of [^{18}F]TFB-PET with [^{18}F]FDG-PET-CT has been proposed as a reasonable strategy to characterize DTC tumor lesions with respect to their differentiation and thereby also individually plan and monitor treatment.[86]

[^{68}Ga]Ga-DOTA.SA-FAPi

[^{68}Ga]Ga-DOTA.SA.FAPi is a promising alternative among the FAPI class of molecules and performed well as compared with standard-of-care radiotracer [^{18}F]F-FDG in the diagnosis of various cancers.[87] Ballal and colleagues in a recent study revealed

head and neck cancers demonstrating the highest SULpeak and average (avg) values similar to the values of [^{18}F]F-FDG [(SULpeak: 15.4 vs 14.2; P-0.680) (SULavg: 8.3 vs 7.9; P-0.783)].

[18]F-Flouride PET-Computed Tomography

[18]F-NaF uptake reflects osteoblastic metabolism, thanks to the physiologic incorporation of fluoride in bone matrix as fluoro-apatite.[88] Fluoride-PET shows an elevated sensitivity for both sclerotic and lytic lesions,[89,90] but this high sensitivity rate outlines the principal drawback of the tracer: ^{18}F-fluoride is not a specific oncological tracer, thus sometimes it can be difficult to differentiate between benign and malignant lesions. ^{18}F-NaF PET-CT can play a role in the identification of bone metastases, in exploring underlying bone metabolism, extent of bone involvement, number of metastatic bone lesions, identifying specific lesions such as impending pathologic fracture site. In posttreatment scenario (post-RAI therapy/local RT/on TSH suppression) follow-up scan, the finding of decrease in SUVmax on fluoride scan with sclerosis in the CT component is a useful finding to detect treatment response (**Fig. 10**).

Medullary Thyroid Carcinoma

MTC represents malignant transformation of neuroectodermally derived parafollicular C cells. Among these, 80% are sporadic and 20% are hereditary. Surgical treatment of MTC includes total thyroidectomy, central compartment lymph node dissection, and ipsilateral modified radical neck dissection. Risk factors for recurrence and death include tumor size, preoperative calcitonin level, advanced age, extrathyroid tumor extension, progression of cervical nodal disease to the mediastinum, extranodal tumor extension and incomplete tumor excision. Serum calctonin levels is measured around 8 to 12 weeks postoperatively to assess the presence of residual disease. For residual local disease a USG of neck and for distant metastatic lesions CT and MRI are considered. The hereditary medullary thyroid carcinoma is not seen in the elderly age group.

PET/Computed Tomography in Medullary Thyroid Cancer

When no disease is detected in the presence of high calcitonin levels molecular imaging that is, scanning with sestamibi, radio-iodinated MIBG, ^{131}I anti-CEA antibody or PET imaging with FDG, ^{68}Ga-DOTATATE/NOC or ^{18}F-DOPA PET-CT is considered to delineate disease burden and further treatment. Multiple studies have now

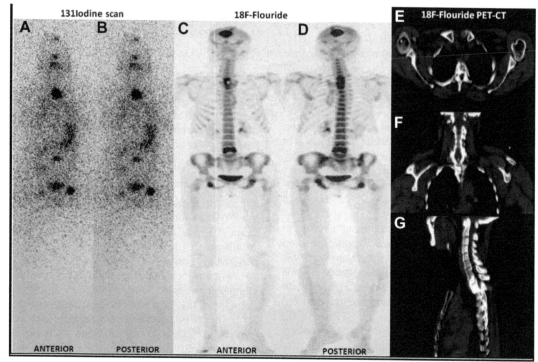

Fig. 10. ¹⁸F-Fluoride PET-CT in evaluating skeletal metastases in DTC. A 60-year-old male post-total thyroidectomy with brain and skeletal metastases, histopathologically follicular carcinoma of thyroid with extrathyroidal extension. Postoperative stimulated Thyroglobulin was 29.37 ng/mL, anterior (A) and posterior (B) whole-body 131-Iodine scan revealed uptake in skull, upper thorax, midline umbilical region, and bilateral proximal femur region; anterior (C) and posterior (D) maximum intensity projection ¹⁸F-Fluoride PET-CT scan and fused fluoride PET/CT axial (E), coronal (F) and sagittal (G) images showing revealed increased osteoblastic activity correlating with radioiodine scan (in skull, D1-D3, L5 vertebra and bilateral ischium with lytic sclerotic changes) suggestive of skeletal metastasis aiding accurate delineation of active skeletal metastasis. Follicular carcinoma of thyroid with metastasis, stimulated Tg postop 29.37 ¹³¹iodine scan revealed uptake in skull, upper thorax, midline umbilical region, and bilateral proximal femur region, and ¹⁸F-fluoride PET scan shows increased osteoblastic activity correlating with 1 mCi scan in skull, D1-D3, L5 vertebra and bilateral ischium with lytic sclerotic changes suggestive of skeletal metastasis aiding accurate delineation of active skeletal metastasis.

reported high sensitivity of PET/CT in MTC [91,92] vis-a-vis the other imaging modalities (**Fig. 11**).

¹⁸F-Fluorodeoxyglucose PET/Computed Tomography in Medullary Thyroid Cancer

Treglia and colleagues[93] in their meta-analysis showed a higher detection rate of recurrent medullary thyroid carcinoma using ¹⁸F-FDG. Bogsrud and colleagues[94] showed the prognostic value of FDG PET/CT in patients with suspected residual or recurrent medullary thyroid carcinoma. They proposed that it is useful if calcitonin ≥ 1,000 ng/L, with a pooled detection rate 75% and low sensitivity if calcitonin < 1,000 ng/L. FDG-PET positive disease had worse prognosis. FDG-PET/CT is useful in suspected residual or recurrent MTC when calcitonin doubling time (CDT) is low and the sensitivity has been reported to be better for sporadic subtype.

¹⁸F-DOPA in Medullary Thyroid Cancer

6-L-¹⁸F-fluorodihydroxyphenylalanine (¹⁸F-DOPA), when available, is frequently the preferred radiopharmaceutical of choice for metabolic imaging of MTC with elevated serum calcitonin level. ¹⁸F-FDOPA demonstrates good diagnostic performance if serum calcitonin level is elevated (>150 pg/mL), with a prolonged CDT. ¹⁸F-FDOPA PET is superior to 18F-FDG PET in the evaluation of metastatic/recurrent MTC, with a higher patient-based sensitivity (64% vs 48%, respectively; range, 38%–83% vs 17%–64%) and lesion-based sensitivity (72% vs 52%, respectively; range, 52%–94% vs 28%–62%).[95,96] The use of this agent is based upon the postulation that ¹⁸F-FDOPA is retained by MTC metastases owing to intracellular decarboxylation, a feature of the cells of neuroendocrine origin in MTC.[91,97] In the cases with negative FDOPA, FDG is often the next PET

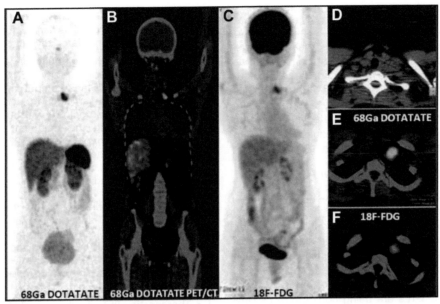

Fig. 11. ¹⁸F-FDG and ⁶⁸Ga-DOTATATE PET-CT in patient of MTC with raised calcitonin. A 56-year-old woman post-total thyroidectomy status, serum Calcitonin: 1500 pg/mL; (*A,B,E*) ⁶⁸Ga-DOTATATE- Anterior maximal intensity projection (*A*) and fused PET/CT(*B*); (*C,F*) 18F-FDG, Anterior maximal intensity projection (*C*) and fused FDG-PET/CT (*F*), CT (*D*). Scan finding reveals tracer avid left supraclavicular lymph node measuring 2.1 cm × 1.7 cm, ⁶⁸Ga-DOTATATE SUVmax 21.27 (Krennings 3) and FDG SUVmax 5.5.

radiopharmaceutical, especially if serum calcitonin and CEA levels are rising rapidly.

Gallium-68-Labeled Somatostatin Analog PET-Computed Tomography in Medullary Thyroid Cancer

PET with a gallium-68 labeled somatostatin analog is another promising approach for investigating MTC patients with elevated serum calcitonin. Conry and colleagues[98] compared ⁶⁸Ga-DOTA-TATE PET/CT and FDG PET/CT in 18 patients with MTC and found that, although the sensitivity was marginally lower for ⁶⁸Ga-DOTA-TATE (72% vs 78%), this difference was statistically insignificant (*P* = 0.056). Treglia and colleagues[99] in the retrospective study compared FDOPA, FDG, and ⁶⁸Ga-somatostatin analog PET/CT in a group of patients with residual or recurrent MTC (*n* = 18) and elevated serum calcitonin levels, found that ⁶⁸Ga-somatostatin analogs had a lower sensitivity than FDOPA PET/CT (33.3% vs 72.2%) and provided no additional information in any patient. Furthermore, they reported that ⁶⁸Ga-somatostatin analog PET/CT missed all liver lesions detected by FDG PET/CT and FDOPA PET/CT, which may be explained by a low lesion-to-background ratio caused by low hepatic tumor expression of somatostatin receptors and physiologic tracer uptake by the liver, thus, concluded that FDOPA PET/CT was superior on both per-

patient and per-lesion analyses. FDOPA was positive in all five patients with known lesions and in eight of 13 patients with negative or inconclusive results on conventional imaging.[99] **Fig. 11** shows ⁶⁸Ga-DOTATATE in the post-operative thyroid bed in a patient of MTC.

Cholecystokinin Receptor Subtype 2/Gastrin Receptors and Gastrin Receptor Scintigraphy

The cholecystokinin receptor subtype 2 is an important promoter of tumor growth. It has been shown to be expressed in normal C cells and over-expressed in numerous NETs, including MTC.[100,101] Two DOTA-minigastrin analogs radio-labeled with ¹¹¹In and ⁶⁸ Ga were evaluated in a preclinical in vivo model and showed higher uptake than ⁶⁸Ga-labeled cyclic DOTA-peptides.[102,103]

¹¹C-Methionine PET in Medullary Thyroid Cancer

¹¹C-Methionine PET was more sensitive for the detection of cervical lymph nodes in MTC when compared with ¹⁸F-FDG, but not better than neck US or a combination of ¹⁸F-FDG PET with neck US.[104] In one study, ¹¹C-Methionine, as well as ¹⁸F-FDG, was more sensitive in cases of elevated calcitonin with a cutoff> 370 pg/mL (1358 pmol/L); however, the high physiologic uptake of ¹¹C-MET in the liver that limits visualization of hepatic metastases.[104]

PET Immunoimaging in Medullary Thyroid Cancer

Using directly labeled antibodies, their fragments, or antibody-derived recombinant constructs has been proposed for the radionuclide targeting of tumors. Immuno-PET using anti-CEA antibodies labeled with ^{111}In, ^{131}I, or ^{68}Ga was reported to be potentially accurate for detecting relapsing MTC.[105] Further studies are required to confirm the accuracy of this new technique.[10,105]

PET-Computed Tomography in Primary Thyroid Lymphoma

PTL is an uncommon malignancy primarily affecting elderly females (age-group: 50–80 years), with increased incidence in the background of Hashimoto's thyroiditis. It comprises of less than 5% of all thyroid malignancies, 1% to 2.5% of all lymphomas, and 2.5% to 7% of all ENLs.[106,107] Most of the PTLs are being non-Hodgkin's lymphoma (NHL) among which greater than two-thirds of the patients have diffuse large B-cell lymphoma followed by follicular (10%), marginal zone or mucosal-associated lymphoid tissue (MALT) (10%), and small lymphocytic lymphoma (3%) subtypes. Like ENLs of other sites, FDG PET/CT has evolved as the state-of-the-art imaging in PTL, playing important role in for initial staging and re-staging, therapy response assessment (interim & end-of-treatment) and follow-up, and aiding in management decisions.[108]

SUMMARY

In summary, PET/CT studies can be potentially useful in elderly thyroid carcinoma patients for exploring the disease biology, especially in metastatic setting and thereby directing appropriate diagnostic and therapeutic management on case-to-case basis, nuclear theranostics, and disease prognostication. With the availability of various PET radiopharmaceuticals, it would be worthwhile to evolve and optimally use the investigational and non-FDG PET/CT tracers as per the clinical need and their utilities in a given case scenario.

CLINICS CARE POINTS

- The elderly patients demonstrate a higher incidence of aggressive histologic subtypes and poor differentiation status and higher documentation of local invasiveness, lateral-sided lymph node involvement in the neck, and vascular invasion.

- An age cutoff of 55 years has been identified as an important predictive factor for disease prognosis in differentiated thyroid carcinoma.

- In patients with thyroglobulin elevation with negative iodine scintigraphy (TENIS), fluoro-deoxyglucose (FDG)-PET/computed tomography (CT) plays an important role in evaluating whole body disease burden and directly impacting the treatment decision-making: (a) patients who on FDG-PET imaging show only active nodal disease can are considered for surgery; (b) those who have been originally planned for empirical radioactive iodine therapy, if FDG-PET/CT shows no definite evidence of disease, further RAI therapy can be deferred and only observation on TSH suppression can be considered; (c) if FDG-PET/CT reveals progressive and extensive inoperable disease, other treatment options (eg, tyrosine kinase inhibitors/radiation therapy) may be considered.

- Theranostic PET-CTs (^{68}Ga-DOTATATE/^{68}Ga-PSMA-11) are employed to assess SSTR/PSMA expression in the lesions in patients with TENIS and evaluated the suitability for targeted radionuclide therapies. Their present status is investigational.

- In medullary thyroid carcinoma, PET-CT imaging with FDG, ^{68}Ga-DOTATATE/NOC or ^{18}F-DOPA is considered to delineate disease burden in the presence of high calcitonin levels and guide further treatment.

DISCLOSURE

The authors have nothing to disclose.

REFERENCES

1. Girardi FM. Thyroid carcinoma pattern presentation according to age. Int Arch Otorhinolaryngol 2017; 21(1):38–41.
2. Noone AM, Howlader N, Krapcho M, et al. In: SEER cancer statistics review, 1975-2015. Bethesda, MD: National Cancer Institute; 2018. Available at: https://seer.cancer.gov/csr/1975_2015/, based on November 2017 SEER data submission, posted to the SEER web site. Accessed 13 September 2022.
3. Fagin JA, Wells SA Jr. Biologic and clinical perspectives on thyroid cancer. N Engl J Med 2016; 375:1054–67.
4. Nixon IJ, Wang LY, Migliacci JC, et al. An international multi-institutional validation of age 55 Years as a cutoff for risk stratification in the AJCC/UICC staging system for well-differentiated thyroid cancer. Thyroid 2016;26(3):373–80.

5. Koshkina A, Fazelzad R, Sugitani I, et al. Association of patient Age with progression of low-risk papillary thyroid carcinoma under active surveillance: a systematic review and meta-analysis. JAMA Otolaryngol Head Neck Surg 2020;146(6): 552–60.

6. Zambeli-Ljepović A, Wang F, Dinan MA, et al. Low-risk thyroid cancer in elderly: total thyroidectomy/RAI predominates but lacks survival advantage. J Surg Res 2019;243:189–97. Epub 2019 Jun 8. PMID: 31185435; PMCID: PMC6773493.

7. Poma AM, Macerola E, Basolo A, et al. Fine-needle aspiration cytology and histological types of thyroid cancer in the elderly: evaluation of 9070 patients from a single referral centre. Cancers (Basel) 2021;13(4):907. PMCID: PMC7926485.

8. Wang Z, Vyas CM, Van Benschoten O, et al. Quantitative analysis of the benefits and risk of thyroid nodule evaluation in patients ≥70 Years old. Thyroid 2018;28(4):465–71. PubMed.

9. Lechner MG, Hershman JM. Thyroid nodules and cancer in the elderly. In: Feingold KR, Anawalt B, Boyce A, et al, editors. Endotext [internet]. South Dartmouth (MA): MDText.com, Inc.; 2000. Available at: https://www.ncbi.nlm.nih.gov/books/NBK278969/.

10. Chereau N, Trésallet C, Noullet S, et al. Prognosis of papillary thyroid carcinoma in elderly patients after thyroid resection: a retrospective cohort analysis. Medicine (Baltimore) 2016;95(47):e5450 [PMC free article] [PubMed].

11. Lin JD, Chao TC, Chen ST, et al. Characteristics of thyroid carcinomas in aging patients. Eur J Clin Invest 2000;30:147–53.

12. Payne RJ, Bastianelli M, Mlynarek AM, et al. Is age associated with risk of malignancy in thyroid cancer? Otolaryngol Head Neck Surg 2014;151(5): 746–50. PubMed.

13. Lennard CM, Patel A, Wilson J, et al. Intensity of vascular endothelial growth factor expression is associated with increased risk of recurrence and decreased disease-free survival in papillary thyroid cancer. Surgery 2001;129(5):552–8.

14. Godballe C, Asschenfeldt P, Jørgensen KE, et al. Prognostic factors in papillary and follicular thyroid carcinomas: p53 expression is a significant indicator of prognosis. Laryngoscope 1998;108(2):243–9.

15. Brierley JD, Gospodarowicz MK, Wittekind C. TNM classification of malignant tumours. 8th ed. Weinheim, Germany: John Wiley & Sons; 2017. p. 69–71.

16. Hay ID, Bergstralh EJ, Goellner JR, et al. Predicting outcome in papillary thyroid carcinoma: development of a reliable prognostic scoring system in a cohort of 1779 patients surgically treated at one institution during 1940 through 1989. Surgery 1993;114(6):1050–7.

17. Davis NL, Bugis SP, McGregor GI, et al. An evaluation of prognostic scoring systems in patients with follicular thyroid cancer. Am J Surg 1995;170(5): 476–80.

18. Ylli D, Burman KD, Van Nostrand D, et al. Eliminating the age cutoff in staging of differentiated thyroid cancer: the safest road? J Clin Endocrinol Metab 2018;103(5):1813–7.

19. Ito Y, Miyauchi A, Jikuzono T, et al. Risk factors contributing to a poor prognosis of papillary thyroid carcinoma: validity of UICC/AJCC TNM classification and stage grouping. World J Surg 2007; 31(4):838–48.

20. Sugino K, Ito K, Nagahama M, et al. Prognosis and prognostic factors for distant metastases and tumor mortality in follicular thyroid carcinoma. Thyroid 2011;21(7):751–7.

21. Halnan KE. Influence of age and sex on incidence and prognosis of thyroid cancer. Cancer 1966;19: 1534–6.

22. Cady B, Sedgwick CE, Meissner WA, et al. Risk factor analysis in differentiated thyroid cancer. Cancer 1979;43:810–20.

23. Orosco RK, Hussain T, Brumund KT, et al. Analysis of age and disease status as predictors of thyroid cancer-specific mortality using the Surveillance, Epidemiology, and End Results database. Thyroid 2015;25(1):125–32.

24. Kauffmann RM, Hamner JB, Ituarte PHG, et al. Age greater than 60 years portends a worse prognosis in patients with papillary thyroid cancer: should there be three age categories for staging? BMC Cancer18 2018;316. https://doi.org/10.1186/s12885-018-4181-4.

25. Natalya Rukhman& Alan Silverberg. Thyroid cancer in older men. Aging Male 2011;14(2):91–8.

26. Ganly I, Nixon IJ, Wang LY, et al. Survival from differentiated thyroid cancer: what has age got to do with it? Thyroid 2015;25(10):1106–14.

27. Ito Y, Kudo T, Takamura Y, et al. Prognostic factors of papillary thyroid carcinoma vary according to sex and patient age. World J Surg 2011;35: 2684–90.

28. Urhan M, Basu S, Alavi A. PET scan in thyroid cancer. PET Clin 2012;7(4):453–61. Epub 2012 Aug 24. PMID: 27157651.

29. Nascimento C, Borget I, Al Ghuzlan A, et al. Postoperative fluorine-18-fluorodeoxyglucose positron emission tomography/computed tomography: an important imaging modality in patients with aggressive histology of differentiated thyroid cancer. Thyroid 2015;25(4):437–44. Epub 2015 Mar 16. PMID: 25633259.

30. Karantanis D, Bogsrud TV, Wiseman GA, et al. Clinical significance of diffusely increased ^{18}F-FDG uptake in the thyroid gland. J Nucl Med 2007;48: 896–901.

31. Nilsson IL, Arnberg F, Zedenius J, et al. Thyroid incidentaloma detected by fluorodeoxyglucose positron emission tomography/computed tomography: practical management algorithm. World J Surg 2011;35(12):2691–7.

32. Ladrón de Guevara HD, Munizaga MC, García SN, et al. Frecuencia de malignidaden incidentalomas tiroideosdetectados con tomografíaporemisión de positrones/tomografíacomputada (PET/CT) con F18-FDG de cuerpoentero [Frequency of malignancy in thyroid incidentalomas detected by whole body 18F-FDG PET/CT]. Rev Med Chil 2020; 148(1):10–6. Spanish. doi: . PMID: 32730431.

33. Soelberg KK, Bonnema SJ, Brix TH, et al. Risk of malignancy in thyroid incidentalomas detected by 18F-fluorodeoxyglucose positron emission tomography: a systematic review. Thyroid 2012;22:918.

34. Sollini M, Cozzi L, Pepe G, et al. [^{18}F]FDG-PET/CT texture analysis in thyroid incidentalomas: preliminary results. Eur J Hybrid Imaging 2017;1(1):3. Epub 2017 Oct 12. PMID: 29782578; PMCID: PMC5954705.

35. Wiebel JL, Esfandiari NH, Papaleontiou M, et al. Evaluating positron emission tomography use in differentiated thyroid cancer. Thyroid 2015;25(9): 1026–32. Epub 2015 Aug 3. PMID: 26133765; PMCID: PMC4560853.

36. Poisson T, Deandreis D, Leboulleux S, et al. ^{18}F-fluorodeoxyglucose positron emission tomography and computed tomography in anaplastic thyroid cancer. Eur J Nucl Med Mol Imaging 2010;37: 2277–85 [Crossref][Medline][Google Scholar].

37. Smallridge RC, Ain KB, Asa SL, et al. American Thyroid Association guidelines for management of patients with anaplastic thyroid cancer. Thyroid 2012;22:1104–39.

38. Schütz F, Lautenschläger C, Lorenz K, et al. Positron emission tomography (PET) and PET/CT in thyroid cancer: a systematic review and meta-analysis. Eur Thyroid J 2018;7(1):13–20. Epub 2017 Oct 24. PMID: 29594049; PMCID: PMC5836193.

39. Pacini F, Castagna MG, Brilli L, et al. Thyroid cancer: ESMO Clinical Practice Guidelines for diagnosis, treatment and follow-up. Ann Oncol 2012; 23:vii110–9.

40. GrabellusF NJ, BockischA SKW, SheuSY. Glucose transporter 1 expression, tumor proliferation, and iodine/glucose uptake in thyroid cancer with emphasis on poorly differentiated thyroid carcinoma. Clin Nucl Med 2012;37:121–7.

41. Kuo CS, Tang KT, Lin JD, et al. Diffuse sclerosing variant of papillary thyroid carcinoma with multiple metastases and elevated serum carcinoembryonic antigen level. Thyroid 2012;22(11):1187–90. View at: Publisher Site | Google Scholar.

42. Giovanella L, Fasolini F, Suriano S, et al. Hyperfunctioning solid/trabecular follicular carcinoma of the thyroid gland. J Oncol 2010;2010:4.

43. Diehl M, Graichen S, Menzel C, et al. F-18 FDG PET in insular thyroid cancer. Clin Nucl Med 2003;28(9): 728–31. View at: Publisher Site.

44. Deandreis D, Al Ghuzlan A, Leboulleux S, et al. Do histological, immunohistochemical, and metabolic (radioiodine and fluorodeoxyglucose uptakes) patterns of metastatic thyroid cancer correlate with patient outcome? Endocrine-Related Cancer 2011; 18(1):159–69. View at: Publisher Site | Google Scholar.

45. Treglia G, Annunziata S, Muoio B, et al. The role of fluorine-18-fluorodeoxyglucose positron emission tomography in aggressive histological subtypes of thyroid cancer: an overview. Int J Endocrinol 2013;2013:856189. Epub 2013 Apr 9. PMID: 23653645; PMCID: PMC3638656.

46. Yadav D, Shah K, Naidoo K, et al. PET/Computed tomography in thyroid cancer. Neuroimaging Clin N Am 2021;31(3):345–57.

47. Treglia G, Bertagna F, Piccardo A, et al. ^{131}I whole-body scan or ^{18}FDG PET/CT for patients with elevated thyroglobulin and negative ultrasound? Clin Translat Imaging 2013;1:175–83 [Crossref] [Google Scholar].

48. Jeong Won L, Sang Mi L, Dae Ho L, et al. Clinical utility of ^{18}F-FDG PET/CT concurrent with ^{131}I therapy in intermediate–to–high-risk patients with differentiated thyroid cancer: dual-center experience with 286 patients. J Nucl Med August 2013; 54(8):1230–6.

49. Khan N, Oriuchi N, Higuchi T, et al. PET in the follow-up of differentiated thyroid cancer. Br J Radiol 2003;76(910):690–5.

50. Razfar A, Branstetter BF4th, Christopoulos A, et al. Clinical usefulness of positron emission tomography-computed tomography in recurrent thyroid carcinoma. Arch Otolaryngol Head Neck Surg 2010;136:120–5.

51. Abraham T, Schoder H. Thyroid cancer: indications and opportunities for positron emission tomography/computed tomography imaging. Semin Nucl Med 2011;41:121–38 [Crossref][Medline][Google Scholar].

52. Saif MW, Tzannou I, Makrilia N, et al. Role and cost effectiveness of PET/CT in management of patients with cancer. Yale J Biol Med 2010;83:53–65 [Medline].

53. Cooper DS, Doherty GM, Haugen BR, et al. Revised American thyroid association management guidelines for patients with thyroid nodules and differentiated thyroid cancer. Thyroid 2009; 19(11):1167–214. View at: Publisher Site | Google Scholar.

54. Robbins RJ, Wan Q, Grewal RK, et al. Real-time prognosis for metastatic thyroid carcinoma based on 2-[18F]fluoro-2-deoxy-D-glucose-positron emission tomography scanning. J Clin Endocrinol Metab 2006;91:498–505.

55. Kebebew E, Greenspan FS, Clark OH, et al. Anaplastic thyroid carcinoma. Treatment outcome and prognostic factors. Cancer 2005;103:1330.

56. Nagaiah G, Hossain A, Mooney CJ, et al. Anaplastic thyroid cancer: a review of epidemiology, pathogenesis, and treatment. J Oncol 2011;2011:542358.

57. Mosci C, Iagaru A. PET/CT imaging of thyroid cancer. Clin Nucl Med 2011;36:e180–5.

58. Treglia G, Muoio B, Giovanella L, et al. The role of positron emission tomography and positron emission tomography/computed tomography in thyroid tumours: an overview. Eur Arch Otorhinolaryngol 2013;270:1783–7.

59. Bogsrud TV, Karantanis D, Nathan MA, et al. ^{18}F-FDG PET in the management of patients with anaplastic thyroid carcinoma. Thyroid 2008;18:713–9.

60. Civan C, Isik EG, Simsek DH. Metastatic poorly differentiated thyroid cancer with heterogeneous distribution of 18F-FDG, 68Ga-DOTATATE, and 68Ga-PSMA on PET/CT. Clin Nucl Med 2021; 46(4):e212–3. PMID: 33156050.

61. Basu S, Parghane RV, Naik C. Clinical efficacy of ^{177}Lu-DOTATATE peptide receptor radionuclide therapy in thyroglobulin-elevated negative iodine scintigraphy: a "not-so-promising" result compared with GEP-NETs. World J Nucl Med 2020;19(3): 205–10. PMID: 33354174; PMCID: PMC7745860.

62. Kiess AP, Banerjee SR, Mease RC, et al. Prostate-specific membrane antigen as a target for cancer imaging and therapy. Q J Nucl Med Mol Imaging 2015;59:241–68.

63. Iwano S, Kato K, Ito S, et al. FDG-PET performed concurrently with initial I-131 ablation for differentiated thyroid cancer. Ann Nucl Med 2012;26(3): 207–13. Epub 2011 Dec 10. PMID: 22160654.

64. Shie P, Cardarelli R, Sprawls K, et al. Systematic review: prevalence of malignant incidental thyroid nodules identified on fluorine-18 fluorodeoxyglucose positron emission tomography. Nucl Med Commun 2009;30:742–8 [Crossref][Medline][Google Scholar].

65. Grünwald F, Menzel C, Bender H, et al. Comparison of [18]FDG-PET with [131]iodine and ^{99m}Tc-sestamibi scintigraphy in differentiated thyroid cancer. Thyroid 1997;7:327–35 [Crossref][Medline][Google Scholar].

66. Freudenberg LS, Antoch G, Jentzen W, et al. Value of [124]I-PET/CT in staging of patients with differentiated thyroid cancer. EurRadiol 2004;14:2092–8.

67. Lubberink M, Abdul Fatah S, Brans B, et al. The role of [124]I-PET in diagnosis and treatment of thyroid carcinoma. Q J Nucl Med Mol Imaging 2008; 52:30–6.

68. Budiawan H, Salavati A, Kulkarni HR, et al. Peptide receptor radionuclide therapy of treatment-refractory metastatic thyroid cancer using (90) Yttrium and (177)Lutetium labeled somatostatin analogs: toxicity, response and survival analysis. Am J Nucl Med Mol Imaging 2013;4:39–52.

69. Versari A, Sollini M, Frasoldati A, et al. Differentiated thyroid cancer: a new perspective with radiolabeled somatostatin analogues for imaging and treatment of patients. Thyroid 2014;24:715–26.

70. Görges R, Kahaly G, Müller-Brand J, et al. Radionuclide-labeled somatostatin analogues for diagnostic and therapeutic purposes in nonmedullary thyroid cancer. Thyroid 2001;11:647–59.

71. Mourato FA, Almeida MA, Brito AE, et al. FDG PET/CT versus somatostatin receptor PET/CT in TENIS syndrome: a systematic review and meta-analysis. Clin Transl Imaging 2020;8:365–75.

72. Chang SS, Reuter VE, Heston WD, et al. Five different anti-prostate specific membrane antigen (PSMA) antibodies confirm PSMA expression in tumor-associated neovasculature. Cancer Res 1999;59:3192–8.

73. Wächter S, Di Fazio P, Maurer E, et al. Prostate-specific membrane antigen in anaplastic and poorly differentiated thyroid cancer-A new diagnostic and therapeutic target? Cancers (Basel) 2021;13(22):5688.

74. Sollini M, di Tommaso L, Kirienko M, et al. PSMA expression level predicts differentiated thyroid cancer aggressiveness and patient outcome. EJNMMI Res 2019;9:93.

75. Folkman J. Tumor angiogenesis. In: Mendelsohn J, Howley P, Liotta L, et al, editors. The molecular basis of cancer. Philadelphia, PA, USA: WB Saunders; 1995. p. 206–32.

76. Ribatti D, Vacca A, Dammacco F. The role of the vascular phase in solid tumor growth: a historical review. Neoplasia 1999;1:293–302.

77. Ramsden J.D. Angiogenesis in the thyroid gland. J. Endocrinol 2000;166:475–80.

78. Sprindzuk MV. Angiogenesis in malignant thyroid tumors. World J Oncol 2010;1:221–31.

79. Mousa SA, Lin H-Y, Tang HY, et al. Modulation of angiogenesis by thyroid hormone and hormone analogues: implications for cancer management. Angiogenesis 2014;17:463–9.

80. De La Torre NG, Buley I, Wass JAH, et al. Angiogenesis and lymphangiogenesis in thyroid proliferative lesions: relationship to type and tumour behaviour. Endocr.-Relat Cancer 2006;13:931–44.

81. Pierotti MA, Bongarzone I, Borello MG, et al. Cytogenetics and molecular genetics of carcinomas arising from thyroid epithelial follicular cells. Genes Chromosomes Cancer 1996;16:1–14.

82. Parihar AS, Mittal BR, Kumar R, et al. ^{68}Ga-DOTA-RGD$_2$ positron emission tomography/computed tomography in radioiodine refractory thyroid cancer: prospective comparison of diagnostic accuracy with ^{18}F-FDG positron emission

tomography/computed tomography and evaluation toward potential theranostics. Thyroid 2020; 30(4):557–67.

83. O'Doherty J, Jauregui-Osoro M, Brothwood T, et al. ^{18}F-Tetrafluoroborate, a PET probe for imaging sodium/iodide symporter expression: whole-body biodistribution, safety, and radiation dosimetry in thyroid cancer patients. J Nucl Med 2017;58(10): 1666–71.

84. Jiang H, DeGrado TR. [18F]Tetrafluoroborate ([18F] TFB) and its analogs for PET imaging of the sodium/iodide symporter. Theranostics 2018;8(14): 3918–31.

85. Samnick S, Al-Momani E, Schmid JS, et al. Initial clinical investigation of [18F]tetrafluoroborate PET/ CT in comparison to [124I]iodine PET/CT for imaging thyroid cancer. Clin Nucl Med 2018;43(3): 162–7. PMID: 29356744.

86. Dittmann M, Gonzalez Carvalho JM, Rahbar K, et al. Incremental diagnostic value of [18F]tetrafluoroborate PET-CT compared with [131I]iodine scintigraphy in recurrent differentiated thyroid cancer. Eur J Nucl Med Mol Imaging 2020;47(11): 2639–46. Epub 2020 Apr 4. PMID: 32248325; PMCID: PMC7515952.

87. Ballal S, Yadav MP, Moon ES, et al. Biodistribution, pharmacokinetics, dosimetry of [68Ga]Ga-DOTA.SA.FAPi, and the head-to-head comparison with [18F]F-FDG PET/CT in patients with various cancers. Eur J Nucl Med Mol Imaging 2021;48(6):1915–31. Epub 2020 Nov 26. PMID: 33244617.

88. Blau M, Nagler W, Bender MA. A new isotope for bone scanning. J Nucl Med 1962;3:332–4.

89. Groves AM, Win Th, Ben Haim S, et al. Non-[18F] FDG PET in clinical oncology. Lancet Oncol 2007; 8:822–30.

90. Even-Sapir E, Metser U, Flusser G, et al. Assessment of malignant skeletal disease with 18F-fluoride PET/CT. J Nucl Med 2004;45:272–8.

91. Beuthien-Baumann B, Strumpf A, Zessin J, et al. Diagnostic impact of PET with [18F-FDG, [18F-DOPA and 3-O-methyl-6-[18F]fluoro-DOPA in recurrent or metastatic medullary thyroid carcinoma. Eur J Nucl Med Mol Imaging 2007;34:1604–9 [Crossref] [Medline][Google Scholar].

92. Kauhanen S, Seppänen M, Ovaska J, et al. The clinical value of [18F]fluoro-dihydroxyphenylalanine positron emission tomography in primary diagnosis, staging, and restaging of neuroendocrine tumors. EndocrRelat Cancer 2009;16:255–65 [Crossref][Medline][Google Scholar].

93. Treglia G, Villani MF, Giordano A, et al. Detection rate of recurrent medullary thyroid carcinoma using fluorine-18 fluorodeoxyglucose positron emission tomography: a meta-analysis. Endocrine

2012;42(3):535–45. Epub 2012 Apr 17. PMID: 22527889.

94. Bogsrud TV, Karantanis D, Nathan MA, et al. The prognostic value of 2-deoxy-2-[18F]fluoro-D-glucose positron emission tomography in patients with suspected residual or recurrent medullary thyroid carcinoma. Mol Imaging Biol 2010;12(5):547–53. Epub 2009 Dec 1. PMID: 19949985.

95. Slavikova K, Montravers F, Treglia G, et al. What is currently the best radiopharmaceutical for the hybrid PET/CT detection of recurrent medullary thyroid carcinoma? Curr Radiopharm 2013;6(2).

96. Verbeek HHG, Plukker JTM, Koopmans KP, et al. Clinical relevance of 18F-FDG PET and 18F-DOPA PET in recurrent medullary thyroid carcinoma. J Nucl Med 2012;53(12):1863–71.

97. Beheshti M, Pöcher S, Vali R, et al. The value of [18F]-DOPA PET-CT in patients with medullary thyroid carcinoma: comparison with [18F]-FDG PET-CT. EurRadiol 2009;19:1425–34 [Crossref][Medline][Google Scholar].

98. Conry BG, Papathanasiou ND, Prakash V, et al. Comparison of ^{68}Ga-DOTATATE and ^{18}F-fluorodeoxyglucose PET/CT in the detection of recurrent medullary thyroid carcinoma. Eur J Nucl Med Mol Imaging 2010;37:49–57 [Crossref][Medline][Google Scholar].

99. Treglia G, Castaldi P, Villani MF, et al. Comparison of [18F]-DOPA, [18F]-FDG and ^{68}Ga-somatostatin analogue PET/CT in patients with recurrent medullary thyroid carcinoma. Eur J Nucl Med Mol Imaging 2012;39:569–80 [Crossref][Medline][Google Scholar].

100. Reubi JC. Targeting CCK receptors in human cancers. Curr Top Med Chem 2007;7(12):1239–42.

101. Bläker M, de Weerth A, Tometten M, et al. Expression of the cholecystokinin 2-receptor in normal human thyroid gland and medullary thyroid carcinoma. Eur J Endocrinol 2002;146(1): 89–96.

102. Von Guggenberg E, Rangger C, Sosabowski J, et al. Preclinical evaluation of radiolabeled DOTA-derivatized cyclic minigastrin analogs for targeting cholecystokinin receptor expressing malignancies. Mol Imaging Biol 2012;14(3): 366–75.

103. Santhanam P, Solnes LB, Rowe SP. Molecular imaging of advanced thyroid cancer: iodinated radiotracers and beyond. Med Oncol 2017;34(12):189. Erratum in: Med Oncol. 2017 Dec 12;35(1):10. PMID: 29086115.

104. Jang HW, Choi JY, Lee JI, et al. Localization of medullary thyroid carcinoma after surgery using (11)C-methionine PET/CT: comparison with

(18)F-FDG PET/CT. Endocr J 2010;57(12): 1045–54.

105. Bodet-Milin C, Faivre-Chauvet A, Carlier T, et al. Immuno-PET using anticarcinoembryonic antigen bispecific antibody and ^{68}Ga-labeled peptide in metastatic medullary thyroid carcinoma: clinical optimization of the pretargeting parameters in a first-in-human trial. J Nucl Med 2016;57(10): 1505–11.

106. Graff-Baker A, Roman SA, Thomas DC, et al. Prognosis of primary thyroid lymphoma: demographic, clinical, and pathologic predictors of survival in 1,408 cases. Surgery 2009;146(6):1105–15.

107. Ruggiero FP, Frauenhoffer E, Stack BC. Thyroid lymphoma: a single institution's experience. Otolaryngol Neck Surg 2005;133(6):888–96.

108. Basu S, Li G, Bural G, et al. Fluorodeoxyglucose positron emission tomography (FDG-PET) and PET/computed tomography imaging characteristics of thyroid lymphoma and their potential clinical utility. Acta Radiol Stockh Swed 1987 2009;50(2):201–4.

Brain PET Imaging
Approach to Cognitive Impairment and Dementia

Matthew Spano, MD[a], Michelle Roytman, MD[a], Mariam Aboian, MD, PhD[b],
Babak Saboury, MD MPH[c], Ana M. Franceschi, MD PhD[d],
Gloria C. Chiang, MD[a,*]

KEYWORDS

- Positron emission tomography • Alzheimer disease • Dementia • Amyloid • Tau
- Neurodegeneration

KEY POINTS

- Specific PET tracers allow for in vivo localization of amyloid and tau, the pathologic hallmarks of Alzheimer disease (AD).
- An understanding of the different distributions of decreased ^{18}F-fluorodeoxyglucose avidity can help differentiate typical AD from AD variants and other common neurodegenerative diseases, such as frontotemporal dementia.
- Several new PET radiotracers are actively being researched and show potential in the diagnosis and management of neurodegenerative diseases.

INTRODUCTION

Alzheimer disease (AD) is the most common cause of dementia, accounting for 50% to 60% of cases and affecting nearly 6 million people in the United States. The prevalence is projected to increase to 14 million people by the year 2050.[1] Despite its prevalence, the diagnosis of AD remains difficult because clinical symptoms are often nonspecific. Definitive diagnosis requires either antemortem brain biopsy or postmortem autopsy. However, clinical neuroimaging has been playing a greater role in the diagnosis and management of AD, and several positron emission tomography (PET) tracers approach the sensitivity of tissue diagnosis in identifying AD pathologic condition. This review will focus on the utility of PET imaging in the setting of cognitive impairment, with an emphasis on its role in the diagnosis of AD.

PATHOPHYSIOLOGY OF ALZHEIMER DISEASE

In 1906, Alois Alzheimer first described the 2 neuropathologic hallmarks of AD: amyloid plaques and neurofibrillary tangles (NFTs). Amyloid plaques are extracellular deposits of beta-amyloid (Aβ) in the brain parenchyma, and NFTs are intracellular hyperphosphorylated paired helical filaments of tau protein.

The amyloid cascade hypothesis remains the most widely accepted theory to explain the pathogenesis of AD, with the deposition of Aβ plaques in the brain inciting a pathological cascade that leads to NFTs, neuronal loss, and cognitive impairment. This hypothesis has formed the basis of the 2018 "ATN" research framework of AD, put forth by the National Institute on Aging and Alzheimer's Association.[2] "ATN" reflects 3 stages of disease, with "A" representing Aβ deposition, "T" tau

---

[a] Department of Radiology, Weill Cornell Medicine, NewYork-Presbyterian Hospital, 525 East 68th Street, Starr Pavilion, Box 141, New York, NY 10065, USA; [b] Department of Radiology, Yale School of Medicine, 330 Cedar Street, New Haven, CT 06520, USA; [c] Department of Radiology and Imaging Sciences, NIH Clinical Center, 10 Center Dr, Bethesda, MD 20892, USA; [d] Department of Radiology, Northwell Health/Donald and Barbara Zucker School of Medicine, Lenox Hill Hospital, 100 East 77th Street, 3rd Floor, New York, NY 10075, USA
* Corresponding author. Division of Neuroradiology
E-mail address: gcc9004@med.cornell.edu

PET Clin 18 (2023) 103–113
https://doi.org/10.1016/j.cpet.2022.09.006
1556-8598/23/© 2022 Elsevier Inc. All rights reserved.

pet.theclinics.com

deposition, and "N" neurodegeneration. Histopathological literature has described characteristic patterns of spread of Aβ and tau. Aβ has been shown to deposit in the neocortex early, before spreading to the allocortex, diencephalic nuclei, striatum, cholinergic nuclei of the basal forebrain, brainstem, and finally cerebellum.[3] However, NFT deposition begins in the transentorhinal cortex, before spreading to the hippocampus and association neocortex,[4] closely tracking synaptic loss and neurodegeneration. NFTs typically spare the motor, somatosensory, and visual cortices until late in the disease course.

Neuroimaging techniques by MR imaging and PET have been developed to track the ATN stages in vivo. In addition, because the complexity of AD has become known, other PET tracers have been developed to explore synaptic function, cholinergic function, dopaminergic function, and neuroinflammation.[5]

CLINICAL STANDARD-OF-CARE IMAGING
MR Imaging

When a patient presents with cognitive symptoms, clinical standard-of-care typically begins with structural MRI to exclude a potentially treatable condition, although uncommon. A 2003 meta-analysis found that 0.9% of dementia cases were secondary to a reversible cause, with 0.6% of cases successfully reversed.[6] Diagnostic considerations for partially or fully reversible dementias may include brain masses, chronic subdural hematomas, adverse drug effects, depression, alcohol use, and systemic endocrine and nutritional deficiencies. Normal pressure hydrocephalus (NPH) is another potentially reversible cause of cognitive impairment, characterized by a classic triad of ataxia, urinary incontinence, and dementia. MR imaging findings of NPH include an acute callosal angle, disproportionate ventricular enlargement, gyral crowding at the vertex, and enlarged Sylvian fissures (**Fig. 1**).[7] When identified early, symptoms can be responsive to ventricular shunt placement.

Beyond excluding reversible causes of cognitive impairment, MR imaging can also be useful in identifying brain atrophy, particularly of the hippocampi, which are commonly affected early in AD. Qualitative MR assessment of hippocampal atrophy can be supplemented with quantitative metrics, such as measuring hippocampal volumes with U.S. Food and Drug Administration (FDA)-approved software such as Neuroquant (Cortechs.ai) (https://www.cortechs.ai/products/neuroquant/), Neuroreader (Brainreader Inc) (https://brainreader.net/), and Icometrix (Icometrix) (https://icometrix.com/). Using such software packages, hippocampal volumes from the patient can be compared with a database of normal controls, matched for age, sex, and intracranial volume. However, there is evidence that visual assessment of medial temporal lobe atrophy has similar accuracy as quantitative hippocampal volumes,[8] and volumes alone do not have high enough accuracies to diagnose AD.[9] One meta-analysis of 33 studies and almost 4000 subjects found that hippocampal volumes had a pooled mean sensitivity and specificity of 73% and 71%, respectively, for diagnosing AD.[9] Atrophy of the medial temporal lobe had a pooled mean sensitivity and specificity of 64% and 65%, respectively, and lateral ventricular volumes had a pooled mean sensitivity and specificity of only 57% and 64%, respectively.

^{18}F-Fluorodeoxyglucose-PET

^{18}F-Fluorodeoxyglucose (FDG) PET is another noninvasive imaging modality commonly used to diagnose AD. FDG-PET assesses cerebral glucose metabolism, which is typically decreased in the posterior cingulate, precuneus, and temporoparietal cortex in AD,[10] due to decreased synaptic density and function. A meta-analysis of 119 studies from 1990 to 2010 showed that FDG-PET has a high accuracy in differentiating AD from normal controls, with 90% sensitivity and 89% specificity, compared with 83% sensitivity and 89% specificity by MR imaging.[11] In clinical practice, FDG-PET is covered by the US Centers for Medicare and Medicaid Services to differentiate AD and frontotemporal dementia (FTD) in individuals who have had cognitive impairment for more than 6 months. Unlike AD, FTD is characterized by decreased FDG avidity in the frontal and temporal lobes.[12]

Beyond visually identifying regional patterns of decreased FDG avidity, quantitative assessment of FDG-PET can be useful clinically to detect more subtle areas of hypometabolism. Automated software packages can be used to coregister FDG-PET images to an atlas of normal brain images from individuals in a similar age range (**Fig. 2**). FDG uptake in atlas-based anatomic regions are then compared between the patient and the normal controls. Z-scores are obtained for each anatomic region, which reflect the degree of decreased FDG avidity in each region, compared with the normal controls. These Z-scores can be used to confirm whether the pattern of decreased FDG avidity is most compatible with AD or FTD (**Figs. 3–5**). Several articles that have investigated whether automated quantitative methods for assessing regional FDG uptake

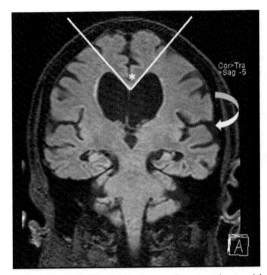

Fig. 1. Coronal T2 FLAIR image in a patient with normal pressure hydrocephalus. The lateral ventricles are dilated out of proportion to sulcal prominence, there is an acute callosal angle (*), and there is widening of the Sylvian fissures (*arrow*).

improve detection of AD have reported an increase in specificities from approximately 58% to 84% for visual assessment to 87% to 98% with quantitative assessment.[13–15] However, sensitivities for detecting AD are similar, ranging from 73% to 85% for visual assessment and 73% to 98% for quantitative assessment.

In addition to differentiating AD and FTD, FDG-PET can be useful in diagnosing atypical forms of AD. For example, patients with posterior cortical atrophy, commonly considered the "visual variant of AD," have decreased FDG avidity in the temporal and parietal lobes, similar to typical AD but also in the occipital lobes (**Fig. 6**).[16] Involvement of the occipital lobes is typically more asymmetric than in dementia with Lewy bodies (**Fig. 7**). Cerebral amyloid angiopathy (**Fig. 8**) would be another entity to consider with occipital lobe involvement and can be seen concomitantly with AD.[17] Patients with logopenic variant primary progressive aphasia (PPA), the "language variant of AD," typically have decreased FDG avidity in the temporal and parietal lobes, but it is typically asymmetric,

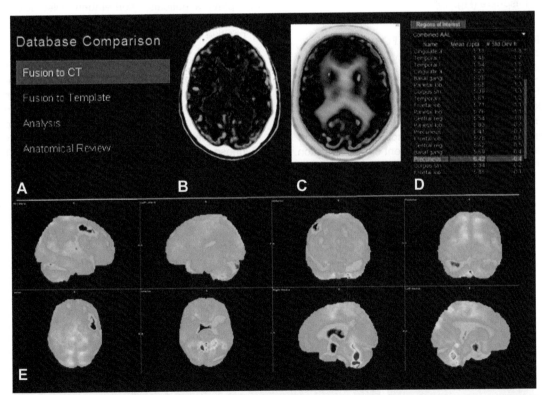

Fig. 2. Typical workflow when comparing a patient's FDG-PET scan with a normative database. Steps (*A*) include fusion of the patient's PET scan with a structural image (*B*), fusion of the patient's structural image to a template image in the same space as the normative images (*C*), and comparison of FDG avidity between the patient and the database across all voxels and regions-of-interest (*D*). Three-dimensional stereotactic surface projection images (*E*) with colors representing the patient's FDG avidity in standard deviations from the normative database.

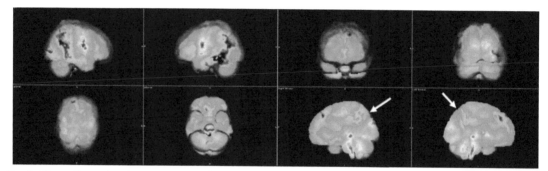

Fig. 3. Three-dimensional stereotactic surface projection images in a patient with AD. The blue color denotes brain regions in which the FDG avidity is at least 3 standard deviations lower than similarly aged healthy controls from a normative database. The distribution of decreased FDG avidity in the temporal and parietal lobes, particularly the precuneus (*arrows*), is typical of AD.

commonly involving the left hemisphere (**Fig. 9**).[18–21] The other 2 subtypes of PPA, nonfluent variant PPA (nfvPPA) and semantic variant PPA (svPPA), are considered clinical syndromes of frontotemporal lobar degeneration. On FDG-PET, nfvPPA typically shows decreased FDG avidity in the frontal and parietal lobes, and svPPA shows decreased FDG avidity in the temporal lobe, commonly preferentially involving the left hemisphere (**Fig. 10**).[18]

RESEARCH PET TRACERS FOR IMAGING ALZHEIMER DISEASE
Amyloid PET

Because Aβ deposition is one of the neuropathologic hallmarks of AD, the use of amyloid PET using the tracer, ^{11}C-Pittsburgh Compound B (PiB), in 2002 was a major advancement in the field in allowing for in vivo assessment of Aβ deposition.[22] Although its 20-minute half-life limits routine

clinical use, due to the need for a cyclotron in proximity, PiB PET remains widely used in AD research studies. Previously, the radiotracer 2-(1-{6-[(2-[fluorine-18]fluoroethyl)(methyl)amino]-2-naphthyl}-ethylidene)malononitrile (^{18}F-FDDNP) was developed to assess amyloid deposition but it fell out of favor because it showed an affinity for both Aβ and tau,[23] lacking specificity.

Currently, there are 3 FDA-approved ^{18}F-labeled radiopharmaceuticals, florbetaben (NeuraCeq), florbetapir (Amyvid), and flutemetamol (Vizamyl). A positive scan shows cortical activity that is greater than or equal to white matter, commonly in the frontal, parietal, and temporal lobes, as well as the posterior cingulate gyrus and precuneus, resulting in loss of gray–white differentiation (**Figs. 11** and **12**). Because healthy controls can have Aβ deposition for years before developing AD,[24] a positive amyloid scan does not definitively diagnose AD. However, a negative amyloid PET scan is useful in excluding AD.

A   **B**

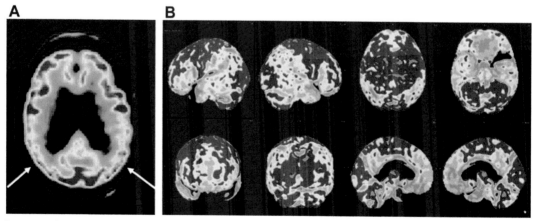

Fig. 4. Axial FDG-PET image (*A*) in a patient with amnestic mild cognitive impairment demonstrates decreased FDG avidity in the parietal lobes bilaterally (*arrows*). Three-dimensional stereotactic surface projection images (*B*) demonstrate decreased FDG avidity in the precuneus, posterior cingulate gyrus, and temporal and parietal lobes bilaterally, suggestive of underlying AD pathologic condition.

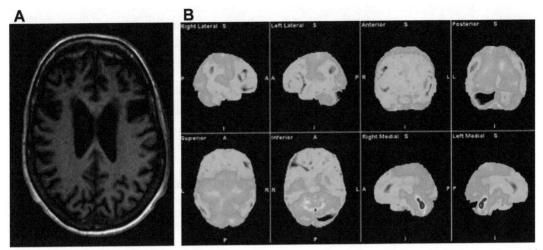

Fig. 5. Axial T1-weighted MR image (*A*) demonstrates marked bilateral frontal lobe atrophy in a patient with behavioral variant frontotemporal dementia (bvFTD). Three-dimensional stereotactic surface projection images (*B*) demonstrate decreased FDG avidity in frontal and temporal lobes bilaterally, a distribution typical of bvFTD.

Identifying the presence of Aβ deposition will become even more important because antiamyloid therapies are being developed. The first, aducanumab (Aduhelm), was FDA approved in June 2021 and is a monoclonal antibody designed to clear Aβ in the brain, in the hopes of slowing the progression of cognitive impairment.[25] In clinical trials, the main adverse effects of aducanumab have been termed amyloid-related imaging abnormalities (ARIA), manifesting as brain edema (ARIA-E), brain hemorrhage (ARIA-H), or a combination of the two.[26] Up to one-third of trial patients receiving aducanumab had one of these adverse events, with 10% of patients having symptoms, such as headache, confusion, vision changes, dizziness, nausea, or vomiting.[27] Amyloid PET scans will be crucial to identify patients with Aβ, who may benefit from this drug, and MR imaging will be crucial to monitoring these patients for edema and hemorrhage.

Tau PET

PET tracers can also be used for in vivo visualization of tau NFT aggregates, the other pathological hallmark of AD. The only FDA-approved tau tracer is [18F]-flortaucipir (AV-1451, trade name: Tauvid), which is considered a first-generation tau tracer (**Fig. 13**). In typical amnestic AD, high [18F]-flortaucipir uptake is seen in the posterior cingulate, precuneus, and lateral temporal and parietal lobes, with sparing of the primary visual, auditory, and sensorimotor cortices.[28] Unlike amyloid PET, which is typically read as positive or negative, [18F]-flortaucipir uptake correlates with severity of cortical atrophy, allowing for AD staging. The

major drawback of the first-generation tracers is off-target binding, especially to the choroid plexus, which can limit accurate quantification of tau deposition in the temporal lobes. Second-generation ligands, such as [18F]-MK6240 (see **Fig. 11**) and [18F]-PI-2620, are actively being tested, and early results have indicated decreased off-target signal with improved binding to tau aggregates.[28]

Of note, several non-AD neurodegenerative diseases are also characterized by tau deposition, including Pick disease, progressive supranuclear palsy, and corticobasal degeneration. However, [18F]-flortaucipir has been shown to have lower affinity for the non-AD tauopathies. However, [18F]-flortaucipir uptake may be seen in chronic traumatic encephalopathy, typically in the superior and dorsolateral frontal cortex early in the disease process, then later involving the temporal and parietal cortices.[29]

FUTURE OF PET IN DEMENTIA

Several new tracers are currently being developed to further characterize pathophysiologic processes underlying dementia using PET.

SV2A (Synaptic Markers)

Loss of normal synaptic density is a well-characterized and consistent pathologic process in AD. Postmortem evaluation in patients with prodromal or mild AD has identified the hippocampus as the site with the most pronounced synaptic loss, with the degree of synaptic loss corresponding to AD severity.[30] PET imaging targeting

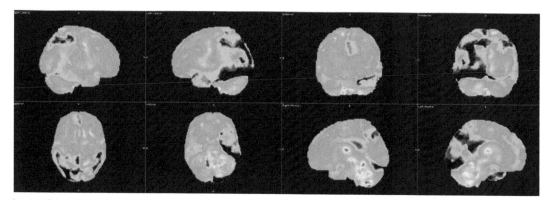

Fig. 6. Three-dimensional stereotactic surface projection images demonstrate decreased FDG avidity in parietal and temporal lobes bilaterally, more pronounced on the left. In addition, there is decreased FDG avidity in the left occipital lobe. The temporoparietal distribution and asymmetric involvement of the left occipital lobe is compatible with posterior cortical atrophy, the visual variant of Alzheimer.

synaptic vesicle glycoprotein 2A (SV2A), which is nearly ubiquitous in presynaptic terminal synaptic vesicles, allows for in vivo examination of synaptic density. Early investigations have shown reductions in SV2A binding with the radiotracer [11C] UCB-J in the mesiotemporal and neocortical regions of the brain in early patients with AD, which was reduced to an even greater extent than the associated gray matter loss.[31] Similar to other ^{11}C PET tracers, the short 20-minute half-life of this tracer limits its use to clinical facilities with onsite cyclotrons. [18F]UCB-H is another radiotracer that targets SV2A, and reduced hippocampal uptake with this tracer, reflective of synaptic loss, has been shown to correlate with cognitive impairment in mild cognitive impairment (MCI) and AD.[32]

Neuroinflammation

Neuroinflammation is another key pathophysiologic process in AD, characterized by activated microglia and astrocytes surrounding Aβ plaques.

To date, the most well-studied avenue to target activated microglia is via the increased expression of the translocator protein (18 kDa; TSPO). In the central nervous system, TSPO is primarily expressed in the outer mitochondrial membrane of steroid-producing cells, such as microglia, astrocytes, and endothelial cells, to transport cholesterol into the mitochondria.[33] TSPO expression can be assessed with [11C]-PK-11195, considered a first-generation TSPO tracer, with increased uptake on PET showing an association with Aβ accumulation in patients with MCI and AD compared with healthy controls.[34]

First-generation TSPO tracers, such as [11C]-PK-11195, demonstrate 2 major drawbacks: their relatively low brain permeability and their high nonspecific or plasma binding, resulting in a low signal-to-noise ratio.[35] To combat these issues, second-generation radiopharmaceuticals have been developed, including [18F]-FEMPA,[36] [18F]-FEPPA,[37] [18F]-DPA-714,[38] and [11C]-PBR28.[39] However, the second-generation TSPO tracers show variable binding affinity that is dependent

A   **B**

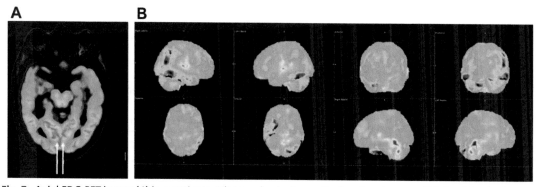

Fig. 7. Axial FDG-PET image (*A*) in a patient with Lewy body dementia showing decreased FDG avidity in the temporal and occipital lobes bilaterally, although with preserved FDG avidity in the medial occipital lobes (*arrows*). Three-dimensional stereotactic surface projection images (*B*) demonstrate decreased FDG avidity in the bilateral temporal and occipital lobes and left parietal lobe.

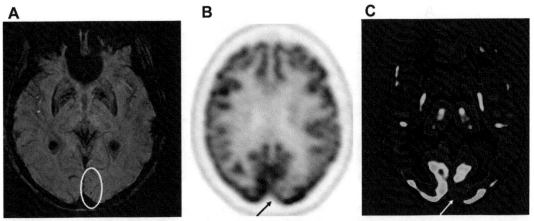

Fig. 8. Axial susceptibility-weighted image (*A*) shows foci of microhemorrhage (*oval*), suggestive of amyloid angiopathy. Axial FDG-PET images (*B, C*) demonstrate decreased FDG avidity (*arrow*) in the left occipital lobe in the region of the microhemorrhages.

on an rs6971 genetic polymorphism, meaning a genetic test must be completed before results can be interpreted.[40] Other tracers, such as [11C]-deuterium-L-deprenyl, bind irreversibly to monoamine oxidase B, which can be an alternative way of identifying neuroinflammation, because MAO-B is overexpressed in activated astrocytes.[40]

Cholinergic Cell Death

Cholinergic cell death underlies both AD and Dementia with Lewy Bodies (DLB), and the degree of cell death strongly correlates with symptom severity.[41] Multiple radiopharmaceuticals have been developed to target the cholinergic system, such as [18F]-fluoroethoxybenzovesamicol (FEOBV)[42] and (-)-(1-(8-(2-[18F]fluoroethoxy)-3-hydroxy-1,2,3,4-tetrahydronaphthalen-2-yl)-piperidin-4-yl)(4-fluorophenyl)methanone ([18F]-VAT),[43] which has high binding affinity for the vesicular acetylcholine transporter, a glycoprotein on the membrane of synaptic vesicles of cholinergic neurons. Studies measuring FEOBV tracer activity have found cortical cholinergic degeneration to be proportional to cholinergic basal forebrain atrophy in AD, suggesting FEOBV may have utility in quantifying cholinergic degeneration.[42] Early studies have also shown FEOBV to be more sensitive for the detection of early AD than certain amyloid tracers.[44] The slow kinetics of FEOBV in the basal ganglia may be disadvantageous clinically, however, because studies may require long scan times.

Dopaminergic Targets

Dopaminergic tracers can be used to differentiate AD from DLB. For example, decreased uptake of the radiotracer 3,4-dihydroxy-6-(18)F-fluoro-l-phenylalanine ([18F]FDOPA), a labeled analog of l-3,4-dihydroxyphenylalanine (L-DOPA), has been reported in the putamen in patients with DLB compared with patients with AD.[45] In one

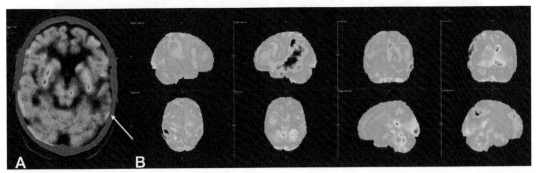

Fig. 9. Axial FDG-PET image fused to the CT of the head (*A*) demonstrating asymmetrically decreased FDG avidity in the left temporal lobe (*arrow*). Three-dimensional stereotactic surface projection images (*B*) demonstrate asymmetrically decreased FDG avidity in the left parietal and temporal lobes, suggestive of logopenic variant primary progressive aphasia, the language variant of Alzheimer.

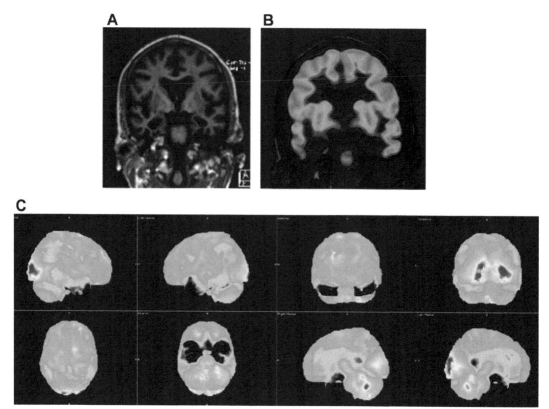

Fig. 10. Coronal T1-weighted MR imaging (*A*), coronal FDG-PET image fused to the MR imaging (*B*), and three-dimensional stereotactic surface projection images (*C*) demonstrating marked bilateral temporal lobe atrophy with associated decreased FDG avidity, compatible with semantic variant primary progressive aphasia.

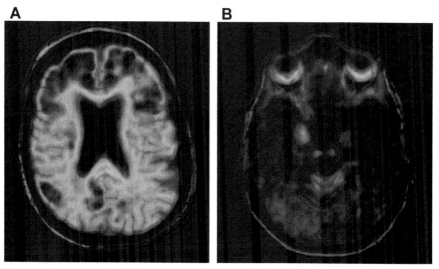

Fig. 11. Axial image from an amyloid PET scan using the tracer, Pittsburgh Compound B, fused to the MR imaging of the head (*A*) demonstrating beta-amyloid deposition in the bilateral frontal lobes and right greater than left parietal lobes. Axial image from a tau PET scan using the tracer, MK6240, fused to the MR imaging of the head (*B*) demonstrating tau deposition in the right uncus.

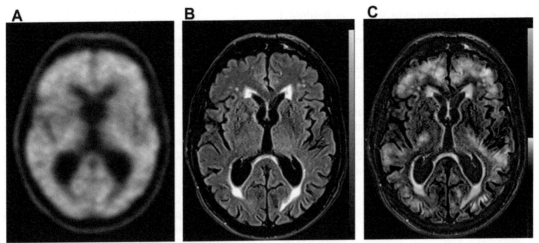

Fig. 12. Axial image from an amyloid PET scan using the tracer, ^{18}F-florbetaben, demonstrating diffuse beta-amyloid deposition (*A*). Axial T2 FLAIR image (*B*) fused to the amyloid PET image (*C*) confirms that the amyloid tracer uptake is in both cortical gray matter and white matter.

retrospective review of 46 cases of suspected DLB on FDG PET/CT, only 6 were still considered DLB after [18F]FDOPA PET/CT.[45] 18F-N-(3-fluoro-propyl)-2β-carboxymethoxy-3β-(4-iodophenyl) nortropane ([18F]-FP-CIT) is another tracer that can be used to measure striatal dopamine transporter activity. Reduced [18F]-FP-CIT has been reported to correlate with occipital Aβ deposition in patients with DLB, possibly contributing to visuospatial dysfunction in these patients.[46]

SUMMARY

Although FDG PET is the most widely used PET tracer in current clinical practice, there are numerous PET radiotracers that allow us to monitor the pathophysiology underlying AD, such as Aβ deposition, tau deposition, loss of synaptic density, neuroinflammation, cholinergic cell death, and decreased monoamine neurotransmission. Currently, there are 3 FDA-approved ^{18}F-labeled radiopharmaceuticals to assess Aβ deposition: flor-betaben (NeuraCeq), florbetapir (Amyvid), and flute-metamol (Vizamyl). These are used in clinical trials but not yet reimbursed for clinical diagnostic use. [18F]-flortaucipir, used to assess tau deposition in staging AD, is similarly FDA-approved but not yet used clinically. As more of these PET radiotracers enter mainstream clinical practice, our ability to diagnose, manage, and potentially treat neurodegenerative disease will improve dramatically.

CLINICS CARE POINTS

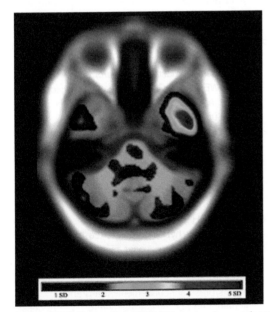

Fig. 13. [18F]-flortaucipir PET-MR imaging in a patient with mild cognitive impairment. Standardized uptake value ratio (SUVR) in a combined region-of-interest, including the entorhinal cortex, amygdala, and inferior temporal cortex, was greater than 1.22 relative to cerebellar cortex, compatible with increased tau deposition.

- Although the imaging evaluation of dementia typically begins with MR imaging, FDG-PET has higher sensitivity for diagnosing AD.
- Automated software packages that compare a patient's FDG avidity against a normative database of FDG images from healthy controls can be helpful in improving the detection of AD.

- There are FDA-approved tracers of amyloid and tau but they are not yet widely reimbursed and therefore typically obtained only in the setting of clinical trials.

DISCLOSURES

Research reported in this publication was supported in part by the following grants: National Institutes of Health/National Institute on Aging R01AG068398 (G.C.), ASNR 2021 Boerger Research Fund for Alzheimer's Disease and Neurocognitive Disorders (A.F.).

REFERENCES

1. Alzheimer's Association. Alzheimer's disease facts and figures. 2019. Available at: https://www.alz.org/media/documents/alzheimers-facts-and-figures-2019-r.pdf. Accessed March 20, 2022.
2. Jack CR Jr, Bennett DA, Blennow K, et al. NIA-AA Research Framework: toward a biological definition of Alzheimer's disease. Alzheimers Dement 2018; 14:535–62.
3. Thal DR, Rub U, Orantes M, et al. Phases of A beta-deposition in the human brain and its relevance for the development of AD. Neurology 2002;58: 1791–800.
4. Braak H, Braak E. Evolution of the neuropathology of Alzheimer's disease. Acta Neurol Scand, Suppl 1996;165:3–12.
5. Kumar ADS. Neuropathology and therapeutic management of Alzheimer's disease - an update. Drugs Future 2008;33:433.
6. Clarfield AM. The decreasing prevalence of reversible dementias: an updated meta-analysis. Arch Intern Med 2003;163:2219–29.
7. Hashimoto M, Ishikawa M, Mori E, et al. Diagnosis of idiopathic normal pressure hydrocephalus is supported by MRI-based scheme: a prospective cohort study. Cerebrospinal Fluid Res 2010;7:18.
8. Persson K, Barca ML, Cavallin L, et al. Comparison of automated volumetry of the hippocampus using NeuroQuant(R) and visual assessment of the medial temporal lobe in Alzheimer's disease. Acta Radiol 2018;59:997–1001.
9. Lombardi G, Crescioli G, Cavedo E, et al. Structural magnetic resonance imaging for the early diagnosis of dementia due to Alzheimer's disease in people with mild cognitive impairment. Cochrane Database Syst Rev 2020;3:CD009628.
10. Mahalingam S, Chen MK. Neuroimaging in dementias. Semin Neurol 2019;39:188–99.
11. Bloudek LM, Spackman DE, Blankenburg M, et al. Review and meta-analysis of biomarkers and diagnostic imaging in Alzheimer's disease. J Alzheimers Dis 2011;26:627–45.
12. Brown RK, Bohnen NI, Wong KK, et al. Brain PET in suspected dementia: patterns of altered FDG metabolism. Radiographics 2014;34:684–701.
13. Frisoni GB, Bocchetta M, Chetelat G, et al. Imaging markers for Alzheimer disease: which vs how. Neurology 2013;81:487–500.
14. Ng S, Villemagne VL, Berlangieri S, et al. Visual assessment versus quantitative assessment of 11C-PIB PET and 18F-FDG PET for detection of Alzheimer's disease. J Nucl Med 2007;48:547–52.
15. Rabinovici GD, Rosen HJ, Alkalay A, et al. Amyloid vs FDG-PET in the differential diagnosis of AD and FTLD. Neurology 2011;77:2034–42.
16. Whitwell JL, Graff-Radford J, Singh TD, et al. (18)F-FDG PET in posterior cortical atrophy and dementia with lewy bodies. J Nucl Med 2017;58:632–8.
17. Bergeret S, Queneau M, Rodallec M, et al. [(18) F] FDG PET may differentiate cerebral amyloid angiopathy from Alzheimer's disease. Eur J Neurol 2021;28: 1511–9.
18. Cerami C, Dodich A, Greco L, et al. The role of single-subject brain metabolic patterns in the early differential diagnosis of primary progressive aphasias and in prediction of progression to dementia. J Alzheimers Dis 2017;55:183–97.
19. Whitwell JL, Jack CR Jr, Kantarci K, et al. Imaging correlates of posterior cortical atrophy. Neurobiol Aging 2007;28:1051–61.
20. Rabinovici GD, Jagust WJ, Furst AJ, et al. Abeta amyloid and glucose metabolism in three variants of primary progressive aphasia. Ann Neurol 2008;64: 388–401.
21. Gorno-Tempini ML, Dronkers NF, Rankin KP, et al. Cognition and anatomy in three variants of primary progressive aphasia. Ann Neurol 2004;55:335–46.
22. Klunk WE, Mathis CA. The future of amyloid-beta imaging: a tale of radionuclides and tracer proliferation. Curr Opin Neurol 2008;21:683–7.
23. Agdeppa ED, Kepe V, Liu J, et al. Binding characteristics of radiofluorinated 6-dialkylamino-2-naphthylethylidene derivatives as positron emission tomography imaging probes for beta-amyloid plaques in Alzheimer's disease. J Neurosci 2001;21: RC189.
24. Hardy JA, Higgins GA. Alzheimer's disease: the amyloid cascade hypothesis. Science 1992;256:184–5.
25. Office of the Commissioner. FDA grants accelerated approval for Alzheimer's drug. U.S. Food and Drug Administration. 2021. https://www.fda.gov/news-events/press-announcements/fda-grants-accelerated-approval-alzheimers-drug. Accessed 20 March 2022.
26. EMERGE and ENGAGE topline results: two phase 3 studies to evaluate aducanumab in patients with early alzheimer's disease. 2019. https://investors.biogen.com/static-files/ddd45672-9c7e-4c99-8a06-3b557697c06f. Accessed 28 April 2022.

27. Tampi RR, Forester BP, Agronin M. Aducanumab: evidence from clinical trial data and controversies. Drugs Context 2021;10:1–9.

28. Mueller A, Bullich S, Barret O, et al. Tau PET imaging with (18)F-PI-2620 in Patients with Alzheimer disease and healthy controls: a first-in-humans study. J Nucl Med 2020;61:911–9.

29. McKee AC, Stern RA, Nowinski CJ, et al. The spectrum of disease in chronic traumatic encephalopathy. Brain 2013;136:43–64.

30. Scheff SW, Price DA, Schmitt FA, et al. Synaptic alterations in CA1 in mild Alzheimer disease and mild cognitive impairment. Neurology 2007;68:1501–8.

31. Mecca AP, Chen MK, O'Dell RS, et al. In vivo measurement of widespread synaptic loss in Alzheimer's disease with SV2A PET. Alzheimers Dement 2020;16:974–82.

32. Bastin C, Bahri MA, Meyer F, et al. In vivo imaging of synaptic loss in Alzheimer's disease with [18F]UCB-H positron emission tomography. Eur J Nucl Med Mol Imaging 2020;47:390–402.

33. Rupprecht R, Papadopoulos V, Rammes G, et al. Translocator protein (18 kDa) (TSPO) as a therapeutic target for neurological and psychiatric disorders. Nat Rev Drug Discov 2010;9:971–88.

34. Parbo P, Ismail R, Hansen KV, et al. Brain inflammation accompanies amyloid in the majority of mild cognitive impairment cases due to Alzheimer's disease. Brain 2017;140:2002–11.

35. Vivash L, O'Brien TJ. Imaging microglial activation with TSPO PET: lighting up neurologic diseases? J Nucl Med 2016;57:165–8.

36. Varrone A, Oikonen V, Forsberg A, et al. Positron emission tomography imaging of the 18-kDa translocator protein (TSPO) with [18F]FEMPA in Alzheimer's disease patients and control subjects. Eur J Nucl Med Mol Imaging 2015;42:438–46.

37. Suridjan I, Pollock BG, Verhoeff NP, et al. In-vivo imaging of grey and white matter neuroinflammation in Alzheimer's disease: a positron emission tomography study with a novel radioligand, [18F]-FEPPA. Mol Psychiatry 2015;20:1579–87.

38. Hamelin L, Lagarde J, Dorothee G, et al. Distinct dynamic profiles of microglial activation are associated with progression of Alzheimer's disease. Brain 2018;141:1855–70.

39. Toppala S, Ekblad LL, Tuisku J, et al. Association of early beta-amyloid accumulation and neuroinflammation measured with [(11)C]PBR28 in elderly individuals without dementia. Neurology 2021;96:e1608–19.

40. Zhou R, Ji B, Kong Y, et al. PET imaging of neuroinflammation in alzheimer's disease. Front Immunol 2021;12:739130.

41. Grothe MJ, Schuster C, Bauer F, et al. Atrophy of the cholinergic basal forebrain in dementia with Lewy bodies and Alzheimer's disease dementia. J Neurol 2014;261:1939–48.

42. Aghourian M, Aumont E, Grothe MJ, et al. FEOBV-PET to quantify cortical cholinergic denervation in AD: relationship to basal forebrain volumetry. J Neuroimaging 2021;31:1077–81.

43. Jin H, Yue X, Liu H, et al. Kinetic modeling of [(18)F]VAT, a novel radioligand for positron emission tomography imaging vesicular acetylcholine transporter in non-human primate brain. J Neurochem 2018;144:791–804.

44. Aghourian M, Legault-Denis C, Soucy JP, et al. Quantification of brain cholinergic denervation in Alzheimer's disease using PET imaging with [(18)F]-FEOBV. Mol Psychiatry 2017;22:1531–8.

45. Emsen B, Villafane G, David JP, et al. Clinical impact of dual-tracer FDOPA and FDG PET/CT for the evaluation of patients with parkinsonian syndromes. Medicine (Baltimore) 2020;99:e23060.

46. Yoo HS, Lee S, Chung SJ, et al. Dopaminergic depletion, beta-amyloid burden, and cognition in lewy body disease. Ann Neurol 2020;87:739–50.

Brain PET and Cerebrovascular Disease

Katarina Chiam[a], Louis Lee, MASc[b], Phillip H. Kuo, MD, PhD[c], Vincent C. Gaudet, PhD[b], Sandra E. Black, MD[d,e], Katherine A. Zukotynski, MD, PhD[f,*]

KEYWORDS

- Cerebrovascular disease • Cognitive impairment • PET • Artificial intelligence

KEY POINTS

- Brain PET may be helpful in the evaluation of patients with cerebrovascular disease.
- Although computed tomography and MR imaging are more commonly used to evaluate stroke/hemorrhage and ultrasound is more commonly used to evaluate carotid artery blockage, brain PET can be very helpful in patients who may have mixed pathologic condition including a combination of vasculopathy and proteinopathy.
- There are several PET radiopharmaceuticals that target metabolism (such as ^{18}F-labeled 2-fluoro-2-deoxy-D-glucose) or a host of proteinopathies; for example, ^{18}F-florbetapir was the first ^{18}F-labeled radiopharmaceutical to target amyloid deposition and was shown to have high sensitivity (87%) and specificity (95%) for distinguishing none-to-sparse from moderate-to-frequent amyloid plaque.
- PET using $H_2^{15}O$ can be used to assess cerebral perfusion, although the process is invasive, requires arterial blood sampling, and is rarely used in clinical practice.
- Machine learning can be useful in brain PET for several applications. Although still in its infancy, on application that is gaining traction is to reduce brain PET acquisition time.

AN INTRODUCTION TO CEREBROVASCULAR DISEASE

Cerebrovascular disease refers to the spectrum of brain diseases caused by impaired vasculature and blood supply. This encompasses a host of pathologic conditions such as stroke, hemorrhage, and other entities associated with vascular narrowing, obstruction, rupture, and inflammation. Vascular disease can involve large and/or small vessels. Although brain disease related to large vessel pathologic condition often manifests with significant abnormalities such as large areas of cerebral infarction or hemorrhage that can be detected with computed tomography (CT), small vessel disease (SVD) may be subtle and more

---

The authors have nothing to disclose.
For the Alzheimer's Disease Neuroimaging Initiative.[1].
[a] Division of Engineering Science, University of Toronto, 40 St. George St., Toronto, ON M5S 2E4, Canada; [b] Department of Electrical and Computer Engineering, University of Waterloo, 200 University Avenue West, Waterloo, ON N2L 3G1, Canada; [c] Departments of Medical Imaging, Medicine, Biomedical Engineering, University of Arizona, 1501 N. Campbell, Tucson, AZ 85724, USA; [d] Departments of Neurology, Sunnybrook Health Sciences Centre, University of Toronto, 2075 Bayview Avenue, Toronto, ON M4N 3M5, Canada; [e] Departments of Medicine, Sunnybrook Health Sciences Centre, University of Toronto, 2075 Bayview Avenue, Toronto, ON M4N 3M5, Canada; [f] Departments of Medicine and Radiology, McMaster University, 1200 Main Street West, Hamilton, ON L9G 4X5, Canada
[1] Data used in preparation of this article were obtained from the Alzheimer's Disease Neuroimaging Initiative (ADNI) database (adni.loni.usc.edu). As such, the investigators within the ADNI contributed to the design and implementation of ADNI and/or provided data but did not participate in analysis or writing of this report. A complete listing of ADNI investigators can be found at: http://adni.loni.usc.edu/wp- content/uploads/how_to_apply/ADNI_Acknowledgement_List.pdf.
* Corresponding author.
E-mail address: katherine.zukotynski@utoronto.ca

easily seen with MR imaging. Manifestations of SVD include subcortical infarcts, lacunes, microbleeds, white matter hyperintensity (WMH), enlarged perivascular spaces, and brain atrophy.[1] The most common subtype of SVD is WMH and is thought to be due to perivenous vasogenic edema from venous collagenosis associated with varying degrees of demyelination.[2,3] Using a T2-weighted or fluid-attenuation inversion recovery MR imaging sequence, WMH often appears as "white" spots, patches, or confluent areas in the periventricular white matter. Often comorbid with cognitive impairment, SVD may be found in association with proteinopathies such as beta-amyloid (Aβ), alpha-synuclein, and TDP43[4,5]; the pathologic cascade leading to the development of these proteinopathies remains enigmatic. Although cerebrovascular disease is commonly imaged using CT and/or MR imaging, PET may play a role, particularly when a patient has cognitive decline.[6] Rarely, PET with $H_2^{15}O$ has been used to measure cerebral blood flow; however, this techniques is invasive, requiring the use of an arterial input function measured with continuous arterial blood sampling, has limitations, and is rarely used in clinical practice.

There are several ways in which vascular disease is associated with cognitive decline. Vascular cognitive impairment (VCI) refers to the spectrum of cognitive deficits associated with cerebrovascular disease; vascular dementia (VaD) refers to dementia of a vascular cause, regardless of the pathogenesis of the vascular disease (ie, ischemic hemorrhagic, solitary, or multiple infarcts).[7] An accurate diagnosis is based on documentation of a cognitive disorder through neuropsychological testing and a history of stroke *or* vascular disease on neuroimaging. VaD can be classified by the type of vessels involved, the range/extent of cerebrovascular disease and the location of resulting brain damage, often due to atherosclerosis, SVD, and/or cerebral amyloid angiopathy (CAA).[8,9] Poststroke dementia, or dementia occurring after a stroke, may develop within 3 months or more following stroke and is estimated to have a 7% incidence at 1 year with 30% prevalence in stroke survivors.[10] Slightly higher neurofibrillary pathologic condition including tauopathy and Lewy bodies may be seen in this setting.[11] Moreover, SVD and CAA may be associated with Alzheimer disease (AD) and mixed pathologic condition is common.[12] PET is helpful to detect changes in brain metabolism and the presence of proteinopathies such as Aβ or tau.

The literature on the association of vascular pathologic condition (particularly SVD), cognitive performance, glucose metabolism, and proteinopathy (ie, Aβ deposition) is mixed. For example, in 1995, DeCarli and colleagues[13] found higher WMH burden was associated with lower frontal lobe metabolism and frontal lobe-mediated neuropsychological test scores. Kim and colleagues[14] showed higher WMH burden was associated with increased apathy and neuropsychiatric symptoms. Iturria-Medina and colleagues[15] suggested vascular dysregulation led to lower Aβ clearance and metabolic dysfunction. Marnane and colleagues[16] found higher WMH burden was linked with higher cerebral Aβ burden and reduced cerebral metabolism. However, Rosenburgh and colleagues[17] concluded WMH and Aβ accumulation were independent but additive processes in their systematic review of WMH burden with cortical Aβ association in healthy elders and individuals with cognitive impairment. It seems likely SVD disrupts white matter networks, decreases integration (longer path length, worse global efficiency), and nodal efficiency (with frontal region predilection).[18,19] Certainly, vascular disease may be linked to cognitive impairment without AD pathologic condition. For example, Kim and colleagues[20] compared patients with pure subcortical VCI to normal controls and found vascular disease alone was associated with cognitive impairment. Ultimately, although vascular disease and Aβ deposition can have an effect on cerebral structure[21] and cognitive performance,[22] the association between them remains unclear.

AGING

Not only do the vascular structures become more tenuous with age leading to risk of stroke and hemorrhage but also cognitive impairment becomes more common. Indeed, cognitive impairment is a spectrum of disease affecting large swaths of the elder population. Clinically, mild cognitive impairment (MCI) affects approximately 7% of subjects aged 60 to 64 years increasing to 25% of subjects aged 80 to 84 years and refers to a state of subjective gradual memory loss for 6 months or more, objective memory loss (clinical memory tests) and preserved activities of daily living. It is estimated that 10% to 15% of subjects with MCI progress to dementia annually with more than 50% progressing to dementia in 5 years.[23,24] According to criteria put forth by the National Institute on Aging and the Alzheimer's Association (NIA-AA) workgroups, a clinical evaluation is key for patients with cognitive impairment; imaging plays a supportive role.[25–28] Recently, it has been suggested that a diagnosis of AD should include biomarker verification of Aβ deposition, hyperphosphorylated tau, and neurodegeneration.[29] It is possible, that with time, this will expand to include a marker of vascular impairment as well.

IMAGING CEREBROVASCULAR DISEASE WITH A FOCUS ON BRAIN PET

Although cerebrovascular disease encompasses a broad spectrum of pathologic condition, brain PET is rarely the first imaging modality used in this setting. Neuroimaging with CT and/or MR imaging is helpful to assess vascular and cerebral structural anatomy. Typically, CT is recommended as part of the evaluation for patients aged younger than 60 years with rapid cognitive function decline, new unexplained symptoms or localizing signs, atypical symptoms/presentation, gait disturbance, urinary incontinence, head trauma, anticoagulant use/history of bleeding, and history of cancer and/or short duration of symptoms. MR imaging is recommended when the requesting specialist thinks additional imaging will provide diagnostic and predictive value; for example, if unsuspected cerebrovascular disease would change clinical management.[28] Moreover, although MR imaging is more sensitive than CT to detect cerebral atrophy and SVD, and may help to stratify and monitor disease, it is often less easily accessible and more expensive depending on the region/nation.

Brain PET may be helpful in the assessment of inflammation such as arteritis (including giant cell arteritis), chronic ischemia (such as Moya Moya) or stroke, among other pathologic conditions, although these indications are rarely seen in routine clinical practice. Moreover, PET may be helpful to assess carotid artery disease such as plaque using ^{18}F-NaF; however, this has yet to gain traction and more commonly evaluation of the carotid arteries is done using ultrasound or CT. Most commonly, brain PET is used in the setting of cerebrovascular disease and cognitive decline to assess cellular metabolism and confirm the presence of proteinopathies. Interestingly, modern PET scanners incorporate CT or MR imaging (ie, PET/CT or PET/MR) and thus provide a yet incompletely realized potential for exquisite real-time multimodality imaging including a dynamic vascular assessment. ^{18}F-labeled 2-fluoro-2-deoxy-D-glucose (^{18}F-FDG) is, currently, the most ubiquitous PET radiopharmaceutical. ^{18}F-FDG-PET/CT or PET/MR is recommended for patients suffering from cerebrovascular disease and cognitive impairment with inconclusive structural imaging (such as CT and MR imaging) and unclear underlying process. For example, ^{18}F-FDG PET may help provide a diagnosis of AD. It is estimated that the sensitivity and specificity of ^{18}F-FDG PET

for diagnosing AD is 90% and 70%, respectively.[30,31] Further, PET radiopharmaceuticals, such as ^{18}F-florbetapir, have high sensitivity (87%) and specificity (95%) for distinguishing none to sparse from moderate to frequent amyloid plaque.[32] Guidelines suggest amyloid PET may be helpful to evaluate patients with cognitive impairment in whom knowledge of amyloid deposition may alter management.[33,34] Although the PET radiopharmaceutical ^{18}F-flortaucipir is approved by the United States Food and Drug Administration for the evaluation of tau neurofibrillary tangles, radiopharmaceuticals that detect tau or other preoteinopathies are rarely available outside of clinical trials.

Currently, there is heated debate on the role of PET in cerebrovascular disease as well as a mechanism to practically implement this relatively expensive and sometimes difficult to access tool. Regardless, it seems likely imaging techniques capable of targeting specific pathologic processes can help with diagnosis, understanding the mechanistic underpinnings of disease, and assessing therapeutic effect.

TECHNOLOGICAL ADVANCES AND A POTENTIAL APPLICATION FOR BRAIN PET

Recent advances in hardware and software have been applied to brain PET in several ways for the purpose of improving image acquisition, interpretation, and outcome prediction. One important application that is currently gaining momentum is the use of machine learning in dementia to improve brain PET quality while minimizing acquisition time and/or patient radiation exposure.[35–39] For the purpose of illustration, we show how a convolutional neural network could be used to decrease noise using a single brain PET acquisition. Specifically, brain PET is acquired as a series of image acquisitions that are averaged to improve the signal-to-noise ratio (**Fig. 1**). A neural network could be designed to reconstruct a single acquisition with minimal noise after using a database of previously acquired brain PET cases with multiple acquisitions for training.

To prove how a neural network would be used to potentially decrease noise associated with shorter brain PET acquisition, we created a database of 215 ^{18}F-Florbetapir brain PET studies derived from the ADNI database (adni.loni.usc.edu); average patient age 75 years, 127 men, and 99 women. Each brain PET study contained 4 consecutive 5-minute acquisitions and was accompanied by a brain MR imaging from the same patient. The raw voxel data was normalized and the images resized to yield a tensor of

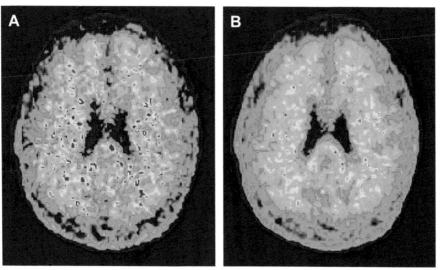

Fig. 1. Comparison between a single-acquisition (*A*) and an average of multiple-acquisitions (*B*) for a brain PET scan. A single pass in a PET machine results in a noisy scan with artifacts. Combining and averaging multiple acquisitions improves the signal-to-noise ratio and reduces artifacts. However, this comes at the expense of increasing scan time.

dimensions 256 × 256 × 1. The data was augmented through reflections in both x-axis and y-axis, as well as a half-rotation. The neural network was a U-Net[40] with several convolutional layers (**Fig. 2**). During the encoding phase, the network begins with the 256 × 256 × 1 input tensor, an axial slice from a single 5-minute brain PET scan (any of the 4 consecutive acquisitions), which passes through a pair of 2D convolutional (conv) layers with 64 filters and 3 × 3 kernel size. Each conv layer is followed by a rectified linear unit (ReLU) activation layer, and after the conv layer couplet, the tensor passes through a batch normalization layer and a 2 × 2 max pooling layer. The encoding phase is described by 4 such pairs of conv layers, each one decreasing the dimensions of the tensor in the x-direction and y-direction and doubling the number of filters. At the

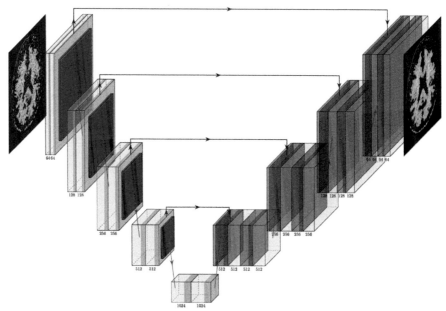

Fig. 2. U-Net structure. The encoding phase comprises the left half of the structure, and the decoding phase follows on the right. The network deconstructs the initial image into numerous low-resolution features, then attempts to reconstruct a noiseless version of the input.

Table 1
Example comparison of standardized uptake value ratios for the 56 regions of interest in one patient, for full 20-min scan and neural network output

	Left		Right	
	20-min Scan	5-min Scan (U-Net)	20-min Scan	5-min Scan (U-Net)
Angular gyrus	1.279	1.203	1.266	1.272
Caudate	0.283	0.301	0.233	0.152
Anterior cingulate gyrus	0.941	0.917	0.931	0.924
Cuneus	1.021	0.980	1.275	1.288
Fusiform gyrus	1.193	1.136	1.037	0.929
Gyrus rectus	1.095	1.214	1.118	1.202
Hippocampus	0.910	1.001	0.947	0.958
Inferior frontal gyrus	1.014	1.010	0.898	0.991
Inferior occipital gyrus	1.446	1.121	1.277	0.981
Inferior temporal gyrus	1.334	1.300	1.147	1.175
Insular cortex	0.980	0.940	0.978	1.048
Lateral orbitofrontal gyrus	0.855	0.814	0.776	0.892
Lingual gyrus	1.232	1.055	1.174	0.947
Middle frontal gyrus	1.017	1.054	0.919	1.055
Middle occipital gyrus	1.340	1.141	1.380	1.281
Middle orbitofrontal gyrus	1.034	1.085	1.031	1.177
Middle temporal gyrus	1.391	1.321	1.239	1.363
Parahippocampal gyrus	0.676	0.702	0.678	0.681
Postcentral gyrus	1.066	1.098	0.850	0.963
Precentral gyrus	1.136	1.228	0.829	0.978
Precuneus	1.065	0.970	0.862	0.855
Putamen	1.411	1.408	1.293	1.477
Superior frontal gyrus	0.923	1.004	0.874	0.872
Superior occipital gyrus	1.185	1.085	1.116	1.027
Superior parietal gyrus	1.106	1.103	0.892	0.939
Superior temporal gyrus	1.120	1.255	0.908	1.021
Supramarginal gyrus	1.106	1.138	0.929	1.030
Posterior cingulate	1.197	1.127	1.240	1.200

Qualitatively, the neural network output is comparable to that of the full scan in all ROIs.

apex of the U-Net, the tensor has dimensions 16 × 16 × 1024. The decoding phase reverts this tensor back to the original dimensions of the image by concatenating each decoding conv layer with the corresponding parallel encoding conv layer. A final conv layer with 1 filter yields an output image with identical dimensions to the input. With the input of an axial slice from a single 5-minute brain PET scan, the output is compared with the axial slice of the 20-minute brain PET scan. The standardized uptake value ratio (SUVR) normalized to cerebellar grey matter was obtained in 56 regions of interest for each of 12 validation studies. A visual qualitative assessment was also performed. **Table 1** shows the SUVR values obtained from a sample validation study. **Fig. 3** shows a comparison of 3 sample validation studies. Overall, image quality generated using 25% of the data (one 5-minute scan) is comparable to the full 20-minute brain PET scan. However, as always, the computer algorithm is not perfect, and the dynamic range may be higher indicating artifacts in certain cases.

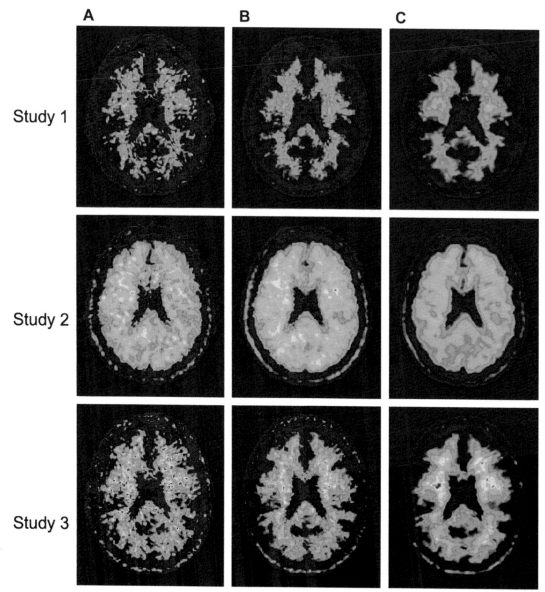

Fig. 3. Comparison of 3 different validation subjects who had brain PET (*A*) a single acquisition, (*B*) an average of 4 acquisitions, and (*C*) a single acquisition run through the neural network. All slices were obtained at the same spatial location.

CLINICS CARE POINTS

Brain PET may be helpful in the evaluation of patients with cerebrovascular disease.-Although the most ubiquitous radiopharmaceutical in clinical practice today is ^{18}F-FDG, other radiopharmaceuticals such as $H_2^{15}O$ may be helpful to assess cerebrovascular disease.-Machine learning algorithms are increasingly being used to improve image acquisition and processing.

DISCLOSURE

P.H. Kuo is an employee of Invicro. He is a consultant and/or speaker for Amgen, Bayer, Chimerix, Eisai, Fusion Pharma, General Electric Healthcare, Invicro, Novartis, and UroToday. He is a recipient of research grants from Blue Earth Diagnostics and General Electric Healthcare. S. Black has received in-kind support from GE Healthcare and Lilly Avid, and has served as Advisor for Roche. K. Zukotynski has been a consultant for GE Healthcare and Invicro. V. Gaudet has received funding from Microsoft Canada and the Natural

Sciences and Engineering Research Council of Canada.

REFERENCES

1. Wardlaw J, Smith E, Biessels G, et al. Neuroimaging standards for research into small vessel disease and its contribution to ageing and neurodegeneration. Lancet Neurol 2013;12:822–38.

2. Keith J, Gao FQ, Noor R, et al. Collagenosis of the deep medullary veins: an unrecognized pathologic correlate of white matter hyperintensities and periventricular infarction? J Neuropathol Exp Neurol 2017;76(4):299–312.

3. Houck AL, Gutierrez J, Gao F, et al. Increased diameters of the internal cerebral veins and the basal veins of rosenthal are associated with white matter hyperintensity volume. AJNR Am J Neuroradiol 2019;40(10):1712–8.

4. Kapasi A, DeCarli C, Schneider JA. Impact of multiple pathologies on the threshold for clinically overt dementia. Acta Neuropathol 2017;134(2):171–86.

5. DeTure MA, Dickson DW. The neuropathological diagnosis of Alzheimer's disease. Mol Neurodegeneration 2019;14(32):1–18.

6. Zukotynski K, Kuo PH, Mikulis D, et al. PET/CT of dementia. AJR 2018;211(2):246–59.

7. Gorelick PB, Scuteri A, Black SE, et al. Vascular contributions to cognitive impairment and dementia: a statement for healthcare professionals from the american heart association/american stroke association. Stroke 2011;42(9):2672–713.

8. Kalaria RN. Neuropathological diagnosis of vascular cognitive impairment and vascular dementia with implications for Alzheimer's disease. Acta Neuropathol 2016;131:659–85.

9. Kalaria RN. Cerebrovascular disease and mechanisms of cognitive impairment. Stroke 2012;43:2526–34.

10. Leys D, Henon H, Mackowiak-Cordoliani MA, et al. Poststroke dementia. Lancet Neurol 2005;4:752–9.

11. Allan LM, Rowan EN, Firbank MJ, et al. Long term incidence of dementia, predictors of mortality and pathological diagnosis in older stroke survivors. Brain 2011;134:3713–24.

12. Thal DR, Grinberg LT, Attems J. Vascular dementia: different forms of vessel disorders contribute to the development of dementia in the elderly brain. Exp Gerontol 2012;47(11):816–24.

13. DeCarli C, Murphy DG, Tranh M, et al. The effect of white matter hyperintensity volume on brain structure, cognitive performance, and cerebral metabolism of glucose in 51 healthy adults. Neurology 1995;45:2077–84.

14. Kim HJ, Kang SJ, Kim C, et al. The effects of small vessel disease and amyloid burden on neuropsychiatric symptoms: a study among patients with subcortical vascular cognitive impairments. Neurobiol Aging 2013;34:1913–20.

15. Iturria-Medina Y, Sotero RC, Toussaint PJ, et al. Early role of vascular dysregulation on late-onset Alzheimer's disease based on multifactorial data-driven analysis. Nat Commun 2016;7:11934.

16. Marnane M, Al-Jawadi OO, Mortazavi S, et al. Periventricular hyperintensities are associated with elevated cerebral amylois. Neurology 2016;86:535–43.

17. Rosenborough A, Ramirez J, Black S, et al. Associations between amyloid β and white matter hyperintenties: a systematic review. Alzheimers Dement 2017;13(10):1154–67.

18. Kim HJ, Im K, Kwon H, et al. Effects of amyloid and small vessel disease on white matter network disruption. J Alzheimers Dis 2015;44:963–75.

19. Kim HJ, Im K, Kwon H, et al. Clinical effect of white matter network disruption related to amyloid and small vessel disease. Neurology 2015;85:63–70.

20. Kim HJ, Ye BS, Yoon CW, et al. Cortical thickness and hippocampal shape in pure vascular mild cognitive impairment and dementia of subcortical type. Eur J Neurol 2014;21:744–51.

21. Kim HJ, Kim J, Cho H, et al. Individual subject classification of mixed dementia from pure subcortical vascular dementia based on subcortical shape analysis. PLOS One 2013;8(10):e75602.

22. Park JH, Seo SW, Kim C, et al. Effects of cerebrovascular disease and amyloid beta burden on cognition in subjects with subcortical vascular cognitive impairment. Neurobiol Aging 2014;35:254–60.

23. Gauthier S, Reisberg B, Zaudig M, et al. Mild cognitive impairment. Lancet 2006;367:1262–70.

24. Petersen RC, Lopez O, Armstrong MJ, et al. Practice guideline update summary: mild cognitive impairment. Neurology 2018;90:1–10.

25. McKhann GM, Knopman DS, Chertkow H, et al. The diagnosis of dementia due to Alzheimer's disease: recommendations from the National Institute on Aging – Alzheimer's Association workgroups on diagnostic guidelines for Alzheimer's disease. Alzheimers Dement 2011;7:263–9.

26. Albert MS, Dekosky ST, Dickson D, et al. The diagnosis of mild cognitive impairment due to Alzheimer's disease: recommendations from the National Institute on Aging – Alzheimer's Association workgroups on diagnostic guidelines for Alzheimer's disease. Alzheimers Dement 2011;7:270–9.

27. Sperling RA, Aisen P, Beckett L, et al. Toward defining the preclinical stages of Alzheimer's disease: recommendations from the National Institute on Aging – Alzheimer's Association workgroups on diagnostic guidelines for Alzheimer's disease. Alzheimers Dement 2011;7:280–92.

28. Gauthier S, Patterson C, Chertkow H, et al. 4th Canadian consensus conference on the diagnosis

and treatment of dementia. Can J Neurol Sci 2012;
39(Suppl 5):S1–8.

29. Jack CR, Bennett DA, Blennow K, et al. NIA-AA research framework: toward a biological definition of Alzheimer's disease. Alzheimers Dement 2017; 14(4):535–62.

30. Hoffman JM, Welsh-Bohmer KA, Hanson M, et al. FDG PET imaging in patients with pathologically verified dementia. J Nucl Med 2000;41:1920–8.

31. Rice L, Bisdas S. The diagnostic value of FDG and amyloid PET in Alzheimer's disease – a systematic review. Eur J Radiol 2017;94:16–24.

32. Clark CM, Pontecorvo MJ, Beach TG, et al. Cerebral PET with florbetapir compared with neuropathology at autopsy for detection of neuritic amyloid-β plaques: a prospective cohort study. Lancet Neurol 2012;11:669–78.

33. Laforce R Jr, Rosa-Neto P, Soucy JP, et al. Canadian Consensus guidelines on use of amyloid imaging in Canada: update and future directions from the specialized task force on amyloid imaging in Canada. Can J Neurol Sci 2016;43:503–12.

34. Minoshima S, Drzezga AE, Barthel H, et al. SNMMI procedure standard/EANM practice guideline for amyloid PET imaging of the brain 1.0. J Nucl Med 2016;57(8):1316–22.

35. Uribe CF, Mathotaarachchi S, Gaudet V, et al. Machine learning in nuclear medicine: part 1—introduction. J Nucl Med 2019;60(4):451–8.

36. Zukotynski K, Gaudet V, Uribe CF, et al. Machine learning in nuclear medicine: part 2—neural networks and clinical aspects. J Nucl Med 2021; 62(1):22–9.

37. Zukotynski K, Gaudet V, Kuo PH, et al. The use of random forests to identify brain regions on amyloid and FDG PET associated with MoCA score. Clin Nucl Med 2020;45(6):427–33.

38. Zhao K, Zhou L, Gao S, et al. Study of low-dose PET image recovery using supervised learning with CycleGAN. PLOS ONE 2020;15(9):e0238455.

39. Wolterink JM, Leiner T, Viergever MA, et al. Generative adversarial networks for noise reduction in low-dose CT. IEEE T Med Imaging 2017;36(12):2536–45.

40. Ronneberger O, Fischer P, Brox T. U-Net: convolutional networks for biomedical image segmentation. MICCAI 2015;234–41.

Brain PET Imaging
Frontotemporal Dementia

Joshua Ward, BS[a], Maria Ly, MD, PhD[a], Cyrus A. Raji, MD, PhD[a,b,*]

KEYWORDS

- Frontotemporal dementia (FTD) • ^{18}F-FDG-PET • MRI • Tau-PET • Amyloid-PET • SPECT
- Alzheimer disease (AD) • Neurodegenerative disorders fused-in-sarcoma protein (FUS)

KEY POINTS

- Diagnostic imaging of frontotemporal demential (FTD), particularly behavioral variant FTD (bvFTD), entails both MR neuroimaging and brain PET.
- Brain MR displays atrophy, a proxy of neurodegeneration, in frontal and temporal lobar areas and FDG-PET shows hypometablism in these regions.
- Additional imaging techniques of interest for FTD include brain SPECT, amyloid, and tau PET but these methods are not as frequently utilized in clinical practice compared to MRI and FDG-PET.

INTRODUCTION

Frontotemporal dementia (FTD) is a term that refers to multiple neurologic syndromes with multiple subclassifications and overlapping symptoms overlying one of several specific protein-based neuropathologies. FTD is the most common cause of early-onset dementia and is primarily characterized by tau protein deposition and frontotemporal lobar degeneration. Currently, FTD has been divided into 3 main presentations: behavioral variant FTD (bvFTD), nonfluent/agrammatic variant primary progressive aphasia (nfvPPA), and semantic variant primary progressive aphasia (svPPA).[1] As bvFTD has an incidence 4 times greater than primary progressive aphasia (PPA) diagnoses and accounts for more than 50% of cases of autopsy-confirmed FTD,[2,3] it will be the focus of this review.

bvFTD was previously called Pick disease (PiD). In 1892, Pick described the first patient with FTD (an svPPA diagnosis). In 1911, Alois Alzheimer coined the term Pick disease,[4] and in 1923, Gans reported "Pick's atrophy" to distinguish cases of patients with frontotemporal atrophy from other similar neurodegenerative phenomena.[5] Just 3 years later, Pick's students Onari

and Patz differentiated "Pick's cells" from "Pick's bodies," reclassifying "Pick's disease" (PiD) as an individual pathologic unit.[5] Subsequent research resulted in a paradigm shift concerning the cause of dementia in the 1970s, moving toward a protein misfolding and deposition focus.[6,7] Today, PiD refers to neurodegeneration displaying Pick bodies associated with tau aggregates; Pick bodies can be seen in all three of the main FTD types. FTD now has subtypes based off of a variety of these protein aggregates, including TAR DNA binding protein (FTLD-TDP) and tau (FTLD-tau).

PET has been used to study dementia since the 1980s and was originally innovated to study normal brain physiology through interrogation of glucose metabolism.[8] This modality has become increasingly used in the diagnosis of neurodegenerative disorders owing to the complexity of presentations and related symptom overlap.

MR IMAGING VERSUS ^{18}F-FLUORODEOXYGLUCOSE-PET: DIAGNOSTIC UTILITY

The utility of both MR imaging and PET in the diagnosis of bvFTD has already been well established,

[a] Division of Neuroradiology, Mallinckrodt Institute of Radiology, Washington University in Saint. Louis, Saint Louis, MO 63130, USA; [b] Department of Neurology, Washington University in St. Louis, 4525 Scott Avenue, St. Louis, MO 63110, USA
* Corresponding author. Division of Neuroradiology, Mallinckrodt Institute of Radiology, Washington University in Saint. Louis, Saint Louis, MO 63130.
E-mail address: craji@wustl.edu

PET Clin 18 (2023) 123–133
https://doi.org/10.1016/j.cpet.2022.09.010

and neuroimaging is required to take a bvFTD diagnosis from "possible" to "probable."[9] Currently, the typical protocol is to first have an MR imaging done and then follow up with a fluoro-deoxyglucose (FDG)-PET to increase sensitivity/specificity[2]; ^{18}F-FDG-PET hypometabolic changes can be visualized before structural changes on computed tomography (CT) or MR imaging in dementia-like disorders and provides superior diagnostic accuracy allowing for earlier and more accurate patient care triage.[10] This section looks at the findings and effectiveness of each imaging technique individually and then in tandem.

Overall, both MR imaging and FDG-PET display atrophy/hypometabolism across similar regions in bvFTD. On MR imaging for a patient with bvFTD, there is typically atrophy of the frontotemporal lobes, and[11,12] the right hemisphere often displays more extensive atrophy than the left side.[13,14] Early in the disease course, von Economo neurons, large spindle-shaped neurons that facilitate faster communication across brain regions, in the anterior insula and anterior cingulate cortex present as the origin point for bvFTD neuropathology[15–17] before it progresses to the frontotemporal lobes. An MR imaging of a person with advanced FTD is shown in **Fig. 1**.

When structural imaging is inconclusive, ^{18}F-FDG-PET can help make a clearer distinction. Although the areas affected are similar, frontotemporal hypometabolism on ^{18}F-FDG-PET is detected earlier and in a comparatively widespread fashion compared with MR atrophy patterns.[18] Frontal lobe hypometabolism specifically targets the medial, dorsolateral, and ventrolateral prefrontal cortex (PFC), as well as the orbitofrontal and anterior cingulate cortex.[19–21] The medial temporal lobe and the anterior and inferior aspect of the temporal lobes are typically affected with hypometabolism extending to the posterior fusiform gyrus.[19,20] Limbic regional hypometabolism is also noted, including the hippocampus, amygdala,[19,20] caudate, and thalamus.[20,21]

These bvFTD PET findings contrast with hypometabolism in other prominent neurodegenerative diseases. In the early stage of Alzheimer disease (AD), frontotemporal hypometabolism that is comparatively less severe than bvFTD can be seen (see **Fig. 3**), and there is frontal, temporal, and parietal hypometabolism in advanced AD. The characteristic FDG-PET finding associated with pathologically confirmed AD is bilateral temporoparietal hypometabolism.[22] Characteristic findings in dementia with Lewy bodies (DLB), corticobasal degeneration (CBD), and AD are shown in **Fig. 2**. By knowing the different regional patterns of hypometabolism, these diseases can be differentiated.

FTD MR imaging and PET findings change as a function of disease severity/duration. As FTD progresses to advanced stages, similar brain regions show increasingly severe and diffuse volume/metabolic loss over time. Hypometabolism on PET progresses[23–25] across multiple regions, including the frontal poles, supplementary motor area, middle temporal gyri, posterior cingulate cortex, precuneus, inferior parietal lobule, lateral superior occipital cortex, and cerebellum.[19,25] Early in the course of FTD, structural MR imaging may detect changes in the temporal region that may not be as apparent on ^{18}F-FDG-PET owing to the differences in anatomic resolution across the techniques. Overall, more metabolic changes than volume changes are noted as FTD progresses year by year. Metabolic decline is also overall more diffuse at both early and late stages.[19]

As imaging findings evolve over time, differences in sensitivity/specificity in PET and MR imaging are also evident with varying stages of disease severity. In patients at early stages of dementia, ^{18}F-FDG-PET outperformed arterial spin-labeled MR in sensitivity as well as volumetric abnormalities.[26] The sensitivity of MR imaging in bvFTD in patients with late-onset behavioral changes is 70%, and the specificity is 93%. ^{18}F-FDG-PET has a sensitivity of 90% and a specificity of 68%. In general practice, MR imaging is ordered first simply because there is greater availability when compared with PET scanners; the American College of Radiology states that MR imaging is usually appropriate in suspected FTD, whereas an FDG-PET "may be appropriate."[27] This delineation may be due to the greater availability, the higher cost of PET, and the patient payment issues. It should be noted, however, that a stand-alone MR imaging with characteristic atrophy is not as sensitive as FDG-PET, and that in order to maximize both sensitivity and specificity, both must be used together. When used together, MR imaging with a follow-up PET has a sensitivity of 96% with a specificity of 73%. In 66% of patients with FTD in which a mutation was the cause of disease, MR imaging did not display the typical frontotemporal atrophy patterns, and a primary psychiatric disorder was the final diagnosis in 40% of cases with a false positive ^{18}F-FDG-PET scan.[2] Thus, it is important to use caution when interpreting neuroimaging results for patients with a genetic history of mutations (such as MAPT or P301L) that are associated with specific PET findings. This care is especially necessary when a primary psychiatric disorder is being

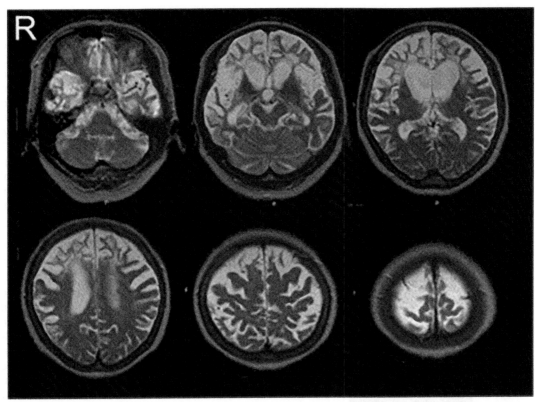

Fig. 1. Structural MR imaging of a person with advanced FTD. There is marked atrophy of the frontotemporal lobes bilaterally. However, the parietooccipital lobe is comparatively preserved.

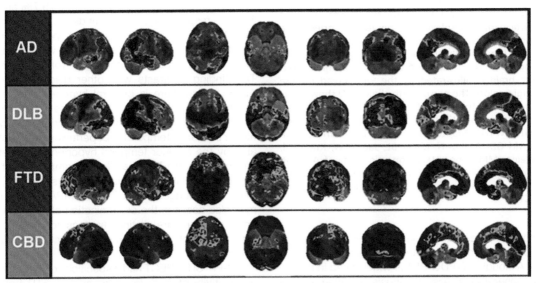

Fig. 2. Differential patterns of hypometabolism on FDG-PET z-score maps in neurodegenerative disease. Blue and purple colors denote areas of the FDG-PET scan that are −2 standard deviations or more below the mean of the control comparison group. There is temporoparietal hypometabolism in AD, marked occipital hypometabolism in DLB, predominantly frontal hypometabolism in FTD, and asymmetric hypometabolism in CBD.[30] *From* Brown RK, Bohnen NI, Wong KK, Minoshima S, Frey KA. Brain PET in suspected dementia: patterns of altered FDG metabolism. Radiographics: a Review Publication of the Radiological Society of North America, Inc. 2014 May-Jun;34(3):684-701.

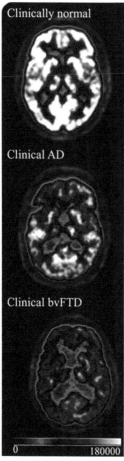

Clinically normal

Clinical AD

Clinical bvFTD

0   180000

Fig. 3. Axial brain FDG-PET uptake in representative participants[31] displayed in neurologic orientation (right side of the image is on reader's right-hand side). The clinically normal participant shows uniform Food and Drug Administration uptake throughout the brain as illustrated by the widespread intense bright colors. The person with clinical AD shows early asymmetric frontal and temporal hypometabolism that is comparatively more advanced in a person with bvFTD. (*Adapted from* Tosun D, Schuff N, Rabinovici GD, Ayakta N, Miller BL, Jagust W, Kramer J, Weiner MM, Rosen HJ. Diagnostic utility of ASL-MRI and FDG-PET in the behavioral variant of FTD and AD. Ann Clin Transl Neurol. 2016 Aug 30;3(10):740-751.)

considered as a diagnosis and ^{18}F-FDG-PET is the sole source of FTD-related imaging findings.

Although ^{18}F-FDG-PET is widely used in neurodegenerative disease diagnosis by differentiating disease subtypes, it remains important to recognize that the landscape for these disorders is rapidly changing because of increasing knowledge. One such set of factors under increasing consideration is comorbidities that can modify risk for FTD. Such FTD risk modifiers include

traumatic brain injury, diabetes mellitus, autoimmune disorders, and a family history of FTD.[28] Prior work has shown that head trauma incidence is significantly higher among patients with FTD than other forms of dementia.[29] Such factors can alter ^{18}F-FDG-PET findings such as asymmetric hypometabolism related to a specific site of head trauma. Atypical patterns on ^{18}F-FDG-PET should therefore be contextualized with known history, including risk modifiers and comorbidities. As AD is frequently considered in the differential diagnosis of FTD, **Fig. 3** demonstrates examples of different FTD-PET patterns on these disorders compared with normal metabolic findings on this modality.

SINGLE-PHOTON EMISSION COMPUTED TOMOGRAPHY

Although ^{99m}Tc-hexamethylpropyleneamine oxime (HMPAO)–single-photon emission computed tomography (SPECT) has been shown to have some diagnostic utility in FTD, ^{18}F-FDG-PET has demonstrated comparatively higher diagnostic utility.[2] Like FDG-PET, SPECT's diagnostic application in FTD comes primarily from distinguishing AD from FTD, but a systematic review has offered support for its utility differentiating FTD from DLB as well.[32] The pooled weighted sensitivity and specificity of ^{99m}Tc-HMPAO-SPECT in a meta-analysis investigating its capacity for distinguishing AD from FTD was 79.7% and 79.9%, respectively.[33] FTD findings in ^{99m}Tc-HMPAO-SPECT include bilateral hypoperfusion that targets the frontal lobes (**Fig. 4**), with asymmetric hypoperfusion of the right frontal lobes. This finding contrasts with other disorders like AD, in which there is bilateral hypoperfusion of the temporal lobes (**Fig. 5**).[34] These disorders can be differentiated not only by the comparatively higher burden of temporal hypoperfusion of AD but also by the anterior temporal hypoperfusion that can be seen in FTD (see **Fig. 5**) compared with the more lateral hypoperfusion in AD (see **Fig. 4**). Prior work suggests that ^{99m}Tc-HMPAO-SPECT may also assist in the discrimination of FTD variants, as there are distinct findings for patients with each of the three-core spectrum FTD disorders.[35]

^{123}I-FP-CIT-SPECT had a specificity of 64% and a sensitivity of 95% for differentiating FTD from DLB.[32] For ^{99m}Tc-HMPAO-SPECT, findings in bvFTD include bilateral frontotemporal hypoperfusion with an absence of posterior changes.[33] **Fig. 6** shows an example of SPECT findings in bvFTD. In general, SPECT in FTD is used more as a supplement to other imaging and clinical

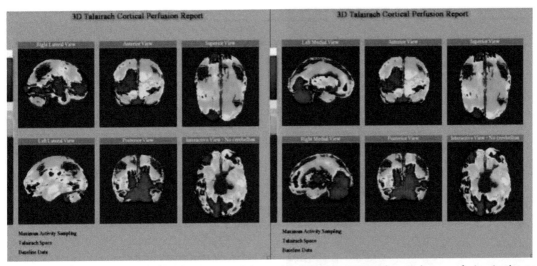

Fig. 4. Visual assessment of brain perfusion in a patient with AD using SPECT. There is hypoperfusion in the parietal lobes bilaterally.[34] (*From* Valotassiou, V, Tsougos, I, Tzavara, C, Georgoulias, P, Papatriantafyllou, J, Karageorgiou, C, Sifakis, N, & Zerva, C (2009). Evaluation of brain perfusion in specific Brodmann areas in Frontotemporal dementia and Alzheimer disease using automated 3-D voxel based analysis. Journal of Instrumentation, 4(05), P05020.)

information particularly when FDG-PET is not readily available. Finally, it should be noted that although most studies suggest PET superiority over SPECT, there is relatively little evidence of SPECT's performance as it pertains to FTD. Further comparative studies will help to clarify SPECT's role in the treatment of these diseases.[36]

AMYLOID PET

Amyloid PET has been shown to have diagnostic utility in FTD.[38] As amyloid-PET imaging typically has no tracer retention in patients with FTD, negative amyloid PET rules out AD.[39,40] This finding is important, as clinical presentations can have considerable overlap, particularly in bvFTD and PPA. PiB-PET, the most commonly used

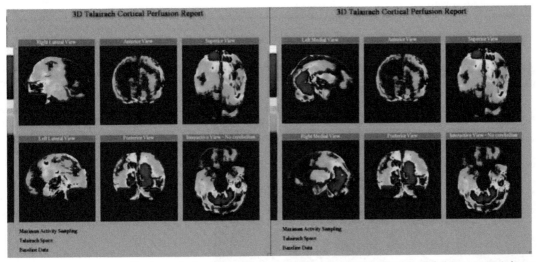

Fig. 5. Visual assessment of brain perfusion in a patient with FTD using SPECT. There is slightly asymmetric hypoperfusion in the frontal lobes, favoring the right side.[34] (*From* Valotassiou, V, Tsougos, I, Tzavara, C, Georgoulias, P, Papatriantafyllou, J, Karageorgiou, C, Sifakis, N, & Zerva, C (2009). Evaluation of brain perfusion in specific Brodmann areas in Frontotemporal dementia and Alzheimer disease using automated 3-D voxel based analysis. Journal of Instrumentation, 4(05), P05020.)

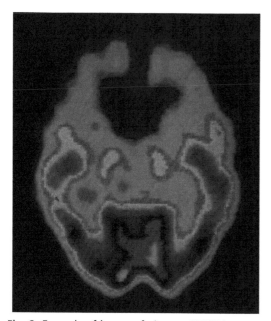

Fig. 6. Example of hypoperfusion on SPECT in a person with bvFTD. There is bifrontal and bitemporal hypoperfusion.[37] *Reprinted from* J Alzheimers Dis. 30(4), Rollin-Sillaire A, Bombois S, Deramecourt V, et al. Contribution of single photon emission computed tomography to the differential diagnosis of dementia in a memory clinic, 833-845. Copyright 2012, with permission from IOS Press. The publication is available at IOS Press through http://dx.doi.org/10.3233/JAD-2012-111067.

amyloid-PET tracer, has been shown to distinguish FTLD from AD with higher sensitivity (89% vs 73%) but relatively lower specificity (83% vs 98%) compared with ^{18}F-FDG-PET.[2] However, it should be noted that although it is relatively rare to have a positive amyloid-PET with a clinical diagnosis of bvFTD, it is possible. On autopsies of patients with a positive amyloid-PET, an FTD syndrome, and typical FTD-like patterns of atrophy/hypometabolism, there have been multiple cases whereby AD and FTD pathologic condition are found to coexist.[41,42] Thus, a positive amyloid-PET should not completely rule out FTD. However, the weight of evidence suggests using amyloid-PET imaging whenever a patient presents with cognitive impairment that creates suspicion for AD. **Fig. 7** shows examples of amyloid deposition and FTD hypometabolism in normal cognition, AD, and FTD variants.

TAU PET

The FTLD-Tau subtypes come in 2 common forms: three-repeat (3R) and four-repeat (4R) tauopathies. 3R and 4R tauopathies refer to tau isoforms that have either 3 microtubule-binding repeat domains (3R-tau) or 4 domains (4R-tau). The only nongenetic 3R tauopathy that primarily occurs with bvFTD is PiD, although svPPA, nfvPPA, and corticobasal syndrome can also occur.[44–46] On the other hand, there are multiple 4R tauopathies that can lead to FTD; the most common by far are progressive supranuclear palsy (PSP), CBD, globular glial tauopathies, argyrophilic grain disease, and PSP and CBD together.[47] These often present as syndromes combined with one of the core spectrum disorders (ie, PSP-bvFTD, CBD-bvFTD, CBD-nfvPPA) to create very complex presentations. As tau-PET findings for these specific subtypes are essentially nonexistent, the findings are mostly based on structural imaging and are not discussed in detail here.

In general, tau-PET has been shown to be useful in differentiating AD pathologic condition from

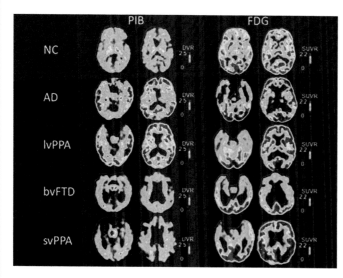

Fig. 7. Amyloid and FDG-PET abnormalities across normal cognition, AD, and FTD variants (lvPPA, logopenic variant primary progressive aphasia; bvFTD, and svPPA). DVR, distribution volume ratio; NC, normal controls; SUVR, standardized uptake value ratio. There is a comparative lack of amyloid uptake in the FTD syndromes.[43] (*From* Laforce R Jr, Rabinovici GD. Amyloid imaging in the differential diagnosis of dementia: review and potential clinical applications. Alzheimers Res Ther. 2011;3(6):31. Published 2011 Nov 10.)

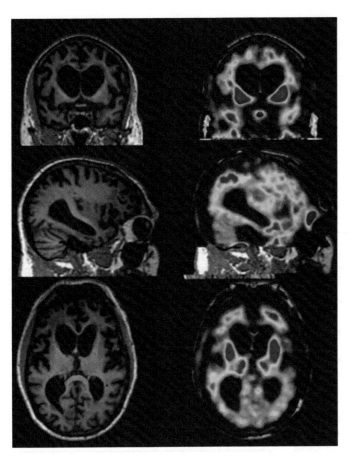

Fig. 8. MR imaging (*left*) and ^{18}F-T807 PET (*right*) brain images from a 56-year-old person with P301L MAPT mutation FTD. Visually apparent frontal and temporal atrophy is noted on MR imaging along with increased tau uptake in the basal ganglia.[55] (*From* Ghetti B, Oblak AL, Boeve BF, Johnson KA, Dickerson BC, Goedert M. Invited review: Frontotemporal dementia caused by microtubule-associated protein tau gene (MAPT) mutations: a chameleon for neuropathology and neuroimaging [published correction appears in Neuropathol Appl Neurobiol. 2015 Jun;41(4):571] [published correction appears in Neuropathol Appl Neurobiol. 2015 Jun;41(4):571]. Neuropathol Appl Neurobiol. 2015;41(1):24-46.)

other types of neuropathology, and it can distinguish AD from FTD syndromes with high accuracy.[48] In a multicenter cross-sectional study comparing the discriminative accuracy of ^{18}F-flortaucipir PET in differentiating AD from other non-AD neurodegenerative disorders, it had a sensitivity of 89.9% and specificity of 90.6%. However, tau-PET is not as useful for delineation of FTLD subtypes, having had mixed results in

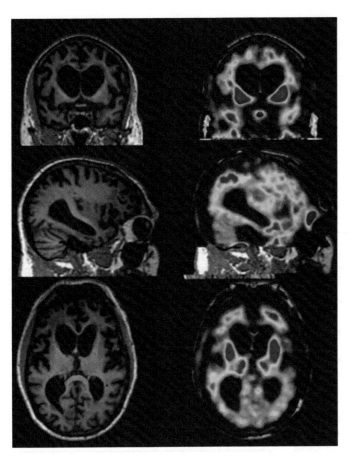

Fig. 9. nTRD22, a novel small molecule that allosterically modulates TDP-43 and may serve as a binding domain for new tau PET tracers.[58] From Rao PPN, Shakeri A, Zhao Y, Calon F. Strategies in the design and development of (TAR) DNA-binding protein 43 (TDP-43) binding ligands. Eur J Med Chem. 2021;225:113753.

distinguishing FTLD pathologic conditions among in vivo studies. It should also be noted that ^{18}F-flortaucipir, the PET tracer most widely used to study tau accumulation in the brain,[49] has yet to demonstrate binding in tauopathies outside of AD and has been shown to bind to several other non-tau targets.[47]

Also, several studies have shown that flortaucipir-PET is elevated in some patients with specific MAPT mutations.[50–53] This elevation occurs in MAPT mutations that result in a mix of 3R/4R tau pathologic condition, but there is variation in the literature, as others have reported data that a mild increase in flortaucipir binding is observed in multiple FTLD-tau subtypes and is therefore not useful in differentiating these subtypes.[54] PET and MR imaging findings in a person with a specific MAPT mutation are shown in **Fig. 8.**

NOVEL RADIOTRACERS

PET imaging with amyloid and tau ligands has been tailored for AD investigation and diagnosis. However, many of these tracers have little to no binding to non-AD tau isoforms and high off-target binding to non-tau structures.[56] This limits

Table 1
Neurodegenerative diseases with respective hypometabolic regions on fluorodeoxyglucose-PET

	PC	Pari	Lat Temp	Med Temp	Fron	Occ	SM	ST	TH	BS
MCI due to AD	↓	↓	→	→ (or ↓)	→	→	→	→	→	→
AD (mild)	↓	↓	↓	→ (or ↓)	→	→	→	→	→	→
AD (moderate)	↓	↓	↓	↓	↓	→	→	→	→	→
DLB	↓	↓	↓	→	↓	↓	→	→	→	→
FTD	→ (or ↓)	→ (or ↓)	↓	↓	→	→	→	→ (or ↓)	→	→
SD	→	→ (or ↓)	↓↓	↓	→	→	→	→	→	→
PSP	→	→	→ (or ↓)	→	↓	→	→	↓	→	↓
CBD (1)	↓	↓	↓	→	↓	→	↓	↓	↓	→
VaD (2)	→ (or ↓)	→ (or ↓)	→ (or ↓)	→ (or ↓)	↓	→	→ (or ↓)	→ (or ↓)	→ (or ↓)	

Abbreviations: (1), asymmetric reduction is characteristic; (2), predominantly frontal metabolic reduction is often demonstrated as well as an infarction region; BS, brainstem; Fron, frontal cortex; Lat, null; lateral, temporal cortex; MCI, mild cognitive impairment; Med, null; medial, temporal cortex; Occ, occipital cortex; Pari, parietal association cortex; PC, posterior cingulate gyrus; SD, semantic dementia; SM, sensorimotor cortex; ST, striatum; TH, thalamus; VaD, vascular dementia; →, preserved; ↓, decreased.
From Ishii K. PET approaches for diagnosis of dementia. AJNR Am J Neuroradiol. 2014 Nov-Dec;35(11):2030-8.[61]

the diagnostic utility of such tracers in non-AD tauopathies.

There remains a need for novel radiotracers that target FTD-associated proteins. Pathologic TDP-43 and tau are involved in ~90% of FTLD cases, with the remaining 10% made up of fused-in-sarcoma protein (FUS).[57] Although multiple PET tau tracers have been developed,[56] there have been efforts to design binding ligands for other proteins, like TDP-43.[59] Discoveries of small molecules such as nTRD22 have brought insights into targets that novel ligands could have (**Fig. 9**). Also, the dopamine transporter (DAT) is an established PET target[49] that has recently been reported to have abnormal findings on DAT-SPECT imaging in some patients with FTD.[59,60] Future research could investigate developing new radiotracers that target TDP-43 as well as FUS, and DAT for PET and SPECT imaging.

SUMMARY OF CLINICAL FINDINGS IN NEUROIMAGING WITH FLUORODEOXYGLUCOSE-PET

In summary, there are key findings for multiple neurodegenerative diseases on FDG-PET. For FTD, there is frontal and temporal hypometabolism. In AD, the most important findings are bilateral temporal and parietal lobe hypometabolism. In DLB, there is frontal and occipital hypometabolism. These differing areas of hypometabolism, as well as their combinations, can be used to differentiate diseases. For example, if there is frontal hypometabolism but the occipital lobe is spared, DLB is less likely. A comparatively anterior temporal hypometabolism advances the differential diagnosis

closer to FTD, whereas AD shows medial temporal and hippocampal hypometabolism. **Table 1** lists areas of hypometabolism of these and other important neurodegenerative diseases.

CLINICS CARE POINTS

- PET scans may not be partial volume corrected for atrophy.[62] Thus, brain MR imaging acquired with PET can be important for PET processing as well as atrophy detection.

- Common mimics of frontotemporal dementia on scans include Alzheimer disease and dementia with Lewy bodies. Thus, interpretations of PET scans should consider related disease presentation, for example, the presence of visual hallucinations in dementia with Lewy bodies versus other dementias as well as the executive dysfunction that predominates in frontotemporal dementia.

- Newer techniques on PET, such as tau PET, hold promise for identifying frontotemporal dementia but are limited by the lack of radioligands that can identify the full range of tau isoforms that can manifest in frontotemporal dementia variants.

DISCLOSURE

The authors have nothing to disclose.

ACNOWLEDGEMENT

Mr. Ward was supported in this work by the Mallinckrodt Institute of Radiology Summer Research Program (Mentor: CA Raji). Dr. Raji is supported in his research by NIA 1RF1AG072637-01 (CA Raji, P.I.). Dr. Raji is a consultant for Brainreader ApS, Neurevolution LLC, Icometrix, and Apollo Health.

REFERENCES

1. Olney RK, Murphy J, Forshew D, et al. The effects of executive and behavioral dysfunction on the course of ALS. Neurology 2005;65(11):1774–7.

2. Duignan JA, Haughey A, Kinsella JA, et al. Molecular and anatomical imaging of dementia with Lewy bodies and frontotemporal lobar degeneration. Semin Nucl Med 2021;51(3):264–74.

3. Uber die Beziehungen der senilen Hirnatrophie zur Aphasie | CiNii Research. Available at: https://cir.nii.ac.jp/crid/1572261550500971008. Accessed June 8, 2022.

4. Alzheimer A. über eigenartige Krankheitsfälle des späteren Alters. Z für die gesamte Neurologie Psychiatrie 1911;4(1):356–85.

5. Thibodeau MP, Miller BL. Limits and current knowledge of Pick's disease: its differential diagnosis". A translation of the 1957 Delay, Brion, Escourolle article. Neurocase 2013;19(5):417–22.

6. Román G. Vascular dementia: a historical background. Int Psychogeriatr 2003;15(Suppl 1):11–3.

7. Ryan NS, Rossor MN, Fox NC. Alzheimer's disease in the 100 years since Alzheimer's death. Brain 2015;138(Pt 12):3816–21.

8. DE K, ME P, EJ H, et al. Initial clinical experience with 18F-2-fluoro-2-deoxy-d-glucose for determination of local cerebral glucose utilization by emission computed tomography. Acta Neurol Scand Suppl 1977;64:192–3. Available at: https://europepmc.org/article/MED/268784. Accessed June 6, 2022.

9. Rascovsky K, Hodges JR, Knopman D, et al. Sensitivity of revised diagnostic criteria for the behavioural variant of frontotemporal dementia. Brain 2011;134(9):2456.

10. Minoshima S, Mosci K, Cross D, et al. Brain [F-18] FDG PET for clinical dementia workup: differential diagnosis of Alzheimer's disease and other types of dementing disorders. Semin Nucl Med 2021;51(3):230–40.

11. Schroeter ML, Raczka K, Neumann J, et al. Towards a nosology for frontotemporal lobar degenerations-a meta-analysis involving 267 subjects. Neuroimage 2007;36(3):497–510.

12. Schroeter ML. Considering the frontomedian cortex in revised criteria for behavioural variant frontotemporal dementia. Brain 2012;135(4):e213.

13. Perry DC, Brown JA, Possin KL, et al. Clinicopathological correlations in behavioural variant frontotemporal dementia. Brain 2017;140(12):3329–45.

14. Whitwell JL, Przybelski SA, Weigand SD, et al. Distinct anatomical subtypes of the behavioural variant of frontotemporal dementia: a cluster analysis study. Brain 2009;132(11):2932.

15. Brown JA, Deng J, Neuhaus J, et al. Patient-tailored, connectivity-based forecasts of spreading brain atrophy. Neuron 2019;104(5):856–68.e5.

16. Seeley WW, Crawford RK, Zhou J, et al. Neurodegenerative diseases target large-scale human brain networks. Neuron 2009;62(1):42–52.

17. Zhou J, Gennatas ED, Kramer JH, et al. Predicting regional neurodegeneration from the healthy brain functional connectome. Neuron 2012;73(6):1216–27.

18. Buhour MS, Doidy F, Laisney M, et al. Pathophysiology of the behavioral variant of frontotemporal lobar degeneration: a study combining MRI and FDG-PET. Brain Imaging Behav 2016;11(1):240–52.

19. Bejanin A, Tammewar G, Marx G, et al. Longitudinal structural and metabolic changes in frontotemporal dementia. Neurology 2020;95(2):e140.

20. Franceschi M, Anchisi D, Pelati O, et al. Glucose metabolism and serotonin receptors in the frontotemporal lobe degeneration. Ann Neurol 2005;57(2):216–25.

21. Diehl-Schmid J, Grimmer T, Drzezga A, et al. Decline of cerebral glucose metabolism in frontotemporal dementia: a longitudinal 18F-FDG-PET-study. Neurobiol Aging 2007;28(1):42–50.

22. Hoffman JM, Welsh-Bohmer KA, Hanson M, et al. Special contributions FDG PET imaging in patients with pathologically verified dementia. J Nucl Med 2000;41:1920–8.

23. Bejanin A, la Joie R, Landeau B, et al. Distinct interplay between atrophy and hypometabolism in Alzheimer's versus semantic dementia. Cereb Cortex 2019;29(5):1889–99.

24. Kanda T, Ishii K, Uemura T, et al. Comparison of grey matter and metabolic reductions in frontotemporal dementia using FDG-PET and voxel-based morphometric MR studies. Eur J Nucl Med Mol Imaging 2008;35(12):2227–34.

25. Jeong Y, Cho SS, Park JM, et al. 18F-FDG PET findings in frontotemporal dementia: an SPM analysis of 29 patients. J Nucl Med 2005;46(2):233–9.

26. Ceccarini J, Bourgeois S, van Weehaeghe D, et al. Direct prospective comparison of 18 F-FDG PET and arterial spin labelling MR using simultaneous PET/MR in patients referred for diagnosis of dementia. Eur J Nucl Med Mol Imaging 2020;47(9):2142–54.

27. Moonis G., Subramaniam R.M., Trofimova A., et al., ACR Appropriateness Criteria® Dementia Expert Panel on Neurological Imaging, J Am Coll Radiol, 17 (5s), 2020, S100-S112.

28. Rasmussen H, Stordal E, Rosness TA. Risk factors for frontotemporal dementia. Tidsskr Nor Laegeforen 2018;138(14). https://doi.org/10.4045/TIDSSKR.17.0763.

29. Kalkonde Yv, Jawaid A, Qureshi SU, et al. Medical and environmental risk factors associated with frontotemporal dementia: a case-control study in a veteran population. Alzheimers Dement 2012;8(3):204–10.

30. Brown RKJ, Bohnen NI, Wong KK, et al. Brain PET in suspected dementia: patterns of altered FDG metabolism. Radiographics 2014;34(3):684–701.

31. Tosun D, Schuff N, Rabinovici GD, et al. Diagnostic utility of ASL-MRI and FDG-PET in the behavioral variant of FTD and AD. Ann Clin Transl Neurol 2016;3(10):740.

32. Brigo F, Turri G, Tinazzi M. 123I-FP-CIT SPECT in the differential diagnosis between dementia with Lewy bodies and other dementias. J Neurol Sci 2015;359(1–2):161–71.

33. Yeo JM, Lim X, Khan Z, et al. Systematic review of the diagnostic utility of SPECT imaging in dementia. Eur Arch Psychiatry Clin Neurosci 2013;263(7):539–52.

34. Valotassiou V, Papatriantafyllou J, Sifakis N, et al. Evaluation of brain perfusion in specific Brodmann areas in frontotemporal dementia and Alzheimer disease using automated 3-D voxel based analysis. J Instrumentation 2009;4(05):P05020.

35. Mamouli D, Stavrakaki S, Iakovou I, et al. SPECT analysis and language profile in Greek speaking patients with subtypes of frontotemporal dementia. Hell J Nucl Med 2022;25(1):43–56.

36. Davison CM, O'Brien JT. A comparison of FDG-PET and blood flow SPECT in the diagnosis of neurodegenerative dementias: a systematic review. Int J Geriatr Psychiatry 2014;29(6):551–61.

37. Rollin-Sillaire A, Bombois S, Deramecourt V, et al. Contribution of single photon emission computed tomography to the differential diagnosis of dementia in a memory clinic. J Alzheimer's Dis 2012;30(4):833–45.

38. Krishnadas N, Villemagne VL, Doré V, et al. Advances in brain amyloid imaging. Semin Nucl Med 2021;51(3):241–52.

39. Shi Z, Fu LP, Zhang N, et al. Amyloid PET in dementia syndromes: a Chinese multicenter study. J Nucl Med 2020;61(12):1814–9.

40. Tan RH, Kril JJ, Yang Y, et al. Assessment of amyloid β in pathologically confirmed frontotemporal dementia syndromes. Alzheimer's Demen Diagn Assess Dis Monit 2017;9(1):10–20.

41. de Leon J, Mandelli ML, Nolan A, et al. Atypical clinical features associated with mixed pathology in a case of non-fluent variant primary progressive aphasia. Neurocase 2019;25(1–2):39–47.

42. Langheinrich T, Kobylecki C, Jones M, et al. Amyloid-PET–positive patient with bvFTD. Neurol Clin Pract 2021;11(6):e952–5.

43. Laforce R, Rabinovici GD. Amyloid imaging in the differential diagnosis of dementia: review and potential clinical applications. Alzheimers Res Ther 2011;3(6). https://doi.org/10.1186/ALZRT93.

44. Choudhury P, Scharf EL, Paolini MA, et al. Pick's disease: clinicopathologic characterization of 21 cases. J Neurol 2020;267(9):2697–704.

45. Piguet O, Halliday GM, Reid WGJ, et al. Clinical phenotypes in autopsy-confirmed Pick disease. Neurology 2011;76(3):253–9.

46. Irwin DJ, Brettschneider J, McMillan CT, et al. Deep clinical and neuropathological phenotyping of Pick disease. Ann Neurol 2016;79(2):272–87.

47. Peet BT, Spina S, Mundada N, et al. Neuroimaging in frontotemporal dementia: heterogeneity and relationships with underlying neuropathology. Neurotherapeutics 2021;18(2):728–52.

48. Ossenkoppele R, Rabinovici GD, Smith R, et al. Discriminative accuracy of [18F]flortaucipir positron emission tomography for Alzheimer disease vs other neurodegenerative disorders. JAMA 2018;320(11):1151.

49. van Waarde A, Marcolini S, de Deyn PP, et al. PET agents in dementia: an overview. Semin Nucl Med 2021;51(3):196–229.

50. Tsai RM, Bejanin A, Lesman-Segev O, et al. 18F-flortaucipir (AV-1451) tau PET in frontotemporal dementia syndromes. Alzheimers Res Ther 2019;11(1). https://doi.org/10.1186/S13195-019-0470-7.

51. Spina S, Schonhaut DR, Boeve BF, et al. Frontotemporal dementia with the V337M MAPT mutation: tau-PET and pathology correlations. Neurology 2017;88(8):758.

52. Smith R, Puschmann A, Schöll M, et al. 18F-AV-1451 tau PET imaging correlates strongly with tau neuropathology in MAPT mutation carriers. Brain 2016;139(9):2372.

53. Jones DT, Knopman DS, Graff-Radford J, et al. In vivo 18F-AV-1451 tau PET signal in MAPT mutation carriers varies by expected tau isoforms. Neurology 2018;90(11):e947.

54. Soleimani-Meigooni DN, Iaccarino L, Joie R la, et al. 18F-flortaucipir PET to autopsy comparisons in Alzheimer's disease and other neurodegenerative diseases. Brain 2020;143(11):3477.

55. Ghetti B, Oblak AL, Boeve BF, et al. Invited review: frontotemporal dementia caused by microtubule-associated protein tau gene (MAPT) mutations: a chameleon for neuropathology and neuroimaging. Neuropathol Appl Neurobiol 2015;41(1):24–46.

56. Beyer L, Brendel M. Imaging of tau pathology in neurodegenerative diseases: an update. Semin Nucl Med 2021;51(3):253–63.

57. Rademakers R, Neumann M, MacKenzie IR. Advances in understanding the molecular basis of frontotemporal dementia. Nat Rev Neurol 2012;8(8): 423–34.

58. Rao PPN, Shakeri A, Zhao Y, et al. Strategies in the design and development of (TAR) DNA-binding protein 43 (TDP-43) binding ligands. Eur J Med Chem 2021;225:113753.

59. Kobayashi R, Kawakatsu S, Ohba M, et al. Dopamine transporter imaging for frontotemporal lobar degeneration with motor neuron disease. Front Neurosci 2022;16. https://doi.org/10.3389/FNINS. 2022.755211/FULL.

60. Morgan S, Kemp P, Booij J, et al. Differentiation of frontotemporal dementia from dementia with Lewy bodies using FP-CIT SPECT. J Neurol Neurosurg Psychiatry 2012;83(11):1063–70.

61. Ishii K. PET approaches for diagnosis of dementia. AJNR Am J Neuroradiol 2014;35(11):2030.

62. Meltzer CC, Kinahan PE, Greer PJ, et al. Comparative evaluation of MR-based partial-volume correction schemes for PET. J Nucl Med 1999;40(12): 2053–65.

Multi-Scale Temporal Imaging: From Micro- and Meso- to Macro-scale-time Nuclear Medicine

Faraz Farhadi, BS[a,b], Jayasai R. Rajagopal, BA[a], Eren M. Veziroglu, MS[b], Hamid Abdollahi, PhD[c], Isaac Shiri, Phd[d], Moozhan Nikpanah, MD[a,h], Michael A. Morris, MD[a], Habib Zaidi, PhD[d,e,f,g], Arman Rahmim, PhD[c,i], Babak Saboury, MD[a,*]

KEYWORDS

- Time • Radiomics • Radiophenomics • Delta radiomics • Multi-scale Temporal Imaging
- Longitudinal imaging studies

INTRODUCTION

Living systems are in constant dynamism to keep the "internal milieu" stable despite the variation of external factors. This continuous change at the molecular and cellular levels aims at preventing a change at a large-scale (principle of homeostasis). In a medical context, there are two processes that can cause change at a large-scale: maladies and aging. Aging is a more gradual process that has been less studied.[1] Time provides a common frame of reference by which different processes of change can be related, and thus, time represents our understanding of change.

The human body is a system that is composed of structure on a range of scales from the nanometer size of amino acids, to the micrometer dimension of cells, to the milimeter length of tissues, to the centimeter proportion of organas.

Properties of these structures can be measured using different imaging technologies. In the spatial domain, these imaging techniques provide characterization in the form of static or structural imaging. For instance electron density of the structure can be evaluated, and the mapping of this characteristics in the space-domain is achieved by CT images (X-Ray Computed Tomography). By comparing these structural snapshots with an expected norm, anatomical pathologies can be diagnosed and treated. In this way, structure can be captured and described as a multi-scale characterization of the spatial domain.

We capture the function and dynamism of an organ or organism via evaluation of the change in structures (like change in volume of left ventricle to measure function of heart as ejection fraction). Function, like structure, can be described as a multi-scale characterization. However, function

This work was originated at: National Institutes of Health (NIH), 9000 Rockville Pike, Bethesda, Maryland 20892, 301-496-4000, TTY 301-402-9612

[a] Radiology and Imaging Sciences, Clinical Center, National Institutes of Health, 9000 Rockville Pike, Building 10, Room 1C455, Bethesda, MD 20892, USA; [b] Geisel School of Medicine at Dartmouth, 1 Rope Ferry Road, Hanover, NH 03755, USA; [c] Department of Integrative Oncology, BC Cancer Research Institute, 675 West 10th Avenue, Vancouver, BC V5Z 1L3, Canada; [d] Division of Nuclear Medicine and Molecular Imaging, Geneva University Hospital, Geneva CH-1211, Switzerland; [e] Department of Nuclear Medicine and Molecular Imaging, University of Groningen, University Medical Center Groningen, 9700 RB Groningen, Netherlands; [f] Department of Nuclear Medicine, University of Southern Denmark, 500 Odense, Denmark; [g] Geneva University Neurocenter, Geneva University, CH-1205 Geneva, Switzerland; [h] Department of Radiology, University of Alabama, 619 19th Street South, Birmingham, AL 35294, USA; [i] Department of Radiology, University of British Columbia, 675 West 10th Avenue, Vancouver, British Columbia V5Z 1L3, Canada

* Corresponding author. Radiology and Imaging Sciences, 10 Center Drive, Bethesda, MD 20892.

E-mail address: Babak.saboury@nih.gov

https://doi.org/10.1016/j.cpet.2022.09.008
1556-8598/23/© 2022 Elsevier Inc. All rights reserved.

could be characterized in the temporal rather than spatial domain:In clinical imaging, time ranges from the seconds of perfusion imaging, to the minutes of ^{18}F-Fluorodeoxyglucose (FDG) kinetics, to the days for ^{177}Lu-PSMA biodistribution, and to the months for tumor growth. If we have dynamic imaging then we can quantify the change to evaluate the function (like glucose metabolism by compartmental modeling in dynamic FDG-PET); however in clinical practice sometimes we only have the temporal snapshots of this dynamism (like static FDG-PET imaging). To interpret the meaning of these snapshots of the function, we have to compare them with the expected status of the dynamic systems at certain times to identify functional pathologies (like 45 second post injection of iodine-based contrast to evaluate arterial perfusion in CT or 60 minutes post injection of 18F-FDG to evaluate metabolic activity in PET).

Change across different time points is a critical factor that is foundational for diagnostic imaging which is the basis of an aphorism in medical imaging community: "the best friend of a radiologist is prior images". This wisdom emphasizes on the superiority of temporal dynamism over static appearance of structure. In this article, we discuss the interrelatedness of "change" and "time", the similarities of "imaging of change" regardless of time-scale, and the scale-dependent difference of "temporal imaging". We first describe the different time scales and the kinds of imaging that take place under those time scales. We then examine the current status of medical imaging literature focused on a macro time scale. We identify strengths and weaknesses of existing evaluations. Finally, we offer some observations and suggestions for future directions of medical imaging research.

TEMPORAL IMAGING AND VARIOUS SCALES OF TIME

The temporal domain can be described over several different time scales. Within the context of medical imaging, we describe three such time scales: micro-, meso-, and macro- time scales.[2] Micro-scale temporal imaging refers to a small temporal window that encompasses a single imaging or acquisition event (session). This can range from the narrow window of beam on-time in a system to repeated scans that occur between when a patient gets on and off the imaging table, including techniques such as dynamic PET and multi-phase CT, or gated imaging. Meso-timescale imaging concerns acquisitions that occur within a short period but as distinct scanning events. Finally, macro-timescale imaging concerns a longer gap between scanning events

extending to months or even years. In both the scientific literature and clinical practice, there has been a greater focus and a better understanding of imaging along the micro- and meso- scales. In this section, we describe the micro- and meso-scales in greater detail. The paper then focuses on macro-scale temporal imaging.

Micro-scale temporal imaging

Beyond routine scanning which is considered along micro-scale time, there are multiple established imaging techniques that utilize a series of scans within a single acquisition period to improve understanding of specific biological and metabolic functions. Examples include kinematic and parametric imaging in nuclear medicine[3–5], multiphase CT for renal and liver lesions[6–9], CT angiography[10], perfusion CT and MRI[11–16], and dynamic and diffusion imaging in MRI[17–19], gated cardiac SPECT and PET imaging, and respiratory gated imaging (for motion tracking or compensation). An important development has been 4D medical imaging technologies, where the three spatial dimensions of volumetric imaging modalities are combined with time to precisely observe temporal change and variation.[20] This concept has been investigated with time resolved CT, SPECT, PET, and MRI.

Meso-scale temporal Imaging

For meso-scale temporal imaging, common techniques include the notion of pre-op and post-op scans for various surgeries[21–24], dosimetry studies in nuclear medicine, and daily scans during the course of a radiation therapy treatment[25–27]. A specific example is radiopharmaceutical therapy (RPT), for which time is a critical factor. Time is a critical factor in radiopharmaceutical therapy (RPT) effectiveness. After the injection of a radiopharmaceutical into the body, radiation dose is deposited to the tumor and normal organs by an exponential decreasing behavior and with a range of a fraction of seconds to months.[28] In this therapeutic approach, time-dependent mechanisms including radionuclide decay and its clearance from the body, determine the tumor and normal organ dose. Accurate estimation of the dose is a complex task and needs specific methodologies. To do so, longitudinal imaging in terms of single photon emission computed tomography (SPECT) is utilized as a practical approach for dosimetry.[29] SPECT images which are obtained at different time points, are used to assess the therapeutic dose. The images can be acquired at different time points, such as before the first cycle of therapy as single-point dosimetry or between the cycles of therapy as multi-point dosimetry methodologies. Although the dose obtained using this method suffers from some uncertainties, it can be considered a patient-specific dose and can be directly converted to a biologically effective dose (BED) or other bioeffect doses.[29,30] On the other hand, positron emission tomography (PET) in terms of dynamic imaging is a time-based imaging modality that can be utilized for predictive dosimetry in RPT. Here the time scale has a range of minutes to hours and the obtained data can simulate dose distribution during the RPT. This short-term longitudinal imaging approach, although has a diagnostic time scale, may mimic the large-scale therapeutic time scale of deposited dose in patients who received RPT. Time-activity curve obtained using whole body dynamic PET/CT acquired form first minutes after injection of the radiopharmaceutical to several minutes to hours after that, can predict therapeutic dose, then this multi-time scale imaging modality will be a feasible approach for patient-specific dosimetry.

Macro-scale temporal Imaging

There has commonly been greater emphasis on the micro-scale and meso-scale temporal imaging in both clinical practice and research, with less focus on questions that are at the macro-scale. Macro-scale temporal imaging is the evaluation of changes over months to years with the prototype example of longitudinal imaging of aging.

LONGITUDINAL DATA IN MEDICAL IMAGING RESEARCH

Thinking on the macro-scale is common in clinical care. When interpreting the images of a particular patient, clinicians often invoke earlier imaging studies or other tests. The specific medical history of that patient is then used to inform medical decision-making. When a specific diagnosis is then made, a clinician can also use the natural history and progression of disease to understand the status of that specific diagnosis. With the advent of personalized medicine, the long-term time focus has become even more important in clinical practice.[31,32] Longitudinal imaging information, along with other specific and deep data including genomics, can help improve clinical outcomes.

Beyond the clinic, there has been research along the macro-scale. The first focus of longitudinal studies was on natural change in the form of development.[33–36] Early studies in radiography studied bone growth in children. With the evolution of medical imaging technology and expansion of imaging capability, there has been an increased interest in brain development which has been studied through PET.

Longitudinal studies focused on the long-term benefits of screening, monitoring of different disease processes, and response to treatments are also represented in the literature. These studies can be grouped into two broader classes based on the type of questions they answer: functional imaging studies, which look at various metabolic processes, and structural imaging studies, which seek to gain increased understanding of the physical features of disease.

Tracking Changes in Metabolic Processes

Many functional imaging longitudinal studies in PET research have focused on tracking changes in metabolic processes to evaluate recovery, assess the impact of treatment options, or track the progression of disease. PET has been used to understand which regions of the brain are associated with aphasia due to subcortical lesions following a stroke. Heiss and colleagues[37] performed a study where they used H_2O^{15}-PET activation patterns to identify brain regions that were associated with language performance in patients with poststroke aphasia at 2 and 8 weeks after stroke and compared their performance with healthy controls. They measured flow changes in the eloquent and contralateral homotopic areas over time to determine the differential capacity of the left and right hemispheres. In a later study by de Boissezon and colleagues[38] that focused on subcortical lesions, H_2O^{15}-PET and a word generation task were used to correlate language performance with change in regional cerebral blood flow over a period of 1 year following strokes. Data across patients were pooled and registered to a standard atlas and then used to calculate correlation between longitudinal change in regional cerebral blood flow and longitudinal change with language performance. Such longitudinal PET studies have inspired similar evaluations with other imaging modalities.[39]

Treatment Response Assessment

Longitudinal PET studies have also been used to assess conditions for certain treatment options and to evaluate the success of those treatments. Tumor hypoxia is an important indicator for the success of radiation therapy treatments as hypoxic cells are more resistant to treatment. As described by Stieb and colleagues,[40] PET is the main clinically validated imaging modality for this purpose and there is an extensive literature base of longitudinal PET studies for tracking the hypoxic status of tumors using a variety of radiotracers. Longitudinal PET studies have also shown potential for monitoring response for metastatic cancers. Hildebrandt and colleagues[41] describe the potential of FDG-PET/CT for evaluation of response in metastatic breast cancer. They first used retrospective data to define a lesion criteria and found that SUL_{peak} to be a useful biomarker of disease fluctuation. In a follow-up prospective study, patients were monitored using PET/CTs where the contrast-enhanced CT scan was used clinically. When comparing PET and CT for determining which method showed disease progression earlier based on final pathology, PET was able to detect the progression first in 50% of the cases. Thus, functional imaging plays an important role in the long-term treatment and response monitoring of disease.

Serial imaging plays a key role in radiotherapy response evaluation. In recent decade, different imaging modalities such as CT, MRI, SPECT, PET, ultrasound, and optical coherence tomography have been used to assess or predict radiation response of both malignant and healthy tissues. Interestingly, as radiation response is a biological process, these kind of imaging carry very rich spatiotemporal biological information, and a number of them may decode biological mechanisms of treatment and also extract a range of (radio)biological parameters that can be used to set biological-guided radiation therapy approaches. For example, serial ^{99m}Tc-dimercaptosuccinic acid (DMSA) SPECT/CT (pre, during, and post-treatment) provided new details of local radiobiological changes following stereotactic ablative body radiotherapy of renal cell carcinoma.[42] In addition, serial ^{18}F-Fluorothymidine PET/CT was used to analyze pattern and radiation-related changes of cellular proliferation in both tumors and bone marrow in non-small cell lung cancer (NSCLC) patients undergoing radiotherapy.[43]

In a comparative study, serial FLT-PET/CT and FDG-PET/CT were analyzed during radical chemoradiotherapy of NSLC, and it was observed that cellular proliferation imaged by PET/CT during therapy is associated with a patient's outcome (survival). It was suggested that therapy planning has to be changed based on these imaging findings, because tumor cell proliferation may reduce radiation-induced tumor cell killing and has a great impact on clinical outcome.[44] Interestingly, a study showed that serial ^{18}F-Fluorocholine PET/CT during chemotherapy in patients with prostate cancer is correlated with changes in circulating cell-free DNA (cfDNA).[45] It is evident that cfDNA is a useful biomarker for tumor profiling and therapy response evaluation. Recently, several radiobiological parameters were extracted from serial PET/CT images in patients with cancer treated with selective internal radionuclide therapy (SIRT) with yttrium-90 (90Y)-microspheres (^{90}Y-SIRT).[46]

In the study, parameters such as cell repopulation time (Tp), kick-off time (Tk), and linear quadratic model parameters (α, α/β) were obtained from serial imaging, dosimetric and clinical data.

Tracking Disease in Neurodegenerative Disorders

Other examples of longitudinal imaging have included studies in neurodegenerative disorders, including normal aging and Alzheimer's disease (amyloid[47] and tau[48] imaging) as well as Parkinson's disease,[49] including both PET and SPECT imaging. These have resulted in publicly available data sets, used extensively for biomarker discovery. Such biomarkers of disease have included disease subtype identification, progression tracking, and predictive modeling.

As an example, functional imaging also plays an important role in monitoring the progression of disease. Li and colleagues[50] describe a longitudinal comparison between two radiotracers, ^{11}C-PE2I and ^{18}F-DOPA, for monitoring Parkinson's disease. In this study, patients were first scanned with each tracer to determine a baseline and then followed up within a period of 2 years. PET findings were correlated with clinical findings quantified as motor severity tests and found that ^{11}C-PE2I showed higher sensitivity to differences in motor severity than ^{18}F-DOPA. In another study looking at aortic dilation in large vessel vasculitis, Muratore and colleagues[51] used FDG-PET/CT to measure the aortic uptake at four different levels at two time points. They found that patients diagnosed with large vessel vasculitis had an increased risk of aortic dilation when compared with controls. Ou and colleagues[52] studied the potential of FDG-PET to be a biomarker for diagnosis of Alzheimer's disease. In this study, a group of patients were recruited, and several biomarkers were tracked over an extended time period. They found that FDG-PET had strong indications for Alzheimer's disease and could be included as an independent biomarker.

Different Modalities Toward Improved Assessments

Longitudinal studies in structural imaging have spanned several different modalities. CT has been used for early detection and characterization of different types of tumors. The National Lung Screening Trial found that periodic CT studies are the imaging modality of choice for identifying the early emergence of lung cancer over time.[53] Similarly, the Response Evaluation Criteria in Solid Tumors (RECIST) use CT.[54] The RECIST criteria were developed to quantitatively assess changes in tumor burden over time. CT is considered one of the most reliable modalities for applying RECIST criteria. RECIST criteria have been applied extensively in clinical trials as a means to define and measure treatment response, and quantify progression-free survival.[55] However, there is need for further demonstrations of machine learning or high-dimensional radiomic analysis as applied to the interpretation of CT changes over time. As an example, in a study by Xu and colleagues[56] on patients experiencing locally advanced NSCLC, a neural network-based model was trained on CT imaging data obtained pretreatment, and 1-, 3-, and 6-month post-radiotherapy treatment. This study is an example of how we can incorporate pretreatment and posttreatment data over multiple time points when training predictive or evaluative algorithms.

Longitudinal studies and clinical standards are also common in radiographic imaging. The Radiographic Assessment of Lung Edema (RALE) score was designed to quantitatively evaluate alveolar opacities on chest radiographs specifically related to pulmonary edema in acute respiratory distress syndrome.[57] It has been shown to have excellent diagnostic performance. An increased RALE score was correlated with worse survival and became adopted as both a prognostic measure and a means of tracking physiologic changes over time that then guide clinical decision-making, such as conservative fluid administration.[58] Another example is mammograms, which are often used for screening for breast cancer. Longitudinal studies of mammographic data have found a connection between breast density and breast cancer risk. Earlier studies were more qualitative in nature, looking at breast imaging reporting & data system (BI-RADS) classifications to assign breast density classifications.[59] More recent works have been more quantitative as they have had an increased emphasis on volumetric classifications.[60]

DEXA scans are the standard for evaluating bone density and hip fracture risk. However, individualized extrapolation of bone densitometry timelines is rarely performed. Instead, an individual's bone density is compared with age- and sex-matched population statistics by a Z-score rather than evaluating how an individual's bone density is changing over time. We are not aware of any scoring methods which evaluate an individual's bone density change over time, yet there are several studies which exemplify individual variations in bone mineralization through space and time perturbations. DEXA scans sensitively evaluate both spatial and temporal changes in bone density. A small study by Iida and colleagues[61] showed that 3 months after hip fracture, greater

and lesser trochanteric bone density increased; contrarily, 3 years postfracture, the greater trochanteric bone density decreased. In another work by Hong and colleagues,[62] a radiomics-based scoring system was correlated with increased risk of hip fracture incidence. These studies exemplify how DEXA scans are capable of both measuring and predicting dynamic changes in physiologic states over space and time.

MR imaging is one of our greatest tools to study the human brain. The human brain is highly dynamic and constantly remodels throughout the course of our growth, development, and later years. MR imaging allows interrogation of the underlying pathologic changes in diseases of cognitive impairment such as dementia. In a study by Smith and colleagues,[63] brain MR imaging with a median comparison time of 5.8 years, the change velocity of specific brain structures/regions was determined and correlated with either healthy or pathologic aging. A recent study led by Cambridge and the University of Pennsylvania aggregated 123,984 MR imaging scans from 101,457 unique people across almost the entire human lifespan. This study sketches a trajectory for brain development over time and proposes a model by which outside images can be compared with the developmental timeline, similar to a pediatric growth chart.[64] However, they explicitly state that the current "brain chart" does not yet support the scoring of a single patient's image as would be desired in a clinical medicine context. Ultimately, we see great potential in the future of quantitative tools for time-series MR imaging analysis especially with regard to understanding brain structure.

Delta Radiomics

The concept of delta radiomics has been introduced to quantify changes typically due to therapies.[65] This information could be extracted from pre-, intra- and post-treatment images.[66] Recently, Shayesteh and colleagues[67] compared treatment response prediction power of MR imaging-based pre-, post-, and delta-radiomic features in locally advanced rectal cancer treated by neoadjuvant chemoradiation therapy. They included 53 patients from two different centers and developed different machine learning algorithms based on these features. They reported that the best performance was achieved by delta-radiomic features which significantly outperformed standalone pre- and post-treatment images-based models, thus confirming that longitudinal changes during treatment sessions could serve as a predictive model. Van Timmeren and colleagues[68] investigated the added value of longitudinal radiomic features in cone-beam CT for prognostic modeling in NSCLC patients. They included patients with at least four imaging sessions and evaluated models on three external data sets and built models using the Cox proportional hazards model using radiomic and clinical features for overall survival and locoregional recurrence prediction. They concluded that longitudinal radiomic features do not improve prognostication in NSCLC.

Longitudinal Imaging in Animal Studies

Longitudinal imaging in animal studies is considered as an important approach to have a deeper look in several diseases as well as aging.[69] Animal models, especially mice, because of similar anatomy and physiology to humans, are a main component of preclinical research. Several animal studies have used longitudinal imaging to study disease such as Alzheimer's, Parkinson's, atherosclerosis, osteoporosis, bone metastasis, lung, and liver cancers. In these studies, special imaging techniques such as micro-CT, micro-MR, PET, SPECT, optical, and microscopy imaging have been used.[69] Furthermore, due to the increasing number of transgenic and disease models available, such imaging approaches enable researchers to test and discover most optimized therapy toward personalized ones. In the realm of nuclear medicine, it is observed that a longitudinal mouse-PET imaging is a reliable method for estimating binding parameters without a reference region or blood sampling.[70] Moreover, longitudinal imaging using PET has a brilliant history in animal studies. For example, micro-FDPA-714 PET was shown as a feasible method to assess translocator protein expression longitudinally in a mouse model of epilepsy with hippocampal sclerosis.[71] Interestingly, longitudinal animal imaging using PET is recruited by several researchers to capture biological information such as cellular growth,[72] apoptosis,[73] activation,[71] and immunologic response.[74]

The natural history of disease offers a final point for the importance of macroscale thinking. As patients are followed over time, change can be contextualized by what was previously observed. As diagnoses have been encountered before and at different stages of disease progression, clinicians are able to refer to these prior documentations or experience to better understand specific diseases and assess treatment options. Natural history for chronic disease is more direct as a particular time point can be compared against the known arc of development for such a disease. For acute diseases, we have a different understanding of change

based on the status of that disease. Both longitudinal and cross-sectional approaches have been used to study disease with this understanding of disease progression and related changes in health over a macroscale time frame.

In the 2022, Cassen Award lecture addressed to the Society for Nuclear Medicine and Molecular Imaging, Simon Cherry advocated for using the temporal domain to our advantage. He describes the human body as a dynamic state of organ-based constituents where many processes go unobserved with modern clinical imaging. Particularly, whole-body PET imaging exemplifies a method which can capture processes within the entire body at the same time point. Furthermore, with improved detector sensitivity, processes occurring at both short (100 ms) and intermediate (days) time scales can now be observed with low radiation exposure. Ultimately, proper leveraging of the temporal domain through dynamic imaging will enable single subject research, that is, personalized medicine.

FOUR CHALLENGES IN QUANTIFYING TIME INTERVAL CHANGES

Different studies of macroscale time in the medical imaging literature were described in the previous section. There are some challenges to expanding the scope and application of these types of studies in the near future. In this section, we identify four challenges, specifically related to (i) data collection, (ii) algorithmic developments, (iii) performance metrics, and (iv) ethical considerations and discuss the need for addressing the key concerns.

The first major challenge is the issue of data. The volume of data that could be used for longitudinal studies is constantly increasing as medical imaging procedures are occurring more often than ever before. For many applications, well curated and extensive data sets are required for the development of algorithms and techniques. Further, the diversity of these data sets is critical to reduce bias in algorithms across all possible patient populations, imaging devices, and acquisition and processing protocols. Increasing access to data is critical for long-term development of techniques and furthering of studies on the macro-scale.

An additional concern with data is the issue of data sparsity. Often, data acquired at different time points and at different institutions do not have perfect concordance with one another. There can be many causes for this across longitudinal studies including technological evolution over time, difference in standards across institutions, variable time points between tests, multicentric data acquisition, missing sessions or specific imaging modality, and only repetition of some imaging tasks. The cumulative effect leads to data sets where certain data points are incomplete. One potential method to address time series data with uneven sampling called the Lomb–Scargle periodogram has already been applied to personalized omics studies and continues to provide quality-controlled insights into temporally relevant biomedical processes.[75,76] The robustness of algorithms to account for this factor is key to the success of long-term studies on the macroscale.

The second major challenge concerns the need for the development of better algorithms. Faster and more efficient algorithms will be needed to handle increasingly larger and more complex data sets. Robustness is important to minimize bias and enable accurate and precise characterization. Currently, there are performance constraints due to both hardware and software challenges. Adding time to current algorithms increases the complexity of the problems being analyzed. Although the development of technologies, such as application specific integrated circuits and various algorithms enable faster processing and handling of larger volumes of data, this problem will continue to require consideration. From the algorithmic perspective, development of future algorithms for longitudinal studies should be done in a way that is specific for the temporal domain and optimized for the analysis of longitudinal data. Time series models which analyze sequence of data points across a period of time by recurrent neural network concepts such as long short-term memory could be used as a tool for the analysis of longitudinal data set.

Quantitative analysis in the longitudinal time frame requires unique solutions. In creating quantitative metrics to represent longitudinal changes, normal and abnormal needs to be distinguished. Both physiologic and pathologic processes display an extraordinary range of temporal behaviors and structural patterns that transcend comprehension based on linear dynamics. In the context of medical imaging, image registration is used to bring images acquired at different times or across modalities into the same frame of reference. Two important characteristics of a registration method for longitudinal data are its robustness and stability (**Fig. 1**). A registration is robust when its performance is not drastically altered by deviations of the input image from the prior knowledge. For example, the algorithm must be able to withstand the presence of imaging artifacts as well as the advent of new imaging discoveries such as new pathologies. A registration is

stable when changes in the input data results in changes in the outcome of registration. Stability is important for longitudinal studies to measure differences that are attributed to temporal anatomic changes.[78] For nonrigid registration algorithms, changes in region/volume of interest due to the registration method should be considered, and using segmentation information for registration is recommended for precise registration.

The third major challenge is the development of performance metrics for algorithms, and the need for the correct metrics to be chosen for each task. With the development of task forces such as the Quantitative Imaging Biomarkers Alliance, standardization and reliability of metrics has taken on a more important role in medical imaging research. Reproducibility along the temporal domain is a particular concern as the change in a metric over time needs to be attributed to the result of change in disease state or a natural process, rather than a difference in acquisition condition or similar factors. In addition, metrics need to be chosen in a task-specific way. The figure of merit for a given task must be selected to reflect the scientific question in mind.

The fourth major challenge is ethical consideration in terms of patient convenience, privacy, and safety. Longitudinal imaging imposes a heavy burden on patients. In addition to time and costs, consecutive imaging exposes patients to a higher level of radiation which increases the chance of cancer risk. However, low dose protocol studies with advanced image reconstruction methods are an advanced solution for imaging centers to reduce the radiation dose effectively.

RECOMMENDATIONS

Information derived from changes over time is central to our understanding of normal physiologic processes, such as development and aging and pathophysiology of diseases. Although medical imaging in both clinical use and research has been focused on localized change, by better understanding the relationship between change and time, we are able to expand our scope. Although most of the longitudinal imaging studies have observations with two or more time points to capture and characterize change over time, methods for investigating time interval changes in medical imaging remain subjective or limited to primitive quantitative techniques. In this section, we outline five main considerations for how medical imaging research can better incorporate ideas of time and change. We offer suggestions for some broader concepts that affect how we think about and understand time as well as some specific

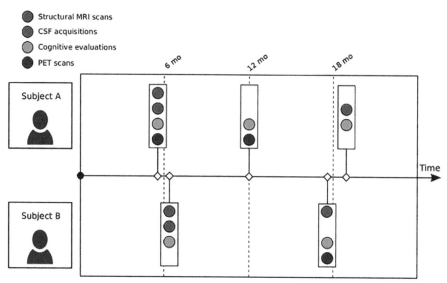

Fig. 1. shows an example of a longitudinal study for two subjects, with multiple data modalities, over a fixed span of time. It illustrates some of the challenges that can appear in a longitudinal, multimodal data study:

1. Each subject can have a different number of acquisitions, leading to an unbalanced data problem. In the figure, Patient B missed the 12th month acquisition for some reasons.
2. There can be missing data due to missing acquisitions from some modalities. In the figure, only patient A at the 6-month follow-up has all the acquisitions.
3. Data are not necessarily acquired at the same time point for different subjects.
4. Time spacing between follow-ups can be variable, even within a single subject.

From Martí-Juan G, Sanroma-Guell G, Piella G. A survey on machine and statistical learning for longitudinal analysis of neuroimaging data in Alzheimer's disease. Comput Methods Programs Biomed. 2020;189:105348.[77]

avenues that require further research and development efforts.

i. *Multiscalar framework*: The development of a multiscalar framework is important for our understanding of change in time. Such a framework would allow us to understand how discoveries in a micro- or meso-scale would affect processes along the macro-scale and vice versa. In physics, multiscalar frameworks are important to understand the relationships between different fundamental forces across a range of size, from the scale of quantum mechanics to cosmological interactions. In biology, we have an understanding of the effects that certain drugs or biological processes have in the microtime or mesotime scales but are only beginning to understand their long-term impacts on the macro-scale. Similarly, we can use medical imaging to study changes in the micro- or meso-scale and relate those to the long-term implications on the macro scale (**Fig. 2**).

Quantitative image analysis of time interval changes can benefit from data of high spatial granularity. Studying population averages, such as averaging voxel values within a lesion, can be misleading due to masking of association between variables that can occur by combining data, a statistical phenomenon known as the Simpson's paradox.[79] Analyzing voxel level data allows for generation of high-resolution landscape information for more accurate characterization of complex biological phenomena. Most of the longitudinal quantitative image analysis research uses voxel-level information to evaluate how experimental variables affect individual voxel engagement. Researchers can explore dispersed patterns of signal activation across several voxels in relation to experimental factors using supervoxel pattern analysis.[80] By increasing spatial resolution for measurement of change, we are able to better characterize disease patterns.

ii. *Backward and forward time*: Time reconstruction is a technique that investigates the fingerprint of change over time by reconstructing the prior conditions of an imaged object of interest. One example can be found in clinical oncology. Cancer cells can evolve over time and adapt to the environment to overcome threats and take advantage of opportunities. Substantial variation

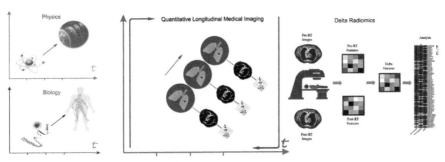

Fig. 2. Time scales in physics and biology have been studied well. In medical imaging, longitudinal imaging would be able to provide more information for personalized medicine. Delta radiomics is an example of quantitative longitudinal imaging.

in gene mutation status and biomarker expression between primary and metastatic lesions limits the successful implementation of personalized cancer therapies.[81] Within a tumor microenvironment, local Darwinian dynamics characteristically produce molecular variations between cells in the same tumor. Regional heterogeneity in molecular features of cancer cells within a tumor or between tumors is known to be induced by branching clonal evolution of cells driven by accumulating mutations. The knowledge of these changes over time can have significant implications in tumor response to treatment and patients outcomes.

Although time reconstruction enables a backwards look at change, the opposite is also possible by looking at *expected* change. Using the known natural history of different diseases, a predictive expectation of disease change can be generated from imaging at a single time point after diagnosis. One application of this concept is using quantitative changes between two imaging studies to train models for predicting future outcomes for improved treatment and surveillance strategies. In a study of renal cell carcinoma in patients with von Hippel–Lindau, Farhadi and colleagues[82] used tumor doubling time based on two CT time points to estimate renal tumor growth rate from baseline MR imaging markers to optimize frequency of imaging for patients on active surveillance. As such, forward projection of time based on a diagnosis can be used for improvement of disease treatment.

iii. *Advanced methods of mapping time relationships*: Another area for improvement is the implementation of new techniques that provide a more nuanced mathematical understanding of time relationships. Recent developments in manifold learning, such as the uniform manifold approximation and projection (UMAP) technique,[83] could enable more complex

processing of medical imaging data. Dimensionality reduction in biological data has been developed and implemented extensively for single-cell multiparametric data analysis. Manifold transformations are commonly used with a method called K-nearest neighbor clustering, where cells are clustered based on their distance from each other in multidimensional space, and then projected onto a lower dimensional space (usually 2D or 3D space). The global architecture of the low-dimensional projection becomes a fingerprint-like representation of cellular qualities in high-dimensional space. Furthermore, cells close in the low-dimensional projection most likely have similar parameters in high-dimensional space, meaning that cell types often self-segregate distinctly.

An example of K-nearest neighbor clustering applied to biological data shows the heterogeneity of leukemic cells within individuals.[84] Furthermore, progression through time in the form of cellular development has been inferred by a similarly based technique termed "Wanderlust."[85] By repeatedly wayfinding between nodes in the graph and then creating an average path, the Wanderlust algorithm produced a trajectory that represented the B cell developmental timeline. Wanderlust extrapolates where a cell sample would be on that timeline without time information being strictly provided. The SCONIFY technique by Burns and colleagues added to dimensionality reduction methods by building the ability to compare differences between biological samples while preserving single-cell resolution.[86] In this case, they compared biological conditions related to cell signaling states. Newer efforts have investigated cell spatial relationships and aimed to compare changes in cell biology over time.[87,88] With advances in computer vision and high-dimensional radiomic analysis of clinical images, we draw an analogy between single cell multiparametric data and superpixels or supervoxels. In this fashion, we propose that existing analytical techniques can be translated to radiologic data where differences in biological states are to be compared, namely the progression through time. Manifold transformations are already being used to approximate a person's progression through biological states and their position along a disease timeline. In a study by Bazzego and colleagues[89], the investigators show a reconstruction of head and neck cancer timelines by PET/CT. Each person's radiomic profile underwent dimensionality reduction and was then annotated by tumor size (TNM staging criteria). The investigators were then able to approximate a trajectory through progression of tumor stage.

iv. *Harmonization techniques*: Different challenges in longitudinal studies could be addressed through new techniques and methodologies. In each center, scanners may change over time as well as acquisition and reconstruction protocols. These changes may lead to variability in image quality and quantitative image-derived metrics. Harmonization techniques could be applied on the images or quantitative indices to tackle these issues. Image-based harmonization using for instance unpaired adversarial neural networks could be used to harmonize images across different scanner and acquisition/reconstruction settings. In addition, for machine learning and deep learning-based models, transfer learning techniques could be applied to adapt developed diagnostic and prognostic models for new settings.

v. *Missing or limited data:* Other issues such as missing sessions or specific imaging modalities for longitudinal studies could potentially be addressed by artificial intelligence-based techniques. Different, deep learning-based models were proposed for image-to-image translation, including MR imaging to CT, MR imaging /CT to PET (and vice versa), and converting different MR imaging sequences to each other. These models could be potentially applied in real clinical situations to generate missing sessions or imaging modality in longitudinal studies. Another issue in longitudinal studies is that a high volume of images might be available collectively in different centers; yet, sharing data between different centers is not straightforward, owing to ethical, legal, and privacy issues. In this context, federated learning frameworks, aiming to develop machine and deep learning models across different centers without sharing data between different centers, could potentially address this challenge for longitudinal studies.

SUMMARY

In medicine, time plays an important role in how we understand the progression of disease and development. Imaging provides a method to characterize this change, and with a focus on different time scales, we are able to contextualize that change and understand the implications for better medical outcomes. The present work focuses on methods and applications beyond only micro- and meso-scales. We discussed strengths and limitations of existing macro-scale (longitudinal) imaging and made recommendation for future advanced imaging efforts integrating this important time scale.

CLINICS CARE POINTS

- Ability to measure change across different time points is critical for diagnostic imaging

- There has commonly been greater emphasis on the micro and meso-scale temporal imaging in both clinical practice and research, than macro-scale.

- Techniques used for quantification of change in one temporal scale can be used in and integrated with other temporal scales (toward multi-scale temporal imaging).

- Challenges associated with longitudinal studies include the need for improved data collection, limitations of current algorithms and performance metrics for studying temporal changes, and ethical considerations.

DISCLOSURE

This research was supported, in part, by the Intramural Research Program of the National Institutes of Health Clinical Center. The opinions expressed in this publication are the author's own and do not reflect the view of the National Institutes of Health, the Department of Health and Human Services, or the United States government. The authors declare no conflicts of interest.

REFERENCES

1. Harman D. The aging process. Proc Natl Acad Sci U S A 1981;78(11):7124–8.

2. Czarnocki BD. Macro-time, Midi-time, and micro-time: a set of Decompositional techniques for making Historical Sense out of longitudinal data. Can J Sociol 1978;3(1):21–39.

3. Kotasidis FA, Tsoumpas C, Rahmim A. Advanced kinetic modelling strategies: towards adoption in clinical PET imaging. Clin Translational Imaging 2014; 2(3):219–37.

4. Gallezot JD, Lu Y, Naganawa M, et al. Parametric imaging with PET and SPECT. IEEE Trans Radiat Plasma Med Sci 2020;4(1):1–23.

5. Wang G, Rahmim A, Gunn RN. PET parametric imaging: Past, present, and future. IEEE Trans Radiat Plasma Med Sci 2020;4(6):663–75.

6. Gakis G, Kramer U, Schilling D, et al. Small renal oncocytomas: differentiation with multiphase CT. Eur J Radiol 2011;80(2):274–8.

7. Foley WD, Mallisee TA, Hohenwalter MD, et al. Multiphase hepatic CT with a multirow detector CT scanner. AJR Am J Roentgenol 2000;175(3):679–85.

8. Itoh S, Ikeda M, Achiwa M, et al. Multiphase contrast-enhanced CT of the liver with a multislice CT scanner. Eur Radiol 2003;13(5):1085–94.

9. Raptopoulos VD, Blake SP, Weisinger K, et al. Multiphase contrast-enhanced helical CT of liver metastases from renal cell carcinoma. Eur Radiol 2001; 11(12):2504–9.

10. Menon BK, d'Esterre CD, Qazi EM, et al. Multiphase CT angiography: a new tool for the imaging triage of patients with acute ischemic stroke. Radiology 2015; 275(2):510–20.

11. Strambo D, Rey V, Rossetti AO, et al. Perfusion-CT imaging in epileptic seizures. J Neurol 2018; 265(12):2972–9.

12. Shen J, Li X, Li Y, et al. Comparative accuracy of CT perfusion in diagnosing acute ischemic stroke: a systematic review of 27 trials. PLoS One 2017;(5): 12. e0176622.

13. Caruso D, Eid M, Schoepf UJ, et al. Dynamic CT myocardial perfusion imaging. Eur J Radiol 2016; 85(10):1893–9.

14. Yan C, Han X, Liang X, et al. Non-invasive evaluation of esophageal varices in patients with liver cirrhosis using low-dose splenic perfusion CT. Eur J Radiol 2022;152:110326.

15. van Dijken BRJ, van Laar PJ, Smits M, et al. Perfusion MRI in treatment evaluation of glioblastomas: clinical relevance of current and future techniques. J Magn Reson Imaging 2019;49(1):11–22.

16. Lapointe E, Li DKB, Traboulsee AL, et al. What have We learned from perfusion MRI in multiple sclerosis? AJNR Am J Neuroradiol 2018 1;39(6):994–1000.

17. Shapiro MG, Atanasijevic T, Faas H, et al. Dynamic imaging with MRI contrast agents: quantitative considerations. Magn Reson Imaging 2006;24(4): 449–62.

18. Michelini G, Corridore A, Torlone S, et al. Dynamic MRI in the evaluation of the spine: state of the art. Acta Biomed 2018;89(1-S):89–101.

19. Baliyan V, Das CJ, Sharma R, et al. Diffusion weighted imaging: technique and applications. World J Radiol 2016;8(9):785–98.

20. Kanaga Anitha. Juliet. 4D medical image analysis: a systematic study on applications, challenges, and future research directions. Advanced Machine Vision Paradigms [Internet]. Available at. https://www.sciencedirect.com/science/article/pii/B9780128192955000044.

21. Chamadol N, Ninpiethoon T, Bhudhisawasd V, et al. The role of CT scan in preoperative staging of colorectal carcinoma. J Med Assoc Thai 2005;88(12): 1847–53.

22. Tranchart H, Gaujoux S, Rebours V, et al. Preoperative CT scan helps to predict the occurrence of severe pancreatic fistula after pancreaticoduodenectomy. Ann Surg 2012;256(1):139–45.

23. Spallone A, Martino V, Floris R. The role of early postoperative CT scan following surgery for herniated lumbar disc. Acta Neurochir 1993;123(1–2): 52–6.

24. Schröder FF, de Graaff F, Bouman DE, et al. The preoperative CT-scan can help to predict postoperative Complications after Pancreatoduodenectomy [Internet]. Biomed Res Int 2015;1–6. https://doi.org/10.1155/2015/824525. Available at.

25. Knight K, Touma N, Zhu L, et al. Journal of medical imaging and radiation Oncology. Implementation daily image-guided Radiat Ther using in-room CT scanner prostate Cancer isocentre localization [Internet] 2009;53:132–8. https://doi.org/10.1111/j.1754-9485.2009.02048.x. Available at.

26. Chen J, Morin O, Aubin M, et al. Dose-guided radiation therapy with megavoltage cone-beam CT. Br J Radiol 2006;1:S87–98, 79 Spec No.

27. Bissonnette JP, Purdie TG, Higgins JA, et al. Cone-beam computed tomographic image guidance for lung cancer radiation therapy. Int J Radiat Oncol Biol Phys 2009;73(3):927–34.

28. Solanki JH, Tritt T, Pasternack JB, et al. Cellular Response to Exponentially Increasing and Decreasing Dose Rates: Implications for Treatment Planning in Targeted Radionuclide Therapy. Radiat Res 2017;188(2):221–34.

29. Ferrari M, De Marco P, Origgi D, et al. SPECT/CT radiation dosimetry. Clinical and Translational Imaging 2014;2(6):557–69.

30. O'Donoghue J, Zanzonico P, Humm J, et al. Dosimetry in Radiopharmaceutical Therapy. J Nucl Med 2022;63(10):1467–74.

31. Chan IS, Ginsburg GS. Personalized medicine: progress and promise. Annu Rev Genomics Hum Genet 2011;12:217–44.

32. Goetz LH, Schork NJ. Personalized medicine: motivation, challenges, and progress. Fertil Steril 2018; 109(6):952–63.

33. Bjork A. Variations in the growth pattern of the human mandible: longitudinal radiographic study by the implant method. J Dent Res 1963;(2):400–11, 42(1)Pt.

34. Shapira L, Tarazi E, Rosen L, et al. The relationship between alveolar bone height and age in the primary dentition. A retrospective longitudinal radiographic study. J Clin Periodontol 1995;22(5):408–12.

35. Jeans WD, Fernando DCJ, Maw AR, et al. A longitudinal study of the growth of the nasopharynx and its contents in normal children. BJR Suppl 1981;54(638):117–21.

36. Keller NB, Liu RW. Prediction of adolescent pelvis development using femoral head and acetabulum growth in a longitudinal radiographic study. Clin Anat 2021;34(5):726–35.

37. Heiss WD, Kessler J, Thiel A, et al. Differential capacity of left and right hemispheric areas for compensation of poststroke aphasia. Ann Neurol 1999;45(4):430–8.

38. de Boissezon X, Démonet JF, Puel M, et al. Subcortical aphasia: a longitudinal PET study. Stroke 2005; 36(7):1467–73.

39. Lahiri D, Ardila A, Dubey S, et al. A longitudinal study of aphasia due to pure Sub-Cortical strokes. Ann Indian Acad Neurol 2020;23(Suppl 2):S109–15.

40. Stieb S, Eleftheriou A, Warnock G, et al. Longitudinal PET imaging of tumor hypoxia during the course of radiotherapy. Eur J Nucl Med Mol Imaging 2018; 45(12):2201–17.

41. Hildebrandt MG, Naghavi-Behzad M, Vogsen M. A role of FDG-PET/CT for response evaluation in metastatic breast cancer? Semin Nucl Med [Internet] 2022;52(5):520–30. https://doi.org/10.1053/j.semnuclmed.2022.03.004. Available at.

42. Jackson P, Foroudi F, Pham D, et al. Short communication: timeline of radiation-induced kidney function loss after stereotactic ablative body radiotherapy of renal cell carcinoma as evaluated by serial (99m)Tc-DMSA SPECT/CT. Radiat Oncol 2014;9(1):253.

43. Everitt S, Hicks RJ, Ball D, et al. Imaging cellular proliferation during chemo-radiotherapy: a pilot study of serial 18F-FLT positron emission tomography/computed tomography imaging for non-small-cell lung cancer. Int J Radiat Oncol Biol Phys 2009; 75(4):1098–104.

44. Everitt S, Ball D, Hicks RJ, et al. Prospective study of serial imaging comparing fluorodeoxyglucose positron emission tomography (PET) and fluorothymidine PET during radical chemoradiation for non-small cell lung cancer: reduction of detectable proliferation associated with worse survival. Int J Radiat Oncol Biol Phys 2017;99(4):947–55.

45. Kwee S, Song MA, Cheng I, et al. Measurement of circulating cell-free DNA in relation to 18F-fluorocholine PET/CT imaging in chemotherapy-treated advanced prostate cancer. Clin Transl Sci 2012; 5(1):65–70.

46. Gholami YH, Willowson KP, Bailey DL. Towards personalised dosimetry in patients with liver malignancy treated with 90Y-SIRT using in vivo-driven radiobiological parameters. EJNMMI Phys 2022;9(1):49.

47. Sojkova J, Zhou Y, An Y, et al. Longitudinal patterns of β-amyloid deposition in nondemented older adults. Arch Neurol 2011;68(5):644–9.

48. Jack CR Jr, Wiste HJ, Schwarz CG, et al. Longitudinal tau PET in ageing and Alzheimer's disease. Brain 2018;141(5):1517–28.

49. Marek K, Jennings D, Lasch S, et al. The Parkinson progression marker Initiative (PPMI). Prog Neurobiol 2011;95(4):629–35.

50. Li W, Lao-Kaim NP, Roussakis AA, et al. 11 C-PE2I and 18 F-Dopa PET for assessing progression rate in Parkinson's: a longitudinal study. Mov Disord 2018;33(1):117–27.

51. Muratore F, Crescentini F, Spaggiari L, et al. Seminars in Arthritis and Rheumatism. Aortic dilatation in patients with large vessel vasculitis: A longitudinal case control study using PET/CT [Internet] 2019;48:1074–82. https://doi.org/10.1016/j.semarthrit.2018.10.003. Available at.

52. Ou YN, on behalf of Alzheimer's Disease Neuroimaging Initiative, Xu W, Li JQ, Guo Y, et al. FDG-PET as an independent biomarker for Alzheimer's biological diagnosis: a longitudinal study [Internet]. Alzheimer's Research & Therapy 2019;11. https://doi.org/10.1186/s13195-019-0512-1. Available at.

53. National Lung Screening Trial Research Team, Aberle DR, Adams AM, et al. Reduced lung-cancer mortality with low-dose computed tomographic screening. N Engl J Med 2011;365(5):395–409.

54. Eisenhauer EA, Therasse P, Bogaerts J, et al. New response evaluation criteria in solid tumours: revised RECIST guideline (version 1.1). Eur J Cancer 2009; 45(2):228–47.

55. Reck M, Rodríguez-Abreu D, Robinson AG, et al. Pembrolizumab versus chemotherapy for PD-L1–Positive non–small-cell lung cancer. N Engl J Med 2016;375(19):1823–33.

56. Xu Y, Hosny A, Zeleznik R, et al. Deep learning predicts lung cancer treatment response from serial medical imaging. Clin Cancer Res 2019;25(11):3266–75.

57. Warren MA, Zhao Z, Koyama T, et al. Severity scoring of lung oedema on the chest radiograph is associated with clinical outcomes in ARDS. Thorax 2018;73(9):840–6.

58. Jabaudon M, Audard J, Pereira B, et al. Early changes over time in the radiographic assessment

of lung edema score are associated with survival in ARDS. Chest 2020;158(6):2394–403.

59. Kerlikowske K, Ichikawa L, Miglioretti DL, et al. Longitudinal measurement of clinical mammographic breast density to improve estimation of breast cancer risk. J Natl Cancer Inst 2007;99(5): 386–95.

60. Krishnan K, Baglietto L, Stone J, et al. Longitudinal study of mammographic density measures that predict breast cancer risk. Cancer Epidemiol Biomarkers Prev 2017;26(4):651–60.

61. Iida Y, Kuroda T, Kitano T, et al. Dexa-measured bone density changes over time after intertrochanteric hip fractures. Kobe J Med Sci 2000;46(1–2): 1–12.

62. Hong N, Park H, Kim CO, et al. Bone radiomics score derived from DXA hip images Enhances hip fracture prediction in older Women. J Bone Miner Res 2021;36(9):1708–16.

63. Smith CD, Van Eldik LJ, Jicha GA, et al. Brain structure changes over time in normal and mildly impaired aged persons. AIMS Neurosci 2020;7(2): 120–35.

64. Bethlehem RAI, Seidlitz J, White SR, et al. Brain charts for the human lifespan. Nature 2022; 604(7906):525–33.

65. Nardone V, Reginelli A, Grassi R, et al. Delta radiomics: a systematic review. Radiol Med 2021; 126(12):1571–83.

66. Yousefirizi F. Pierre Decazes, amyar A, Ruan S, Saboury B, Rahmim A. AI-based detection, classification and prediction/Prognosis in medical imaging:: towards Radiophenomics. PET Clin 2022;17(1): 183–212.

67. Shayesteh S, Nazari M, Salahshour A, et al. Treatment response prediction using MRI-based pre-, post-, and delta-radiomic features and machine learning algorithms in colorectal cancer. Med Phys 2021;48(7):3691–701.

68. van Timmeren JE, van Elmpt W, Leijenaar RTH, et al. Longitudinal radiomics of cone-beam CT images from non-small cell lung cancer patients: evaluation of the added prognostic value for overall survival and locoregional recurrence. Radiother Oncol 2019;136:78–85.

69. Dall'Ara E, Boudiffa M, Taylor C, et al. Longitudinal imaging of the ageing mouse. Mech Ageing Dev 2016;160:93–116.

70. Wimberley C, Nguyen DL, Truillet C, et al. Longitudinal mouse-PET imaging: a reliable method for estimating binding parameters without a reference region or blood sampling. Eur J Nucl Med Mol Imaging 2020;47(11):2589–601.

71. Nguyen DL, Wimberley C, Truillet C, et al. Longitudinal positron emission tomography imaging of glial cell activation in a mouse model of mesial temporal lobe epilepsy: toward identification of optimal treatment windows. Epilepsia 2018;59(6):1234–44.

72. Ishikawa TO, Kumar IP, Machado HB, et al. Positron emission tomography imaging of DMBA/TPA mouse skin multi-step tumorigenesis. Mol Oncol 2010;4(2): 119–25.

73. Hu S, Kiesewetter DO, Zhu L, et al. Longitudinal PET imaging of doxorubicin-induced cell death with 18F-Annexin V. Mol Imaging Biol 2012;14(6):762–70.

74. Islam A, Pishesha N, Harmand TJ, et al. The Journal of Immunology. Converting Anti-Mouse CD4 Monoclonal Antibody into scFv Positron Emission Tomography Imaging Agent Longitudinal Monit CD4 T Cells [Internet] 2021;207:1468–77. https://doi.org/ 10.4049/jimmunol.2100274. Available at.

75. Chen R, Mias GI, Li-Pook-Than J, et al. Personal omics profiling reveals dynamic molecular and medical phenotypes. Cell. 2012;148(6):1293–307.

76. Zheng M, Piermarocchi C, Mias GI. Temporal response characterization across individual multiomics profiles of prediabetic and diabetic subjects. Sci Rep 2022;12(1):12098.

77. Martí-Juan G, Sanroma-Guell G, Piella G. A survey on machine and statistical learning for longitudinal analysis of neuroimaging data in Alzheimer's disease. Comput Methods Programs Biomed 2020;189:105348.

78. Sotiras A, Davatzikos C, Paragios N. Deformable medical image registration: a survey. IEEE Trans Med Imaging 2013;32(7):1153–90.

79. Simpson EH. The interpretation of interaction in contingency tables. J R Stat Soc 1951;13(2):238–41.

80. Davis T, LaRocque KF, Mumford JA, et al. What do differences between multi-voxel and univariate analysis mean? How subject-, voxel-, and trial-level variance impact fMRI analysis. Neuroimage 2014;97: 271–83.

81. Zhang C, Guan Y, Sun Y, et al. Tumor heterogeneity and circulating tumor cells. Cancer Lett 2016; 374(2):216–23.

82. Farhadi F, Nikpanah M, Paschall AK, et al. Clear Cell Ren Cell Carcinoma Growth Correlates Baseline Diffusion-weighted MRI Von Hippel–Lindau Dis [Internet]. Radiology 2020;295:E10. https://doi.org/ 10.1148/radiol.2020204010. Available at.

83. McInnes L, Healy J, Melville JUMAP. Uniform manifold approximation and projection for dimension reduction [Internet]. arXiv [stat.ML] 2018. Available at. http://arxiv.org/abs/1802.03426.

84. Amir EAD, Davis KL, Tadmor MD, et al. viSNE enables visualization of high dimensional single-cell data and reveals phenotypic heterogeneity of leukemia. Nat Biotechnol 2013;31(6):545–52.

85. Bendall SC, Davis KL, Amir EAD, et al. Single-cell trajectory detection uncovers progression and regulatory coordination in human B cell development. Cell. 2014;157(3):714–25.

86. Burns TJ, Nolan GP, Samusik N. Continuous visualization of differences between biological conditions in single-cell data [Internet]. bioRxiv 2018;337485. Available at. https://www.biorxiv.org/content/10.1101/337485 [cited 2022 Aug 17].

87. Ji AL, Rubin AJ, Thrane K, et al. Multimodal analysis of Composition and spatial architecture in human Squamous cell carcinoma. Cell. 2020;182(6):1661–2.

88. Rozenblatt-Rosen O, Regev A, Oberdoerffer P, et al. The human tumor atlas network: Charting Tumor Transitions Across Space Time Single-cell Resolution Cell. 2020;181(2):236–49.

89. Bizzego A, Bussola N, Salvalai D, et al. Integrating deep and radiomics features in cancer bioimaging [Internet]. bioRxiv 2019;568170. Available at. https://www.biorxiv.org/content/biorxiv/early/2019/03/05/568170 [cited 2022 Aug 17].

Aging Muscles, Myositis, Pain, and Peripheral Neuropathies: PET Manifestations in the Elderly

Sanaz Katal, MD, MPH[a], Kim Taubman, MD[a], Jess Han[b],
Ali Gholamrezanezhad, MD[b],*

KEYWORDS

- Positron emission tomography (PET) • Aging • Peripheral nerve system (PNS) • Sarcopenia
- Myositis • Idiopathic inflammatory myopathy (IIM) • Sporadic inclusion body myositis (sIBM)
- Molecular imaging

KEY POINTS

- Early experiences with PET in pain imaging have shown promising results to localize pain generators which can improve outcomes for patients by guiding clinical management.
- Recent studies suggest that the metabolic information from PET may complement that gain from CT for the evaluation and management of age-related sarcopenia.
- The presence of amyloid and tau proteins in Sporadic inclusion body myositis (sIBM) makes these proteins a potential target for PET imaging using Alzheimer's biomarkers.

INTRODUCTION

Advancing age significantly affects the structural and functional characteristics of organs and tissues, including the peripheral nervous system (PNS) and musculoskeletal system. PET molecular imaging systems offer the ability to assess the metabolic and quantitative effects due to nerve and muscle injuries, which has the potential to impact clinical management of aged subjects. PET molecular imaging also enables recognition of age-related changes to the PNS and skeletal muscle system at the molecular and cellular level, which can provide valuable information regarding knowledge, prevention, and management of conditions such as pain and nerve injuries, age-related sarcopenia, and myositis. Here, we aim to describe some features of molecular imaging PET systems using different tracers and methods of imaging in musculoskeletal disorders and peripheral neuropathies commonly seen in elderly patients.

Pain and the Peripheral Nervous System

Aging causes notable morphologic and functional changes in the PNS.[1] Several structural, biochemical, and functional changes have been reported in peripheral nerves of older adults. Morphological studies have demonstrated a slow, progressive loss of neurons and nerve fibers in aged populations, in which age-related decrease in regenerative and reinnervating capabilities of nerve fibers causes irreversible damage. Aging also influences several functional and electrophysiologic features of the PNS, including a decline in nerve conduction velocity, sensory discrimination, muscle strength, and autonomic responses. In a study by Kawabuchi

---

The authors have nothing to disclose.
[a] Saint Vincent's Hospital Medical Imaging Department, Melbourne, Victoria, Australia; [b] Keck School of Medicine, University of Southern California (USC), Los Angeles, CA, USA
* Corresponding author. Department of Diagnostic Radiology, Keck School of Medicine, University of Southern California (USC), 1520 San Pablo Street, Los Angeles, CA.
E-mail address: ali.gholamrezanezhad@med.usc.edu

and colleagues,[2] the process of muscle reinnervation after sciatic nerve crush was assessed in both young and old rats. They found that the older rats had a reduced rate of reinnervation with greater number of abnormal nerve bundles postcrush. These age-related PNS deficits might explain the reduced functional reserve capacity of the neuropathic systems in elderly populations. One clinical implication of such a deficit might be that aged subjects are more likely to be vulnerable to pain-associated events with resultant decreased quality of life due to inadequate pain management.

Pain is a major issue affecting elderly people.[3] Chronic pain in older patients often occurs in the setting of multiple comorbidities, limited treatment options, psychological changes, and environmental issues, all of which complicate pain management in elderly populations. However, despite such a high clinical burden, the diagnosis and characterization of pain remains challenging, especially in the elderly. Generally, the diagnosis of peripheral nerve injuries or peripheral neuropathies is based on clinical history, physical examination, electrophysiological tests, and specific imaging methods. Clinical assessment of pain is often highly subjective because it depends on the patient's self-analysis and experience. Pain imaging systems, although reliable in their ability to capture structural abnormalities contributing to the experience of pain, are incomplete tools for holistically assessing pain. Potential anatomical abnormalities detected on pain imaging may be nonspecific because these structural variations can be found in healthy subjects. Consequently, neuropathic pain remains underrecognized and untreated in most chronic pain sufferers, resulting in poor quality of life for patients and substantial health-care costs that are burdensome to society. Hence, there is a great need for more sophisticated, consistent quantitative imaging tools to functionally elucidate pain-related nociceptive activity. Very recently, early experience with molecular imaging PET has shown promise in the detection of pain-generating pathologic conditions.

[18F] Fluorodeoxyglucose: It is well studied that fluorodeoxyglucose (FDG) PET has the potential to identify pain-generating locations, due to increased glucose metabolism by neurons in high-energy consumption states, such as inflammation or overstimulation. Therefore, uptake of glucose analog, FDG, can be considered a marker of neural activity. Early rat studies have found an increase in FDG uptake in injured nerves as well as in the denervated calf musculature on the affected limb.[4] Additionally, there was no increase in FDG uptake in the contralateral, uninjured limb, or control animals. These studies suggest PET can image increased spontaneous activity and metabolic changes in injured nerves, both of which are mechanisms implicated in contributing to the symptoms of neuropathic pain.

Similar findings have been reported using FDG PET scan in human subjects with neuropathic pain syndromes. In a case report by Cheng and colleagues,[5] FDG PET scanning of a 78-year-old man with progressive difficulty walking showed diffusely increased FDG uptake along the lower spinal cord and sciatic nerves. Subsequent nerve biopsy confirmed a neuropathy. In another study, Biswal and colleagues[6] used FDG PET/MR imaging to localize pain to affected nerves in 6 patients suffering from chronic neuropathic pain of the lower extremities (4 complex regional pain syndrome [CRPS], 1 chronic sciatica, and 1 neuropathic pain). Of the 6 patients who underwent FDG PET/MR imaging, 5 patients showed focal increased FDG uptake in affected nerves and muscle (uptake greater than 2–4 times normal). Consequently, the radiologist was able to localize the symptoms in these patients, which altered clinical management of these chronic pain sufferers.

Similarly, Cipriano and colleagues[7] investigated the role of FDG PET/MR imaging in identifying mediators of pain in chronic sciatica. They found FDG-avid lesions not only in the impinged spinal nerves but also in nonspinal regions, such as facet joint degeneration, pars defects, or a presumed scar neuroma. Interestingly, they also reported increased FDG uptake in leg muscles without any structural abnormalities on MR imaging, which may be explained by each of these causes: neuropathic changes in muscle such as edema or atrophy, primary problem with the muscle itself, or alterations in mechanics of voltage-gated channels. More studies are required though to clarify and validate these potential nonspinal pain-generating sources.

In a recent study using FDG PET/MR imaging in patients with CRPS, increased FDG uptake was depicted in the symptomatic painful areas, reflective of increased metabolism due to the inflammatory response causing the pain.[8] Thus, in patients with CRPS of the extremities, PET may be a potent tool to demonstrate muscular, neurovascular, and skin abnormalities (**Fig. 1**). They also found that metabolic examination with FDG PET may detect CRPS-induced changes earlier than MR imaging, therefore potentially promoting early and effective management of CRPS to secure better outcomes.

In summary, FDG PET/MR imaging has the potential to correctly localize sites of increased neuronal/muscular activity and inflammation in painful neuropathies in the elderly. Areas of increased FDG uptake relates to neurogenic

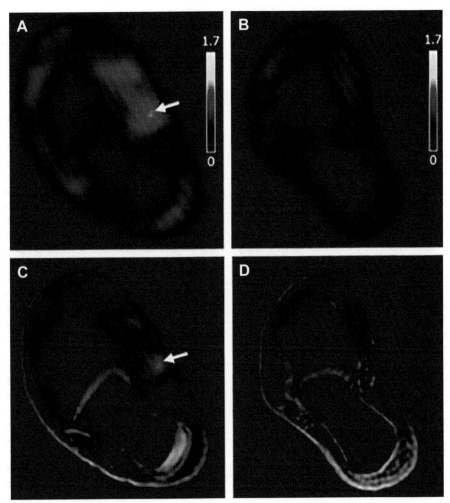

Fig. 1. *FDG uptake in neurovascular bundles at the pain site in CRPS.* Locally increased FDG uptake (*white arrow*) is demonstrated on the tibial neurovascular bundle passing through the scar tissue at the ankle of a CRPS patient (*A*: PET-only and *C*: PET/MR imaging coregistered images), compared with a healthy control subject where the PET-only (*B*) and PET/MR imaging coregistered (*D*) images show no abnormalities at the same site. The same color scale (0–1.7) was used for all subfigures for PET.[8] (*From* Yoon D, Xu Y, Cipriano PW, et al. Neurovascular, Muscle, and Skin Changes on [18F]FDG PET/MRI in Complex Regional Pain Syndrome of the Foot: A Prospective Clinical Study. Pain Med. 2022;23(2):339–346. Figure reproduced under the CC BY- NC 4.0 license)

sources of pain, which can be applied to guide clinical management in chronic pain sufferers to improve patient outcomes. The hybrid FDG PET/MR imaging system offers the chance to combine the metabolic interrogation by FDG PET with the high-resolution anatomic information by MR imaging to locate the pain-inducing inflammatory changes within the culprit lesions. Additionally, it offers noninvasive monitoring of the distribution and progression of inflammatory changes associated with pain-generative conditions, offering an alternative to the current management of pain.

MR imaging, PET/MR imaging: Direct MR imaging of pain relies on tracking macrophages with ultrasmall superparamagnetic particles of iron oxide. Inflammatory cells, in particular macrophages, are critical components of the response to peripheral nerve injury and pain. In animals with neuropathic pain, there was increased trafficking of ultrasmall superparamagnetic iron oxide (USPIO)-tagged macrophages to the nerve injury site.[9] Thus, USPIO-MR imaging is a promising in vivo imaging tool to study the role of macrophages in the development of neuropathic pain.

Moreover, MR imaging provides high-resolution morphological imaging of peripheral nerves.[10] The inflammation around nerves is usually manifested as a high signal on fat-suppressed T2-weighted images. Sometimes, fat-suppressed T1-weighted can also be used for morphology and to differentiate injured nerves from blood vessels. MR imaging has been used to identify and locate entrapment neuropathies, nerve compression syndromes, and plexus injuries.[11] Given its exceptional contrast resolution and multiplanar abilities, MR imaging provides important additional information on neuropathic pain. However, although MR imaging offers high-resolution imaging of peripheral nerve abnormalities, it still suffers from low specificity to identify sites of nerve inflammation or injury. Hybrid PET-MR imaging modalities would overcome such a limitation by combining PET molecular information to localize neuropathic pain with morphological information provided by MR imaging to assess nerve inflammation sites with both high specificity and high anatomical resolution. As mentioned above, early experiences with hybrid PET-MR imaging in chronic neuropathic pain showed promising results, with increased FDG uptake in the affected nerves, which altered clinical management of pain sufferers leading to improved patient outcomes.

Beyond FDG (Non-FDG PET tracers in pain imaging): Non-FDG-PET novel tracers have also been increasingly examined to localize pain-related activity, including [11C] PK11195 to image activated microglia and macrophages in neuroinflammation and [18F] FTC-146, a marker of sigma-1 receptors (S1R) to directly image signaling pathways involved in pain.[12]

[11C] PK11195: Studies have reported enhanced [11C] PK11195 uptake in the lumbar spinal cord of rats with neuropathic pain.[13] Microglial activation plays a role in the development and persistence of neuropathic pain after nerve injury. PK11195 specifically binds to the translocator protein (TSPOs) expressed by these activated microglia and therefore has implications in elucidating pain mechanisms by illustrating the role of microglia in neuroinflammation or nerve injuries. Furthermore, application of PK11195 can be better studied to investigate drugs against neuropathic pain that inhibit glial activation.

[18F] FTC-146: There is increasing evidence linking sigma 1 receptors (S1R) dysregulation to various neurologic conditions, including neuropathic pain, Alzheimer disease (AD), and addiction. Previous animal PET studies have reported specific binding of [18F] FTC-146 to S1R in vivo, indicating the role of FTC PET imaging to directly investigate the signaling pathways involved in pain disorders.[14,15] As these studies suggest, the enormous potential of [18F] FTC-146 as an in vivo S1R imaging agent deserves further investigation. Noninvasive imaging S1Rs via PET could serve as a useful means to identify S1R-related disorders and to monitor therapeutic response. Moreover, S1R PET could help us gain more information about the in vivo role of S1Rs in different neuropsychological conditions and improve our understanding of the underlying pathology of such conditions. Safe for human use, FTC-146 PET-MR imaging is currently being used in various studies to better understand its role in various disease pathologic conditions.

[18F] Sodium Fluoride: Many studies have evaluated the potential role of sodium fluoride (NaF) PET/CT in evaluating age-related degeneration and osteoarthritis of the spine. Degenerative changes are associated with altered osteoblastic activity, and therefore, imaging modalities sensitive to such molecular changes are potential tools for clinical assessment, disease prophylaxis, and monitoring early therapy response. PET/CT imaging using NaF can detect spinal lesions with high diagnostic accuracy in aged subjects with back pain. NaF PET images bone remodeling, and therefore, it has the potential to show osseous changes before fractures develop. Previous studies have found that NaF PET/CT can diagnose the cause of back pain in adolescents presenting with back pain as an isolated complaint with high accuracy.[16] Other studies have examined the potential usefulness of NaF PET/CT in detecting age-associated changes in adult populations with a broad age spectrum. For example, Gammie and colleagues[17] found abnormal NaF uptake in the spine of 84% of the patients. Park and colleagues[18] demonstrated that aging is associated with increased NaF uptake in the cervical spine, which may be related to osteoblastic activity coupled with degeneration. They reported a significant difference in NaF uptake in younger groups compared with older groups for both sexes at the C5-C7 vertebrae. Thus, NaF PET can assess the sources of neck and back pain in the elderly while also measuring degenerative changes in the aging spine.

Given the novelty of imaging pain and using hybrid-imaging modalities, more research on human subjects with a larger number of patients is still warranted. A detrimental factor would be the long-term consequences associated with their use such as radiation exposure; however, as with much medical imaging, the potential gain needs to be weighed against the potential risks.

Age-Related Skeletal Muscle Disorders

Skeletal muscle is the most abundant tissue in the human body, providing the fundamental basis for locomotion, thermogenesis, energy supply, and respiration.[19] To ensure these essential functions, skeletal muscles must have sufficient mass and quality.

Aging manifests as a time-related progressive loss of tissue and function over time.[20] One of the most serious consequences of aging is its effects on skeletal muscles. As the human body ages, muscle mass and strength considerably decrease. After the age of 30 years, approximately 0.1% to 0.5% of muscle mass is expected to be lost every year, with dramatic acceleration after 65 years.[21,22] This age-related muscle deconditioning is a geriatric syndrome called "sarcopenia," which contributes to a significant impairment in functional capacity, disability, poor life quality, and death within the elderly population. Apart from sarcopenia, there are a variety of other skeletal muscle diseases affecting aged subjects, including myosteatosis, idiopathic inflammatory myopathies (IIMs) or myositis, adult-onset congenital myopathies and dystrophies, toxic and endocrine myopathies, and polymyalgia rheumatica (**Fig. 2**).

Inevitably, as populations around the world are aging, the impact of such age-related disorders on public health will continue to grow, which will place a heavy burden on health-care costs. As a result, the identification of cost-effective interventions to maintain muscle mass, muscle strength, and physical performance in the elderly remains a major public health challenge. It requires understanding of the cellular and molecular mechanisms as well as the underlying systemic pathways involved in these muscular disorders. Molecular imaging of biological processes offers significant potential to recognize some of these changes at the molecular level and may provide valuable insight into the pathophysiology and management of these conditions.[23] Here we aim to discuss some of the main PET imaging features of these age-related muscle disorders.

Sarcopenia

Sarcopenia is a quantitative and qualitative muscle disorder associated with advancing age, which leads to a significant influence on activities of daily living. Multiple factors contribute to sarcopenia, such as low physical activity, diet, chronic diseases, and the aging process itself. The overall estimate of sarcopenia prevalence is about 10% in

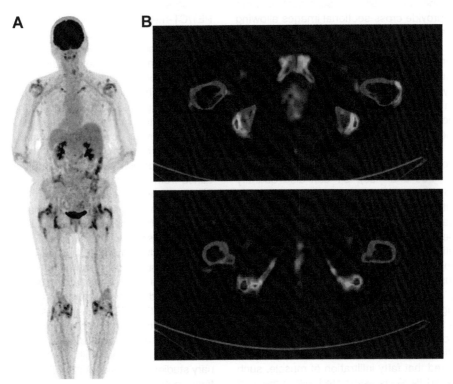

Fig. 2. *FDG distribution in polymyalgia rheumatica (PMR)* in a 70-year-old woman with weight loss and proximal weakness. Schema representing (*A*) MIP PET and (*B*) PET/CT fused axial slices. Increased periarticular FDG uptake is identified around the acromioclavicular, glenohumeral, costoclavicular, sternoclavicular, hip, knee, and wrist joints, in keeping with arthritis. Additionally, there is extra-articular FDG uptake in the greater trochanters, interspinous bursae, ischiogluteal bursae, and praepubic regions (bursitis and enthesitis). MIP, maximum intensity projection.

men and women aged older than 60 years.[24] Muscle fiber loss occurs gradually with almost 50% of fibers lost by the age of 80 years.[25] Sarcopenia has significant socioeconomic and health implications, including osteoporosis, falls, fractures, hospitalization, major postoperative complications, and death.[26]

During recent decades, sarcopenia has garnered increasing interest among clinicians and has become a heavily researched topic. Due to its growing prevalence and clinical implications, physicians would benefit from awareness of sarcopenia and its manifestations. Although the primary diagnosis is suspected via specific questionnaire filling and clinical tests, imaging and nonimaging tools play a determinant role in confirming the diagnosis by estimating muscle quality and quantity. Diverse methods are utilized to evaluate muscle mass and body composition, including anthropometry, bioelectrical impedance analysis, and medical imaging modalities (whole-body dual-energy X-ray absorptiometry [DEXA], computed tomography [CT], MR imaging, and ultrasonography).[27] Currently, MR imaging together with CT, is considered the gold-standard technique for body composition assessment, as both methods provide cross-sectional images allowing for segmental and total measures of fat and lean mass.[28]

CT scans have the capability to provide information on muscle quantity and composition based on the ability to discriminate among different tissues based on their different X-ray attenuation. Normal attenuation values for muscle density are 40 to 100 HU. Higher muscle fat contents (fatty infiltration of muscles, which occurs during aging) result in low attenuation (low muscle density with HU values between −200 and −35). CT can also quantify the amount of intramuscular adipose tissue (IMAT) with postprocessing analysis, using muscle segmentation with HU density threshold.[29] Apart from research purposes, CT quantitative muscle composition analysis provides an additional tool to diagnose sarcopenia in aged patients who are already undergoing CT studies for other reasons, such as oncologic diseases. As sarcopenia is increasingly recognized as an important independent risk factor for adverse health outcomes, CT-measured muscle metrics can be utilized as a prognostic tool in these patients. For example, it is suggested that fatty infiltration of muscle, such as increased IMAT, is associated with increased morbidity and mortality in patients with cancer.[30] Therefore, it might be helpful to consider muscle analysis in CT examination of aged subjects who are already undergoing routine CT examinations for other medical reasons. Muscle is routinely included in radiologic examinations, and therefore, such an analysis as a potential prognostic biomarker for sarcopenia deserves further investigation, for example, on PET/CT for patients undergoing these scans for other reasons especially in oncology or rheumatologic diseases.

MR imaging has some advantages over CT scan. The ability to depict qualitative abnormalities such as edema, muscle disruption, or the presence of IMAT and fibrosis at the same time, with no exposure to ionizing radiation, makes MR imaging the most advanced, reliable method for assessing body composition. MR imaging also provides several quantitative techniques for precise measurements of muscle volume and degree of fat infiltration. However, the high cost and low availability relative to CT are the main drawbacks of MR imaging, limiting its use to primarily research settings.

PET/CT: The role of PET-only imaging in the assessment of sarcopenia has not been well studied yet. Nevertheless, it is proposed that the PET-derived muscle metrics can add some complementary information to CT measures for prognostic implications. For example, Foster and colleagues[31] have studied the association of FDG PET/CT-measured muscle indices with health outcomes and serum biomarkers in patients with soft-tissue sarcoma. They evaluated the association between imaging metrics and pretherapy levels of serum biomarkers (C-reactive protein [CRP], creatinine, hemoglobin, and albumin), as prior studies suggested that patients with age-related muscle wasting may have high serum CRP, low hemoglobin levels, low serum albumin, and lower creatinine. The authors found that the metabolic information from FDG PET may complement that obtained from CT for the characterization of skeletal muscles. For example, they stated that although a higher HU mean (less IMAT) correlated with lower recurrence-free survival (LRFS), increased PET SUV of muscle was associated with decreased overall survival and LRFS. They also found that muscle measurements obtained on routine FDG PET/CT are associated with some serum biomarkers and overall outcome in patients with sarcoma. FDG PET/CT images are routinely performed for cancer evaluation, with the primary focus being on the evaluation of the primary tumor and the extent of malignant spread. Given preliminary studies correlating FDG PET/CT data with patient outcomes in sarcoma, opportunistically measuring muscle metrics during routine cancer evaluation seems worthwhile to provide further insight into cancer-related cachexia and prognosis.

Ultimately, PET/CT biomarkers can provide insight into the mechanisms of sarcopenia to help researchers and clinicians identify disease targets or therapies. Additionally, by using volumetric measures from both CT and PET, large parts of the body can be surveyed in a single PET/CT examination. These volumetric measures would be more robust and reproducible compared with cross-sectional area measures (similar to those from L3 and L4 cross-sections in CT-based analysis). As Foster suggested, imaging measures from a single axial section (as used in CT-bases analysis) may not be representative of measures derived using volumetric analyses (as used in PET/CT-based analysis). Volumetric measures should be pursued because they have more associations with health outcomes and prognostic implications than cross-sectional area measures.

Apart from the possible complementary role of PET information in muscle assessment studies, the role of low-dose or attenuation correction CT (LDCT) component of PET/CT has also been investigated compared with high-dose or diagnostic CT (HDCT). It is suggested that LDCT is a possible accurate alternative for measuring abdominal fat and muscles in clinical practice. LDCT is a safe, accurate, and precise method for the measurements of the skeletal muscle, visceral, and subcutaneous adipose tissue. Low-dose measurements have been reported to be reproducible and correlate closely with HDCT, providing another reason to consider PET/CT-derived muscle metrics in clinical settings. As prior studies suggest, LDCT has significant potential to act as a surrogate for sarcopenia assessment, with several clinical advantages, such as the possibility to have both metabolic and morphological information from the same tool (PET/CT), reduced radiation exposure, and sarcopenic measurements available immediately after scanning.[32]

In summary, sarcopenia is a condition that becomes more prevalent with advancing age, and it is increasingly recognized as an independent risk factor for adverse health outcomes. However, despite its important clinical and prognostic implications, sarcopenia is often underrecognized and undertreated. Although the role of PET-only imaging in the assessment of sarcopenia has not been well studied yet, there is increasing evidence that the metabolic information from FDG PET may complement that gained from CT for anatomic correlation and characterization of skeletal muscles. FDG PET/CT examinations are routinely acquired for oncologic evaluations in patients with cancer to survey large parts of the body in a single examination. Concurrently, important muscle metrics should be derived from both the PET and CT components during routine cancer evaluation to guide future research, clinical management of sarcopenia, and patient prognostication.

Myositis

IIMs, generally referred to as myositis, are a group of immune-related heterogeneous muscle disorders. They are considered systemic in nature and often present with weakness, elevated muscle enzymes, and inflammatory infiltrates on biopsy. Apart from muscle inflammation, which is the disease hallmark, they can display other systemic manifestations such as arthritis, interstitial lung disease, and characteristic skin involvement.[33] These disorders can be broadly subdivided into 5 phenotypes: dermatomyositis (DM), polymyositis (PM), sporadic inclusion body myositis (sIBM), necrotizing autoimmune myopathy, and antisynthetase syndrome.[34]

Imaging plays an important noninvasive role in the diagnosis, biopsy guidance, management, monitoring, and follow-up of patients with myositis.[35] Recently, there is increasing interest in the use of PET for the evaluation of myositis patients. PET/CT provides useful metabolic information for diagnostic purposes, determining the myositis phenotype, characterizing muscular and extramuscular involvement, measuring disease activity, and malignancy screening.[36,37] There is a well-known association between myositis and malignancy, and PET/CT can be used as a reliable screening tool. A retrospective study by Li and colleagues[38] with 38 patients evaluated the role of FDG PET/CT in detecting malignant tumors, muscle activity, and interstitial lung disease in patients with various myositis phenotypes. In this study, FDG PET/CT correctly detected 7 cases of malignant tumors (18.4%). In addition, muscle FDG uptake was higher in myositis patients compared with controls. Moreover, PET/CT findings showed a good correlation with creatine kinase values, muscle weakness, and detection of interstitial lung disease. These findings highlight the potential utility of PET/CT imaging in the clinical course of diagnosing and managing inflammatory myositis.

In terms of selecting appropriate PET tracers, the suspected myositis subtype should be considered, as there are heterogeneous metabolic pathway involvements in various myositis subtypes. For example, carbohydrate metabolism is increased in DM or PM cases, whereas in IBM, this pathway is depressed.[39] Thus, if IBM seems more likely, neurodegeneration markers are more appropriate. In IBM, the presence of vacuoles with amyloid and tau proteins is detected by PET tracers usually used in AD, including 11C-Pittsburgh Compound B (PIB) and 18F-florbetapir (amyloid markers),[40] and [18F] THK5317 (tau marker). Increased activity in muscle after the injection of such neurodegenerative markers suggests the diagnosis of IBM with high specificity. All other types of IIMs may display increased FDG activity in muscles, but to a variable extent, which negatively affects diagnostic sensitivity.[41,42] It should be noted that false-positive errors may also happen, which reduces specificity, as increased FDG activity can be seen in other clinical situations such as postrecent trauma or biopsy sites.[43]

In addition, whole-body PET, particularly if coupled to CT or MR imaging, allows the investigation of other organs involved in IIMs and may contribute to the diagnosis. It also allows detection of interstitial lung diseases[44] or malignancies (whose prevalence is 2 to 5 times increased in IIMs).[45] The FDG PET and PET/CT scans also offer the ability to provide semiquantitative objective monitoring of muscle lesions[46] while being cost-effective.[47]

In summary, although PET imaging, combined with MR imaging or CT, is not always sufficiently sensitive to allow the diagnosis of IIM on its own, it allows follow-up monitoring of muscular lesions detected in myositis. There is increasing interest in this technique due to its ability to predict, detect, and monitor associated extramuscular lesions, particularly tumors and malignancy. Currently, however, the lack of large multicenter studies does not allow for a formal recommendation of this technique in cases of IIM. Even though, when the typical patterns are seen, it merits comment.

As sIBM is the most frequent progressive muscle disease associated with aging, we will briefly review some of the main PET features associated with this disorder.

Sporadic inclusion body myositis sIBM is described as an uncommon, distinct, progressive, inflammatory myopathy, mostly involving patients aged older than 50 years.[48] Quadriceps and forearm flexors are the most commonly affected muscles. A pathological hallmark of sIBM is the accumulation of multiple protein aggregates within muscle fibers with the presence of inclusion bodies. Even though several criteria have been proposed for sIBM diagnosis, missed diagnoses occur in patients with sIBM with atypical features due to the lack of diagnostic criteria sensitivity.[49] Needle electromyography approaches are sometimes challenging as the amplitude of motor units can be large in sIBM. Similarly, autoantibodies to cytosolic 5'-nucleotidase 1A (anti-cN1A) cannot be used reliably for diagnosis as they test positive in other myositis subsets. Untargeted muscle biopsy presents its own challenges, such as sampling error occurring in some cases. It is, therefore, suggested that noninvasive molecular imaging tools with novel radiotracers can be an effective approach in these conditions.

It has been previously shown that a variety of abnormal protein deposits in sIBM muscle fibers are similar to those in the brains of patients with AD, such as β-amyloid and phosphorylated tau proteins. Recent studies have revealed that molecular imaging PET can show abnormal deposition proteins in muscles, which is helpful for early diagnosis as well as differential diagnosis of rimmed vacuolar myopathy. Thus, muscle Amyloid-PET or tau-PET imaging can be applied to make a diagnosis of sIBM when biopsy or other conventional diagnostic approaches are difficult or equivocal.

Amyloid PET: The rimmed vacuoles detected in muscle biopsy of sIBM patients are rich in neurodegenerative proteins, including β-amyloid. β-Amyloid protein is the main feature of amyloid plaques found in the brains of patients with AD.[50] PET imaging using novel amyloid tracers can measure amyloid pathologic condition in vivo and play an important role in research, clinical trials, diagnosis, and monitoring of AD.[51] Due to similarities in pathologic conditions of AD and IBM, amyloid PET imaging may provide value in the assessment of patients with IBM. In this regard, [11C] PIB and [18F] Florbetapir PET have been investigated in a few recent preliminary studies.

[11C] PIB PET: [11C] PIB, is an 11C-labelled substituted benzothiazole PET biomarker, which has been evaluated clinically for in vivo analysis of amyloid plaques in patients with AD. AD patients typically show marked PIB retention in areas of association cortex known to contain large amounts of amyloid deposits.[52] As β-amyloid is also accumulated and misfolded in sIBM, it can be expected that [11C] PIB PET may have the potential to elucidate β-amyloid in the skeletal muscles of patients with IBM.

Previously, Maetzler and colleagues[53] suggested that [11C] PIB-PET can potentially detect abnormal muscular deposits of β-amyloid proteins in sIBM patients in vivo. In that study, they measured [11C] PIB-SUV in 4 muscles (deltoid, finger flexors, gastrocnemius, and vastus lateralis muscles) and found a significant increase of the median [11C] PIB-SUV only in the gastrocnemius muscle of 7 patients with sIBM compared with those of non-IBM patients. These results suggested that the measurement of [11C] PIB retention may be of diagnostic value in the early diagnosis and differentiation of sIBM. However,

s-IBM -9
(81 years old, female)

IIM-3
(79 years old, female)

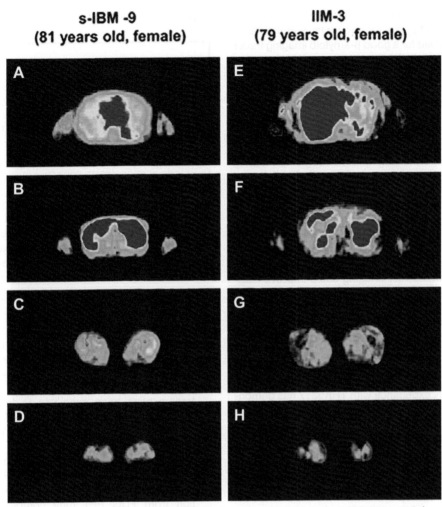

Fig. 3. *[11C] PIB muscle uptake in IBM.* PIB uptake in limb and trunk muscles of an IBM patient. Higher mean [11C] PIB-SUVs are noted in each muscle group of an IBM patient in comparison with a patient with IIM. Upper arm muscle group: 0.30 versus 0.18 (*A, E*), forearm muscle group: 0.31 versus 0.21 (*B, F*), trunk muscle group: 0.32 versus 0.24 (*B, F*), thigh muscle group: 0.40 versus 0.26 (*C, G*), lower leg muscle group: 0.30 versus 0.24 (*D, H*).[54] [11C] PIB-PET can potentially detect abnormal muscular deposits of β-amyloid proteins in sIBM patients in vivo. SUV, standardized uptake values. (*From* Noto YI, Kondo M, Tsuji Y, et al. Diagnostic Value of Muscle [11C] PIB-PET in Inclusion Body Myositis. Front Neurol. 2020;10:1386. Published 2020 Jan 17. Figure reproduced under the CC BY license)

there was no correlation between uptake level and clinical severity of the involved muscles.

In another study by Noto and colleagues,[54] sIBM patients had significantly higher levels of [11C] PIB retention in their muscles, especially forearm and lower-leg muscles, compared with other subtypes of IIM. In this study, 9 patients with sIBM and 4 patients with other types of IIM were included. All patients underwent PIB-PET of body muscles and the standardized uptake values (SUVs) were measured in 16 muscles. They found that the mean SUV of all muscles in sIBM patients was higher than in other patients, with a significant difference in SUVs of the forearm and lower-leg

muscle groups in sIBM. Yet, there was still no correlation between SUVs and clinical parameters in patients with sIBM. To validate the utility of this novel method, further studies with larger patient populations are necessary (**Fig. 3**).

[18F] Florbetapir PET: Recently, a study by Lilleker and colleagues[40] suggested that another amyloid PET imaging, which detects amyloid using the radioactive tracer [18F] Florbetapir, can also be helpful for the differential diagnosis of IBM and PM. [18F] Florbetapir is a good marker for detecting amyloid disease, suggesting utility in the use of [18F] Florbetapir PET for IBM and PM diagnosis. More importantly, only a small minority

of PET scanner sites have the on-site capability of producing [11C]-labeled products, and therefore, there is a need for a good β-amyloid imaging tracer with wider availability such as [18F]-labeled agents. In a small study by Pinal-Fernandez and colleagues, [18F] Florbetapir PET was performed in 10 patients with sIBM and compared the findings with those of 6 patients with PM. The Florbetapir SUV was significantly higher in those with sIBM, yielding a sensitivity of 80% and specificity of 100% for sIBM diagnosis. Although the initial results are encouraging, additional studies with larger patient series are still warranted to determine the real efficacy and practicality of such novel applications of PET imaging as a complementary tool for the diagnosis of sIBM or optimal selection of sites for muscle biopsy.[55]

Tau PET: Recent molecular studies have suggested that tau-PET imaging could improve diagnostic efficiency for AD. In vivo studies using [18F] THK5317 on patients with AD have shown considerable cortical uptake and temporal lobe retention, compared with healthy control individuals.[56] Given the similarities between pathologic features of sIBM and AD, it is assumed that tau protein imaging may be an interesting tool in sIBM. Early experience with THK5317 has demonstrated promising results regarding the application of tau-PET imaging in the diagnosis of sIBM. For example, Zhang and colleagues[57] reported the usefulness of [18F] THK5317 PET/MR imaging in a case that was pathology-confirmed sIBM through muscle biopsy. They found a significantly increased tau uptake within involved muscles, reflecting the ability of [18F] THK5317 PET to depict muscular tau deposits in vivo. This case confirmed that the involved muscles of sIBM patients can show tau-tracer binding in vivo. They also found higher THK5317 SUV levels within quadriceps muscles compared with other involved muscles, consistent with the clinical severity of involvement. These results illustrate usefulness of tau-PET imaging in visually evaluating tau deposition in the IBM muscles and reflecting the severity of muscular involvement. More importantly, the advantage of PET imaging is its ability to assess tau deposition within all skeletal muscles during single whole-body imaging.

Finally, tau PET has the potential to identify muscular tau deposition in vivo, providing a novel noninvasive imaging tool for IBM diagnosis. Additionally, it may provide the opportunity to monitor the progression of tau pathologic condition along with muscle impairment. However, further studies with this PET biomarker are still needed before drawing a definite conclusion on its usefulness in sIBM diagnosis and surveillance.

CLINICS CARE POINTS

> PET imaging using FDG and novel non-FDG tracers might be a promising tool in addressing musculoskeletal disordes in the elderly, such as imaging pain and peripheral neuropathies, sarcopenia (age-related muscle loss), and myositis.

SUMMARY

In this article, we briefly reviewed the clinical implications of PET imaging using FDG and non-FDG novel tracers in addressing a few musculoskeletal disorders in elderly subjects, such as imaging pain and peripheral neuropathies, sarcopenia (age-related muscle loss), and myositis. In summary,

1. PET has the potential to correctly localize pain-generating locations, which can improve outcomes for pain sufferers by guiding clinical management. Early experiences with hybrid PET-MR systems in imaging pain have shown increased FDG uptake in the affected nerves and muscles. Moreover, a few non-FDG-PET tracers have been examined to localize the pain-related activity, including [11C] PK11195 to image activated microglia and [18F] FTC-146, which target S1R.

2. In sarcopenia, the role of PET-only imaging has not been well studied yet; however, there is increasing evidence that the metabolic information from FDG PET may complement that gained from CT for the muscle analysis, which has significant prognostic implication. As FDG PET/CT examinations are routinely acquired for oncologic reasons in patients with cancer, muscle metrics from both the PET and CT components should be concurrently acquired to guide future research and clinical management of sarcopenia.

3. sIBM is a common progressive muscle disease in older people. Although FDG is not a suitable tracer for IBM imaging, the presence of amyloid and tau proteins in IBM makes these proteins a good target for PET imaging using Alzheimer biomarkers, including 11C-PIB and 18F-florbetapir (amyloid markers), and [18F] THK5317 (tau marker).

Finally, it should be emphasized that given the novelty of PET applications in all the above topics, further studies with larger numbers of patients are necessary before drawing a definite conclusion in the utility of these PET features for clinical purposes.

REFERENCES

1. Verdú E, Ceballos D, Vilches JJ, et al. Influence of aging on peripheral nerve function and regeneration. J Peripher Nerv Syst 2000;5(4):191–208.

2. Kawabuchi M, Chongjian Z, Islam AT, et al. The effect of aging on the morphological nerve changes during muscle reinnervation after nerve crush. Restor Neurol Neurosci 1998;13(3–4):117–27.

3. Gibson SJ, Farrell M. A review of age differences in the neurophysiology of nociception and the perceptual experience of pain. Clin J pain 2004;20(4):227–39.

4. Behera D, Jacobs KE, Behera S, et al. (18)F-FDG PET/MRI can be used to identify injured peripheral nerves in a model of neuropathic pain. J Nucl Med 2011;52:1308–12.

5. Cheng G, Chamroonrat W, Bing Z, et al. Elevated FDG activity in the spinal cord and the sciatic nerves due to neuropathy. Clin Nucl Med 2009;34(12):950–1.

6. Biswal S, Behera D, Yoon DH, et al. [18F]FDG PET/MRI of patients with chronic pain alters management: early experience. EJNMMMI Phys 2015;2:A84.

7. Cipriano PW, Yoon D, Gandhi H, et al. 18F-FDG PET/MRI in chronic sciatica: early results revealing spinal and nonspinal abnormalities. J Nucl Med 2018;59(6):967–72.

8. Yoon D, Xu Y, Cipriano PW, et al. Neurovascular, muscle, and skin changes on [18F] FDG PET/MRI in complex regional pain syndrome of the foot: a prospective clinical study. Pain Med 2022;23(2):339–46.

9. Ghanouni P, Behera D, Xie J, et al. In vivo USPIO magnetic resonance imaging shows that minocycline mitigates macrophage recruitment to a peripheral nerve injury. Mol Pain 2012;8:49.

10. Kogan F, Fan AP, Gold GE. Potential of PET-MRI for imaging of non-oncologic musculoskeletal disease. Quant Imaging Med Surg 2016;6(6):756–71.

11. Ohana M, Moser T, Moussaouï A, et al. Current and future imaging of the peripheral nervous system. Diagn Interv Imaging 2014;95(1):17–26.

12. Yoder JS, Kogan F, Gold GE. Applications of PET–computed tomography–magnetic resonance in the management of benign musculoskeletal disorders. PET Clinics 2019;14(1):1–5.

13. Imamoto N, Momosaki S, Fujita M, et al. [11C] PK11195 PET imaging of spinal glial activation after nerve injury in rats. Neuroimage 2013;79:121–8.

14. Hjørnevik T, Cipriano PW, Shen B, et al. Biodistribution and radiation dosimetry of 18F-FTC-146 in humans. J Nucl Med 2017;58:2004–9.

15. James ML, Shen B, Nielsen CH, et al. Evaluation of sigma-1 receptor radioligand 18FFTC-146 in rats and squirrel monkeys using PET. J Nucl Med 2014;55:147–53.

16. Ovadia D, Metser U, Lievshitz G, et al. Back pain in adolescents: assessment with integrated 18F-fluoride positron-emission tomography-computed tomography. J Pediatr Orthop 2007;27(1):90–3.

17. Gamie S, El-Maghraby T. The role of PET/CT in evaluation of Facet and Disc abnormalities in patients with low back pain using (18) F-Fluoride. Nucl Med Rev Ent East Eur 2008;11:17–21.

18. Park PSU, Raynor WY, Khurana N, et al. Application of 18F-NaF-PET/CT in assessing age-related changes in the cervical spine. Quant Imaging Med Surg 2022;12(6):3314–24.

19. Brioche T, Pagano AF, Py G, et al. Muscle wasting and aging: Experimental models, fatty infiltrations, and prevention. Mol Aspects Med 2016;50:56–87.

20. Flatt T. A new definition of aging? Front Genet 2012;3:148.

21. Morley JE, Baumgartner RN, Roubenoff R, et al. Sarcopenia J Lab Clin Med 2001;137(4):231–43.

22. Liguori I, Russo G, Aran L, et al. Sarcopenia: assessment of disease burden and strategies to improve outcomes. Clin interventions Aging 2018;13:913.

23. Katal S, Maldonado A, Carrascoso J, et al. Theranostic agents in musculoskeletal disorders. PET Clinics 2021;16(3):441–8.

24. Shafiee G, Keshtkar A, Soltani A, et al. Prevalence of sarcopenia in the world: a systematic review and meta- analysis of general population studies. J Diabetes Metab Disord 2017;16:21.

25. Bisyri K, Lambrou GI. The assessment of sarcopenia using magnetic resonance imaging. JRPMS 2022.

26. Boutin RD, Yao L, Canter RJ, et al. Sarcopenia: current concepts and imaging implications. Am J Roentgenol 2015;205(3):W255–66.

27. Lee K, Shin Y, Huh J, et al. Recent issues on body composition imaging for sarcopenia evaluation. Korean J Radiol 2019;20(2):205–17.

28. Messina C, Maffi G, Vitale JA, et al. Diagnostic imaging of osteoporosis and sarcopenia: a narrative review. Quant Imaging Med Surg 2018;8(1):86–99.

29. Heymsfield SB, Gonzalez MC, Lu J, et al. Skeletal muscle mass and quality: evolution of modern measurement concepts in the context of sarcopenia. Proc Nutr Soc 2015;74:355–66.

30. Malafarina V, Uriz-Otano F, Iniesta R, et al. Sarcopenia in the elderly: diagnosis, physiopathology and treatment. Maturitas 2012;71(2):109–14.

31. Foster B, Boutin RD, Lenchik L, et al. Skeletal muscle metrics on clinical 18F-FDG PET/CT predict health outcomes in patients with sarcoma. J Nat Sci 2018;4(5):e502.

32. Albano D, Camoni L, Rinaldi R, et al. Comparison between skeletal muscle and adipose tissue measurements with high-dose CT and low-dose attenuation correction CT of 18F-FDG PET/CT in elderly Hodgkin lymphoma patients: a two-centre validation. The Br J Radiol 2021;94(1123):20200672.

33. Dalakas MC. Inflammatory muscle diseases. N Engl J Med 2015;372:1734–47.

34. Selva-O'Callaghan A, Pinal-Fernandez I, Trallero-Araguás E, et al. Classification and management of adult inflammatory myopathies. Lancet Neurol 2018;17:816–28.

35. Katal S, Gholamrezanezhad A, Nikpanah M, et al. Potential applications of PET/CT/MR imaging in inflammatory diseases: Part I: musculoskeletal and gastrointestinal systems. PET Clinics 2020;15(4): 547–58.

36. Katal S, Gholamrezanezhad A, Kessler M, et al. PET in the diagnostic management of soft tissue sarcomas of musculoskeletal origin. PET Clinics 2018; 13(4):609–21.

37. Selva-O'Callaghan A, Gil-Vila A, Simó-Perdigó M, et al. PET scan: nuclear medicine imaging in myositis. Curr Rheumatol Rep 2019;21(11):1–8.

38. Li Y, Zhou Y, Wang Q. Multiple values of 18F-FDG PET/CT in idiopathic inflammatory myopathy. Clin Rheumatol 2017;36(10):2297–305.

39. Liu D, Zuo X, Luo H, et al. The altered metabolism profile in pathogenesis of idiopathic inflammatory myopathies. Semin Arthritis Rheum 2020;50(4): 627–35.

40. Lilleker JB, Hodgson R, Roberts M, et al. [18F] Florbetapir positron emission tomography: identification of muscle amyloid in inclusion body myositis and differentiation from polymyositis. Ann Rheum Dis 2019; 78(5):657–62.

41. Pipitone N, Versari A, Zuccoli G, et al. 18F-Fluorodeoxyglucose positron emission tomography for the assessment of myositis: a case series. Clin Exp Rheumatology-Incl Supplements 2012;30(4):570.

42. Owada T, Maezawa R, Kurasawa K, et al. Detection of inflammatory lesions by f-18 fluorodeoxyglucose positron emission tomography in patients with polymyositis and dermatomyositis. The J Rheumatol 2012;39(8):1659–65.

43. Van De Vlekkert J, Maas M, Hoogendijk JE, et al. IN. Combining MRI and muscle biopsy improves diagnostic accuracy in subacute-onset idiopathic inflammatory myopathy. Muscle & nerve 2015;51(2): 253–8.

44. Cao H, Liang J, Xu D, et al. Radiological characteristics of patients with anti-MDA5–antibody-positive dermatomyositis in 18F-FDG PET/CT: a pilot study. Front Med 2021;8:779272.

45. Selva-O'Callaghan A, Martinez-Gómez X, Trallero-Araguás E, et al. The diagnostic work-up of cancer-associated myositis. Curr Opin Rheumatol 2018;30(6):630–6.

46. Matuszak J, Blondet C, Hubelé F, et al. Muscle fluorodeoxyglucose uptake assessed by positron emission tomography–computed tomography as a biomarker of inflammatory myopathies disease activity. Rheumatology 2019;58(8):1459–64.

47. Kundrick A, Kirby J, Ba D, et al. Positron emission tomography costs less to patients than conventional screening for malignancy in dermatomyositis. In-Seminars Arthritis Rheum 2019;49(1):140–4. WB Saunders.

48. Catalan M, Selva-O'Callaghan A, Grau JM. Diagnosis and classification of sporadic inclusion body myositis (sIBM). Autoimmun Rev 2014;13:363–6.

49. Hilton-Jones D, Brady S. Diagnostic criteria for inclusion body myositis. J Intern Med 2016;280:52–62.

50. Pruitt JN 2nd, Showalter CJ, Engel AG. Sporadic inclusion body myositis: counts of different types of abnormal fibers. Ann Neurol 1996;39:139–43.

51. Su Y, Flores S, Wang G, et al. Comparison of Pittsburgh compound B and florbetapir in cross-sectional and longitudinal studies. Alzheimer's & Dementia: Diagnosis. Assess Dis Monit 2019;11(1): 180–90.

52. Klunk WE, Engler H, Nordberg A, et al. Imaging brain amyloid in Alzheimer's disease with Pittsburgh Compound-B. Ann Neurol 2004;55(3):306–19.

53. Maetzler W, Reimold M, Schittenhelm J, et al. Increased [11C]PIB-PET levels in inclusion body myositis are indicative of amyloid beta deposition. J Neurol Neurosurg Psychiatr 2011;82:1060–2.

54. Noto YI, Kondo M, Tsuji Y, et al. Diagnostic value of muscle [11C] PIB-PET in inclusion body myositis. Front Neurol 2020;10:1386.

55. Pinal-Fernandez I, Mammen AL. Amyloid-PET: a new tool for diagnosing IBM? Nat Rev Rheumatol 2019; 15:321–2.

56. Saint-Aubert L, Almkvist O, Chiotis K, et al. Regional tau deposition measured by [18F] THK5317 positron emission tomography is associated to cognition via glucose metabolism in Alzheimer's disease. Alzheimer's Res Ther 2016;8(1):1–9.

57. Zhang Y, Li K, Pu C, et al. A novel application of tau PET in the diagnosis of sporadic inclusion body myositis: a case report. Medicine 2020;99(31).

Printed and bound by CPI Group (UK) Ltd, Croydon, CR0 4YY

03/10/2024

01040363-0015